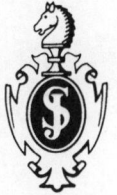

Francis Brunelle, Danièle Pariente and
Pierre Chaumont

Liver Disease in Children

An Atlas of Angiography and Cholangiography

With 181 Figures

Springer-Verlag London Ltd.

Francis Brunelle
Professor of Radiology, Service de Radiologie, Hôpital des Enfants Malades,
149 rue de Sevres, 75743 Paris Cedex 15, France

Danièle Pariente MD
Chef de Service, Service de Radiopediatrie, Hôpital de Bicetre,
78 rue du Gal Leclerc, 94270 Le Kremlin Bicetre, France

Pierre Chaumont MD
Consultant, former Chef de Service, Service de Radiopediatrie, Hôpital de Bicetre,
78 rue du Gal Leclerc, 94270 Le Kremlin Bicetre, France

Cover illustrations. Halftone: Caroli's Disease. Percutaneous cholangiography shows multiple cystic dilatations of the intrahepatic bile ducts. *Line drawings*: Ch. 2, Fig. 1. Normal anatomy and variations.

ISBN 978-1-4471-3824-2

British Library Cataloguing in Publication Data
Brunelle, Francis
    Liver Disease in Children: Atlas of
    Angiography and Cholangiography
    I. Title
    618.92
ISBN 978-1-4471-3824-2
Library of Congress Cataloging-in-Publication Data
Brunelle, Francis, 1949–
    Liver disease in children : an atlas of angiography and
cholangiography / Francis Brunelle, Daniele Pariente, and Pierre
Chaumont.
        p.   cm.
    Includes bibliographical references and index.
    ISBN 978-1-4471-3824-2   ISBN 978-1-4471-3822-8 (eBook)
    DOI 10.1007/978-1-4471-3822-8

    1. Liver—Diseases—Diagnosis—Atlases. 2. Angiography—Atlases.
3. Bile ducts—Radiography—Atlases. 4. Children—Diseases—
Diagnosis—Atlases. I. Pariente, Daniele. II. Chaumont, Pierre.
III. Title.
RJ456.L5B78   1993   93–33451
618.92' 362' 07572—dc20   CIP

© Springer-Verlag London 1994
Softcover reprint of the hardcover 1st edition 1994

Typeset by Expo Holdings, Malaysia
12/3830-543210 Printed on acid-free paper

Foreword

In recent years, developments in ultrasound, computed tomography and magnetic resonance imaging have made important changes in the practice of diagnostic radiology. Concomitantly, invasive radiology for both diagnostic and therapeutic purposes has grown into a rapidly evolving subspecialty.

This text represents a landmark in paediatric radiology. The three authors are distinguished radiologists who, over the past two decades, have greatly contributed to paediatric hepatology. Their pioneering work in the area of splanchnic angiography and diagnostic as well as therapeutic cholangiography was facilitated by their close day-to-day interaction with the Paediatric Liver Disease Unit at Hôpital Bicêtre. The contents and the format of this "atlas" are testimony to their knowledge of clinical hepatology and to their wide experience in invasive paediatric radiology. The outstanding quality of the images is enhanced by appropriate clinical descriptions which will help the reader understand the indications for these procedures, their accuracy and limitations.

Although non-invasive organ imaging has reduced the need for diagnostic angiography in diseases of the liver, pancreas and retroperitoneum, selective angiography still has an important place for vascular lesions, tumours, and portal hypertension. It remains a necessary complement to non-invasive imaging before and during interventional procedures such as liver transplantation. If percutaneous cholangiography has become a primary radiological procedure in paediatric hepatology, it is largely due to the innovative work of Doctors Chaumont, Brunelle and Pariente. They have truly shown the way to the rest of the world by stressing the value of the procedure as well as its relative simplicity and speed.

We are deeply grateful to the authors for this exceptional collection of clinical and radiological data which constitutes a wonderful tribute to their clinical skills, timeless efforts and dedication to the welfare of children with hepatobiliary diseases.

C. Roy
D. Alagille

Preface

This book presents all the aspects of angiography and cholangiography in liver diseases in children. It represents more than 20 years' experience (1969–1993). During this period the techniques have evolved. Splenoportography was largely used during the initial years, then cut films arteriographies and now DSA.

The technical aspects of angiography are fully described – the need to use small catheters and heparin to reduce the number of complications is emphasised.

Anaesthetic aspects and special problems in patients with liver diseases are mentioned as appropriate.

We have stressed normal anatomy and variations as a basis for analysing pathological features.

We have described in detail the venous anatomy of the pancreas to allow percutaneous venous samplings in hyperinsulinism.

The wide experience of our radiological team in the field of portal hypertension in children should make Chapter 3 a valuable tool for any radiologist involved in the pre- and postoperative work-up of these patients. Ultrasonographers will find in our illustrations clues to an accurate and rapid assessment of this condition.

Many rare diseases, such as congenital hepatic fibrosis, are fully described and illustrated. Original and previously unpublished data are presented in the difficult area of liver angiomas. As treatment differs according to the precise type of angioma, accurate and detailed diagnosis is mandatory. An algorithm is given for an optimal diagnostic approach.

Such a clinicoradiological approach is also used for hepatomas, adenomas and other rare tumours.

In the difficult area of bile duct disease our wide experience of percutaneous opacifications allows us to give a precise anatomical description of intrahepatic bile duct involvement in biliary atresia and of intrahepatic lymphatics in chronic biliary cirrhosis. Sclerosing cholangitis is described.

The functional anatomy of choledochal cysts is given.

The increased number of liver transplantations in children is taken account of in Chapter 7 which is dedicated to this difficult area. Angiography and percutaneous diagnostic as well as therapeutic procedures are discussed.

In addition to diagnostic angiography we present an extensive description of interventional procedures.

The vascular radiological anatomy of liver disease provides an essential basis for a detailed understanding of new imaging methods such as magnetic resonance imaging and Doppler ultrasound.

1993

F. B.
D. P.
P. C.

Acknowledgements

All this work was done in very close collaboration with the Paediatric Hepatology Department created and directed by Professor Daniel Alagille. Their clinical and scientific work served as a base for our radiological studies.

Our secretaries, Marie-Lise, Sylvie, Fabienne, Nathalie and Dominique deserve our deep thanks. Their work starts when ours finishes. Their efficient management of patients' files was a great assistance in our work.

Our technicians participated in every single examination. They were indispensable and appreciated companions. We owe to them the quality of our films. They helped us by their continuing advice and remarks.

Anaesthesiologists and their nurses worked in close collaboration with us. It is thanks to their skills that we could achieve good quality examinations in complete security. They are too numerous all to be listed; they are keenly aware of our friendship.

During 25 years, many radiologists contributed to the realisation of angiographies. Among the members of the medical team of the Bicêtre Pediatric Radiology department, one must first mention Francis Brunelle: his intelligence, his shrewdness constantly devoted to his young patients, his qualities as a teacher are acknowledged by all. He was the initiator of the project which could not have been done without him as a driving force. At present he works and teaches in Hôpital des Enfants-Malades. Daniele Pariente, first as his resident and then as my associate with her deep knowledge of paediatric radiology and the scientific accuracy of her medical activity, is now directing the department in Bicêtre.

We owe special thanks to Jean-Yves Riou whose competence in cardiovascular radiology was inestimable for the completion of many of the exams. Gerard Harry was also a precious collaborator in this field. We must also quote the names of G. Kalifa, J. P. Montagne, P. Douillet and E. Urvoas and many residents and students who helped us.

I also want to thank Marc Savary with whom I started my career in vascular radiology.

P. Chaumont

Contents

1 Technique

Angiography

Anaesthesia

It is generally necessary to anaesthetise children under 10–12 years of age as this is the only way to assure apnoea during the injections. This is even more important when using digital subtraction angiography (DSA). The puncture of small vessels also necessitates complete immobility of the child.

Technique

In order to reduce irradiation rapid films and screens were used with standard angiographic equipment, namely a small focus X-ray tube (0.1, 0.3 or 0.9 mm). Exposure time must be as short as possible (less than 20 ms). Direct magnification is often obtained by removing the grid, especially in small infants. When using digital subtraction equipment the number of exposures is reduced as much as possible.

For 10 years we have used stereographic films (0.3 mm focus). This technique does not increase the number of films and allows 3D visualisation of angiographies. Only rarely are lateral views used. However, this technique is now less important since the introduction of computed tomography (CT) and magnetic resonance imaging (MRI). A C-arm equipment is necessary when interventional radiology is routinely performed because oblique views may be necessary for needle punctures and opacifications.

Arterial Accesses

Femoral Artery

This is the most commonly used artery because it is superficial, easy to puncture and to compress for haemostasis after angiography.

We prefer puncture at the level of the crural crux or just below because the artery is less mobile at this level. A low puncture is preferred by some but there is a risk of puncturing the deep femoral artery. Although we have not encountered pelvic haematomas, they are said to be associated with this high puncture. The puncture is performed with one hand, the fingers of the other hand being on the artery. One must feel both the artery and the needle within the subcutaneous tissues.

The artery must be transfixed even if a reflux during the puncture is noted. The needle is then removed and the catheter slowly withdrawn. A "click" is perceived when the catheter enters the lumen of the artery and a free systolic reflux is obtained.

A guide-wire is then introduced, the catheter withdrawn over it and replaced by the catheter. Entry into the artery is achieved by slowly pushing and rotating the catheter. If resistance is felt, turning the catheter will general overcome it. Simply pushing the catheter could kink the guide-wire within the subcutaneous tissue.

A good fit of the diameter of the guide-wire with the lumen of the catheter is a key to smooth and easy entry into the vessel lumen. Silicone oil or Vaseline is useful to prevent artery spasm.

Dilation of the needle track with a slightly larger catheter needle can be used for small arteries and a test injection of contrast medium can be used to check the diameter of the artery.

Lateral Puncture. Continuous reflux without systolic pulses and without perception of a click usually means that the artery has been punctured laterally and that reflux is through a haematoma. It will then be impossible to introduce a guide-wire. A second attempt is then better than to introduce the guide-wire by force.

Femoral Artery Spasm. After an initial but abortive attempt, the femoral artery may be difficult to feel. This can be due to a spasm or a small haematoma around the artery. Percutaneous xylocaine cream and gentle massage of the region will generally reestablish a good pulsation. If not, another artery should be used.

Non-Palpable Femoral Artery. Occasionally it may be necessary to puncture a non-palpable femoral artery. This can happen in obese children, in aortic coarctation or aortic valve stenosis. The artery should then be punctured with the help of fluoroscopic landmarks. The femoral artery should be punctured on the femoral head (as defined with the fluoroscope) at the union of the first inner third and medial third. Doppler ultrasound can also be used.

If the femoral vein is entered by mistake the catheter needle should be slowly withdrawn as it could have been punctured when lying behind the artery. A systolic reflux will then be observed after the continuous-flow venous reflux.

Left Femoral Artery Puncture. The left femoral artery is easily punctured if a corresponding approach to that described for the right femoral artery is used.

Upper Extremities Arteries

The humeral, brachial or axillary artery can also be used in children. These arteries are extremely mobile and easily go into spasm. The puncture should be as far as possible done in one attempt. The left arm should be used for descending aortic access. The right arm is less often used as it can be difficult to gain access to the abdominal aorta by this route.

Carotid Arteries

Direct puncture of the carotid artery is exceptionally needed for abdominal angiography. In very rare occasions retrograde puncture of the carotid artery allows access to the abdominal aorta.

Umbilical Artery

In newborns the umbilical artery can be used to catheterise or embolise selectively abdominal arteries. A 3F or smaller catheter should be used.

Heparin

After the puncture with the needle, before introducing the catheter, heparin is injected in a bolus of 0.7–1 mg kg^{-1} (70–100 U kg^{-1}), unless there is a known coagulation disorder. We prefer this type of heparinisation, which allows strict control of the injected dose, to heparinisation via a saline flush. In our experience, heparin greatly helps to avoid femoral artery thrombosis.

Introducer Sheath

Nowadays, 3F and 4F sheaths are available. It is our practice to use them every time an embolisation or a change of catheter is planned. They protect the femoral artery from excessive catheter manipulation and provide continuous vascular access.

Venous Punctures

Femoral Vein Puncture

The right femoral vein is easily punctured medial to the femoral artery, during abdominal compression. The latter manoeuvre dilates the femoral vein and thus facilitates catheter entry. The left hand is used for abdominal compression after the position of the femoral artery has been checked.

Venous reflux occurs during puncture and when the catheter is withdrawn. Femoral vein puncture can be difficult especially in small infants or in dehydrated children.

One technique is to puncture a visible vein on the foot and to opacify the femoral vein with a small amount of contrast medium and then puncture the vein under fluoroscopy. Sometimes as the guide-wire is entered a resistance is felt after a few centimetres have been introduced, which may mean that the ascending lumbar vein has been entered. Manipulation of the guide-wire or use of a J guide-wire will overcome the problem. A test injection should be performed if the inferior vena cava (IVC) is to be opacified before the full test is started. If the tip of the catheter has entered the ascending lumbar vein, rupture of this vein may occur. Severe spasm of the femoral vein may also occur.

Jugular Vein Puncture

Retrograde internal jugular vein puncture or brachial vein puncture may be needed when IVC or hepatic vein opacification is intended but an IVC thrombosis is present.

Material and Flow Rates

Catheter Needle

The size of the catheter needle has to be adapted to the femoral artery or other diameter. The appropriate size must be matched to the child's weight as indicated in Table 1.1. A rule of thumb is to adapt the catheter needle to the catheter diameter as the puncture hole diameter will be that of the size of the catheter. It will be impossible to introduce a 5 F catheter after a 22 G catheter needle puncture. Using a 3 F catheter after an 18 G catheter needle puncture will lead to bleeding around the catheter.

Table 1.1. Relationship between catheter size and weight of child

Catheter needle	External diameter (mm)	Weight of child (kg)	Catheter
24 G	0.7	2–3	3 F
22 G	0.9	3–10	3 F–3.7 F
20 G	1.1	8–30	4 F
18 G	1.3	>25	5 F

Catheter Size

The catheter should be adapted to the child's weight and also to the flow rate needed and to the size of the artery to be entered. For example a 4 F catheter is sufficient in a 35 kg child when selective injections are needed.

Problems are encountered when high flow is necessary in low weight babies. This is the case in newborns with hepatic angiomas. The high flow would necessitate a large catheter, whereas the small size of the femoral artery limits the size of the catheter. The use of DSA has improved this problem.

Catheter Shape and Side Holes

Multipurpose catheters are used. The curve is simple and its diameter should be 110%–120% the aortic diameter. Side holes are useful to increase the flow. A side hole catheter should not be used when embolisation is performed.

Guide-Wire

Soft tip guide-wires are used. The tip shape can be modified to enter tortuous vessels. The soft part of the guide-wire should be short to selectively catheterise arteries in children.

Flow Rate

The flow rate should be adapted to the injected artery and body weight as indicated in Table 1.2.

This table is only a guide: flow rate greatly depends on the vascularity of the lesion, the size and the repartition of the vessels. About 30% iodinated contrast media may be used for arterial injection. With conventional arteriography techniques the total volume and the flow rate have to be increased by about 50% for selective injection and 100% for aortogram.

Table 1.2. Flow rate for abdominal angiography: using contrast media with 30% of iodine and DSA technique

	Flow rate ($ml\,kg^{-1}\,s^{-1}$)	Total volume ($ml\,kg^{-1}$)	Duration of injection (s)
Abdominal aorta	0.4	1	2–2.5
Celiac trunk	0.15–0.2	0.5–0,7	2–5
Mesenteric artery			
Arterial run	0.15	0.5	2–4
Portography run	0.15	1	6–8

Portal Phase of Mesenteric Artery Injection. A good opacification of the portal system is obtained when 1 ml kg^{-1} of contrast medium is used. Injection of a vasodilatator prior to opacification allows an early and good opacification of the portal system. Papaverin (1 mg kg^{-1}) should be diluted in 10–20 ml (1 mg cm^{-3}) of saline and slowly injected into the mesenteric artery in 30 s. The injection of contrast medium must be started shortly after. The portal vein is opacified at about 10 s, the parenchymal liver phase at 15–20 s and the hepatic veins are seen at 20–30 s.

Percutaneous Transhepatic Access

Whatever the structures to be punctured in the liver the landmarks are the same. The liver is punctured on the mid-axillary line at the 9th or 10th intecostal space. Care should be taken to avoid puncturing the pleural space using fluoroscopy to check.

The catheter needle is aimed horizontally towards the superior plateau of the eleventh vertebra along the eleventh rib. The eleventh rib indicates the posterior projection of the hepatic hilum. The tip of the catheter needle should not pass over the right aspect of the spine. A firm resistance can be felt when hilar structures are punctured.

A gentle vacuum is maintained with a syringe while the catheter is withdrawn. Bile and blood can be obtained. Hepatic vein blood is darker than portal blood due to the difference in oxygen concentration.

Occasionally hepatic artery branches can be punctured.

Splenic Portography

Splenic puncture is performed in order to opacify the splenic vein. The splenic puncture is done on the mid-axillary line in the tenth intercostal space; the puncture track is oblique parallel to the inner limit shadow of the spleen. A test injection is done and a run is performed with 30% contrast medium and DSA. The dose injected is 1 ml kg^{-1} in 6–8 s.

Cholangiography

Percutaneous Transhepatic Cholangiography

Dilated Bile Ducts. The same technique is used as for any transhepatic approach. A 20G catheter needle is used. A gentle aspiration is maintained as the catheter is withdrawn. When bile is obtained a small amount of contrast is injected to check the position of the sheath. A 25 guide-wire is introduced and a side hole catheter (4F)

is exchanged with the needle sheath. A desilet sheath (4 to 6F) can be used if a balloon catheter has to be used.

Left Lobe Approach. In special cases direct access to the left lobe of the liver is necessary. In this case a vertical or oblique puncture in the region of the xyphoid after ultrasonic guidance can be used.

Non-Dilated Bile Ducts

Transhepatic Cholangiography

Even when the intrahepatic bile ducts are not dilated it is possible to opacify them. However, the rate of success is low (between 50% and 60%). A thin needle (Chiba, 21 or 23G) is used with the same transhepatic approach. A connecting tube is adapted to the needle. Very small amounts of contrast are injected while the needle is withdrawn. Hepatic parenchymatous injection is recognised by an irregular mottled area of opacification. Opacification of hepatic portal vein or hepatic artery branches is easily recognised. Bile duct opacification is also easily recognised (Chapter 5).

Percutaneous Cholecystography

When the bile ducts are not dilated it is possible to opacify them by a percutaneous approach to the gallbladder. We first used this technique in 1983 to opacify the intrahepatic bile ducts in sclerosing cholangitis cases. The gallbladder is punctured through the anterior edge of the liver in its extraperitoneal portion. A side-hole catheter is placed in the lumen of the gallbladder and contrast medium is injected. The contrast–bile mixture is aspirated at the end of the examination to prevent abdominal pain due to gallbladder distension, and bile leak around the gallbladder. When the gallbladder is small, opacification of the bile ducts can be obtained through a catheter needle, without placement of a side-hole catheter which could be difficult.

Bibliography

Antonovic R, Rösch J, Dotter CT (1976) The value of systemic arterial heparinization in transfemoral angiography: a prospective study. AJR 127: 223–225

Brunelle F, Chaumont P (1984) Percutaneous cholecystography in children. Ann Radiol 27: 111–116

Chaumont P, Doyon D, Blonstein R, Harry G, Mouzon A (1974) Agrandissement au foyer 0.1 Application en pédiatrie. J Radiol Electrol 55: 660–661

Garel L, Belli D, Grignon A, Roy CC (1987) Percutaneous cholecystography in children. Radiology 165: 639–641

Garel L, Pariente D (1991) Pediatric non vascular hepatobiliary interventions. Semin Interventional Radiol 8: 217–223

Weitzman JJ, Stanley P (1978) Splenoportography in the pediatric age group. J Pediatr Surg 13: 707–712

2 Normal Anatomy and Variations

An understanding of arterial variations is based on the concept that all variations are due to preferential flow in normal arterial structures.

During the development some arterial pathways develop and some involute. The same concepts that explain abnormal aortic arch developments can be used for hepatic arterial or venous variations.

Embryologically, the liver bud derives from the duodenum, in parallel to the development of the pancreas. This explains why the bile duct is vascularised by branches of the gastroduodenal artery. As the liver develops the hepatic artery flow increases. The hepatic artery can then be considered as a collateral of the gastroduodenal artery.

Because of the presence of a marginal vessel parallel to the digestive tube between the left gastric, gastroduodenal, inferior diaphragmatic and superior mesenteric arteries, it is possible that the hepatic artery can haemodynamically derive from any of these vessels (Fig. 2.1).

A replaced right hepatic artery is the most common variation. Because of the rotation of the digestive system this artery is often posterior to the portal vein, making up the posterior inferior gastroduodenal arch. The replaced left hepatic artery defines the take off of the hepatic artery from the left gastric artery.

This explains why it is possible to find a gastroduodenal artery which takes off from the inferior diaphragmatic artery (1 case in our series). Veins are satellites of the arteries. There are thus venous equivalents of these variations. They will be described in the chapter on pancreatic venous sampling (Chapter 6) and that on portal vein thrombosis (Chapter 3) as they appear as collaterals opacified during angiography.

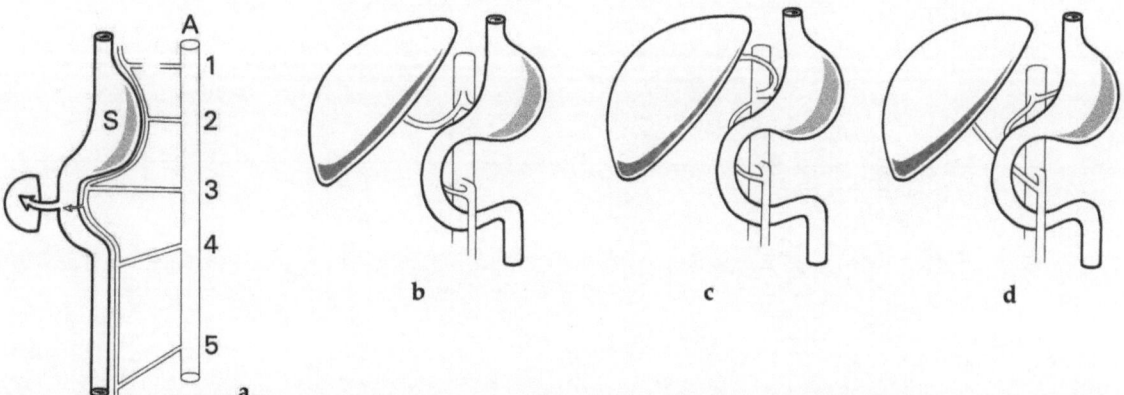

Fig. 2.1. Normal anatomy and variations **a** Embryologically the digestive tube is vascularised by five major arteries: 1, inferior diaphragmatic (or cardial); 2, left gastric; 3, gastroduodenal; 4, superior mesenteric; 5, inferior mesenteric. **b** Normal anatomy: the hepatic artery is derived from the gastroduodenal artery. **c** Replaced left hepatic artery: the hepatic artery (or the left branch only) is derived from the left gastric. **d** Replaced right hepatic artery: the hepatic artery (or the right branch only) is derived from the superior mesenteric artery.

3 Portal Hypertension

Introduction

Portal hypertension is defined as elevation of the corrected portal pressure above 10 cm H_2O (portal pressure minus IVC pressure) or of the absolute portal pressure above 20 cm H_2O. On a practical point of view the portal pressure can be measured by direct transhepatic portography or by splenoportography. The clinical consequence is splenomegaly, the spleen acting as a reservoir for splanchnic venous blood. Development of collaterals between the portal venous system and the caval systemic venous system is common. Some of these collaterals are submucosal in the digestive tract: oesophagus, duodenum and rectum. These collaterals and only these can carry the risk of bleeding. The other collaterals shunt the portal system to the vena cava and rarely lead to portal encephalopathy in children. These collaterals per se are extremely rarely sufficient to allow a normalisation of the portal pressure.

Radiological work-up includes ultrasound which, in our experience, allows a complete positive and aetiological diagnosis. Angiography is necessary only when surgery is contemplated or when a more precise anatomical diagnosis is needed.

The most common aetiology for portal hypertension in our series was portal vein thrombosis (222 cases) followed by non-biliary cirrhosis (79 cases), biliary cirrhosis (171 cases), congenital hepatic fibrosis (30 cases), Budd–Chiari syndrome and hepatic vein occlusion (27 cases).

Portal Vein Thrombosis
(222 cases)

Definition

Portal vein thrombosis may involve any portion of the portal system resulting in prehepatic portal hypertension. Usually, thrombosis progresses in a retrograde fashion, that is cases with an isolated splenic obstruction with normal portal trunk and mesenteric vein are exceptional.

The causes are various. Many cases remain classified as "idiopathic", probably because of poor medical recording during the early life of the babies. Most of these cases were caused by catheterisation of the umbilical vein, a cause that is now diminishing in frequency as umbilical vein catheterisation is less often used in the newborn. Other causes include surgery, infection, dehydration, diffuse thrombotic disease and retroperitoneal fibrosis. Some cases are associated with diseases in which it is difficult to establish a relationship to portal vein thrombosis: oesophageal atresia, cardiopathies, duodenal atresia, Budd–Chiari syndrome, spontaneous perforation of the biliary duct, Turner's syndrome.

Clinical Findings

The most common clinical finding is isolated splenomegaly. The liver is small due to diminished portal flow. Digestive haemorrhage can reveal the portal hypertension, which is usually

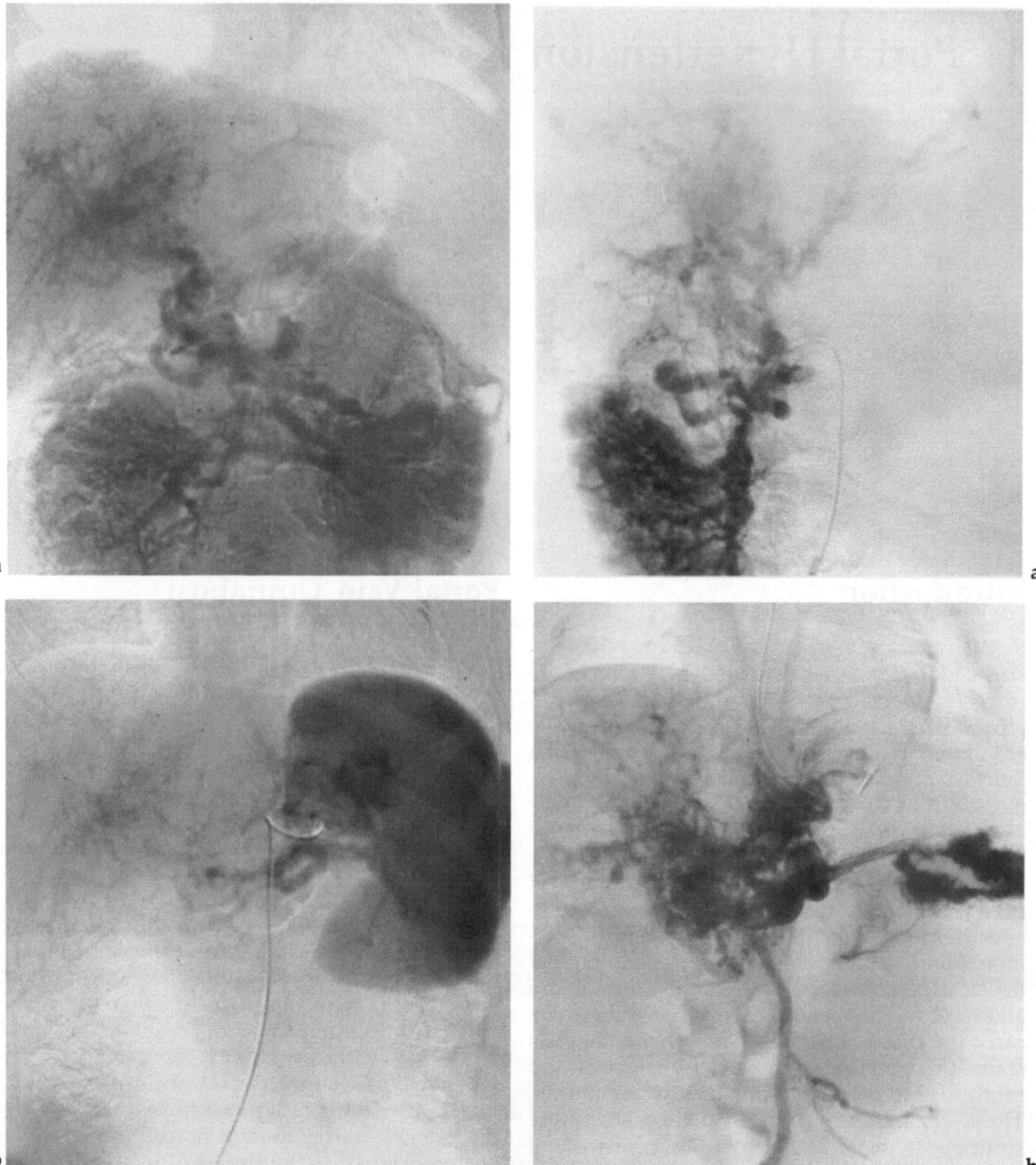

Fig. 3.1. Umbilical catheterisation at birth. Portal vein thrombosis. 7 years of age. **a** Venous return after superior mesenteric artery injection. There is a complete thrombosis of the superior mesenteric vein, portal trunk and distal portion of splenic vein. Multiple pancreatico-duodenal collaterals are seen, revascularising the liver. **b** Venous return after splenic artery injection. The medial third of the splenic vein is thrombosed with multiple intrapancreatic collaterals.

Fig. 3.2. Portal vein thrombosis, 7 years of age. **a** Venous return of a superior mesenteric artery injection. The thrombosis is extensive including the superior mesenteric vein and portal trunk. Multiple pancreaticoduodenal collaterals are seen. There is a reflux toward oesophageal varices. **b** Spleno-portogram. Only the proximal third of the splenic vein is patent. There is a reflux in the inferior mesenteric vein. Multiple collaterals are seen in the region of the hepatic hilum. Note opacification of perigallbladder veins.

triggered by the absorption of aspirin. In our series it has been observed early in life and also in late childhood.

Diagnosis

The diagnosis is now made by ultrasound only. Upper gastrointestinal endoscopy will show the oesophageal varices and grade the severity of portal hypertension, and the risk of digestive haemorrhage.

Angiographic Findings

Technique

The preoperative work-up includes superior mesenteric arteriogram, which usually shows at the venous phase the entire portal vein system. When the splenic vein is not seen, it can be visualised with DSA at the venous phase of the splenic arteriogram or by splenoportography.

Cavography is also performed to detect any associated anomaly of the IVC.

Findings (Figs. 3.1–3.22)

The portal vein thrombosis may involve the intrahepatic branches only (hilar thrombosis) ($n=8$), the portal trunk, the splenomesenteric confluence, the origin of the superior mesenteric vein, the splenic vein or the whole splanchnic venous system, in rare cases of diffuse portal vein thrombosis ($n=8$).

Presence of portal vein thrombosis leads to development of hepatopetal and hepatofugal collaterals.

Hepatopetal Collaterals. Peribiliary veins represent the most common and important collaterals in portal vein thrombosis. They include choledochal, cystic and pancreaticoduodenal veins. They may be responsible for an apparent portal vein duplication, or triplication when a portal vein remnant (12 cases) is present. Indeed, in few cases, the portal vein, although atretic, may still be patent. In case of splenic vein thrombosis, the transverse pancreatic vein may serve as a collateral responsible for the appearence of a double splenic vein.

As in the extrahepatic portal venous system, development of peribiliary veins in the liver may be responsible for intrahepatic portal vein duplications ($n=8$).

Hepatofugal Collaterals. Obstruction of the portal vein increases the portal pressure and leads to the opening of portosystemic collaterals. These collaterals are the consequence of the dilatation of normal anatomic communications between the portal and the caval system and they divert the portal blood toward the caval system. They are summarised in Fig. 3.23.

The most common diversion is the presence of oesophageal varices fed by the left gastric vein, which arises from the portal vein or the spleno-mesenteric confluence, or by the short or posterior gastric veins. They drain in the azygos vein system. In one case opacification of bronchial veins has been observed.

Splenorenal anastomosis can be direct or by the following pathway: posterior gastric vein or cardial veins, inferior diaphragmatic vein, adrenal vein, and left renal vein. The splenorenal shunts even where large are rarely sufficient to normalise the portal pressure.

The inferior mesenteric vein can divert the blood flow into the hypogastric veins via the superior rectal veins, and may be responsible for bleeding from the rectum.

A patent paraumbilical vein has never been observed in our series of portal vein thrombosis, as the obstruction is located upstream from the umbilical vein.

Cholangiographic Findings

Dilatation of intrahepatic bile ducts has been demonstrated in about 8% of our cases. They usually present with mild anomalies of the laboratory tests, but in one case biliary cirrhosis was evident on liver biopsy.

These dilatations, which do not involve the choledochus, are thought to be due to compression of the bile ducts by the hepatopetal veins, as regression has been observed after surgical portocaval shunt.

Cirrhosis

Definition

Cirrhosis is defined histologically as a replacement of the normal hepatic structure by regenerative nodules which are surrounded by prominent fibrous tissue. The main pathophysiological effects are impaired hepatic function due to loss of hepatocytes, and portal hypertension due to a post-sinusoïdal block.

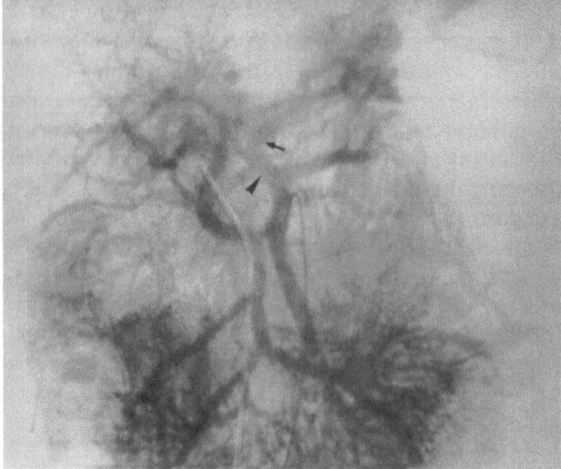

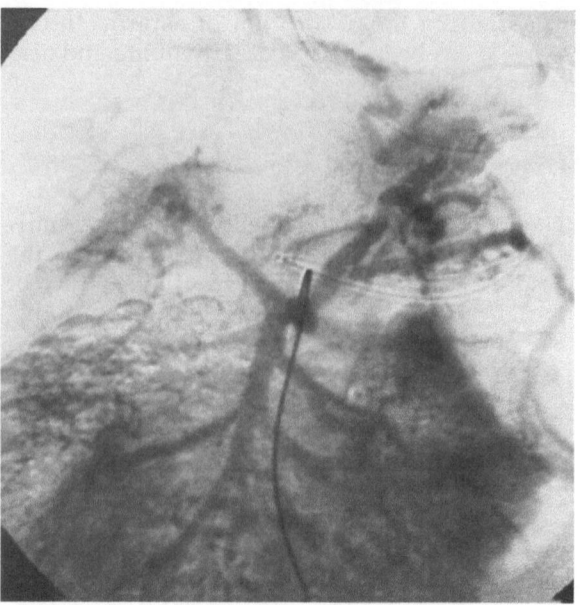

Fig. 3.3. Neonatal meningitis. 3 years of age. Venous return of a superior mesenteric artery injection. There is an aspect of duplication of the superior mesenteric vein due to the selective drainage of the jejunal blood into the left gastric vein and splenic vein. The blood from the ileum is draining into a pancreaticoduodenal vein. One catheter (white) is in the inferior vena cava. Portal vein (*arrowhead*). Left gastric vein (*arrow*).

Fig. 3.5. Age: 9 months. Congenital cardiac malformation (patent foramen ovale and interventricular communication) and pulmonary sequestration. Costal anomalies: synostosis and dorsal hemivertebrae. Venous return of a superior mesenteric artery injection. This thrombosis is limited to the hilum of the liver. The superior mesenteric vein and the splenic vein are patent. Note reflux in the left gastric vein.

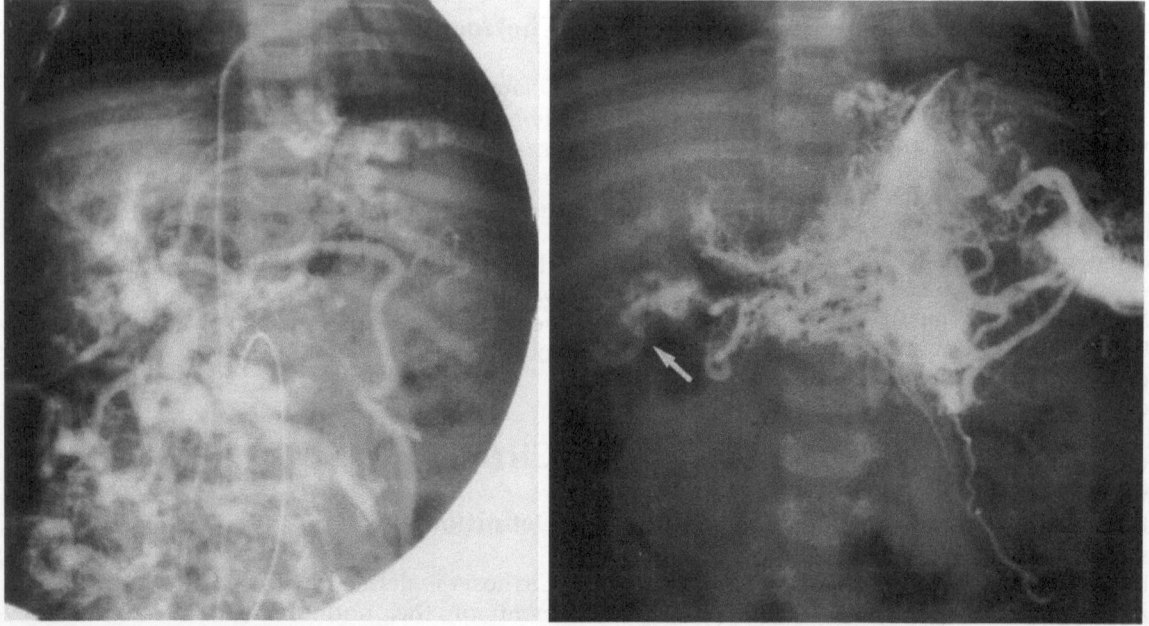

a   b

Fig. 3.4. Extensive portal vein thrombosis. 2 years of age. **a** Venous return of a superior mesenteric artery injection. **b** Splenoportogram. There is no recognisable vein. Multiple pancreaticoduodenal, pancreatic collaterals are seen. The cystic veins are opacified (*arrow*). There is a reflux in a probable left colic vein.

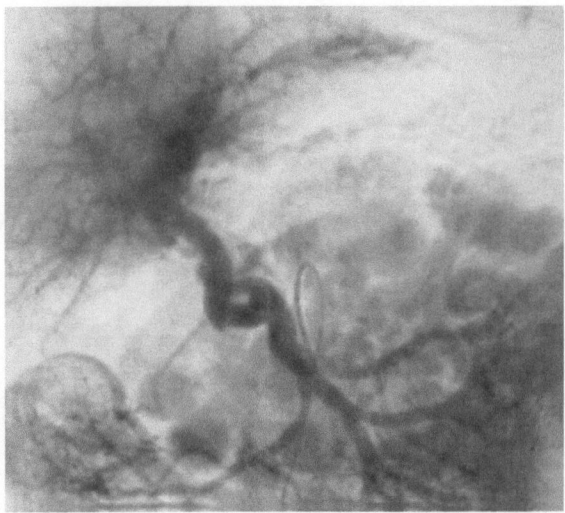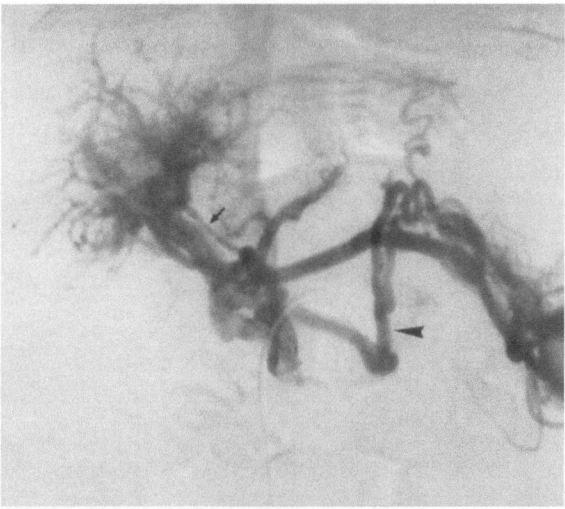

a

b

Fig. 3.6. Portal venous thrombosis: 5 years of age. **a** Venous return of a superior mesenteric artery injection. **b** Spleno-portography. The thrombosis is limited to the portal bifurcation with an atretic remnant of portal trunk (*arrow*). The splenic vein is patent as is the superior mesenteric vein below the third portion of duodenum. The liver is opacified through pancreaticoduodenal collaterals. There is a spontaneous spleno-adreno-renal shunt (*arrowhead*) with opacification of the inferior vena cava.

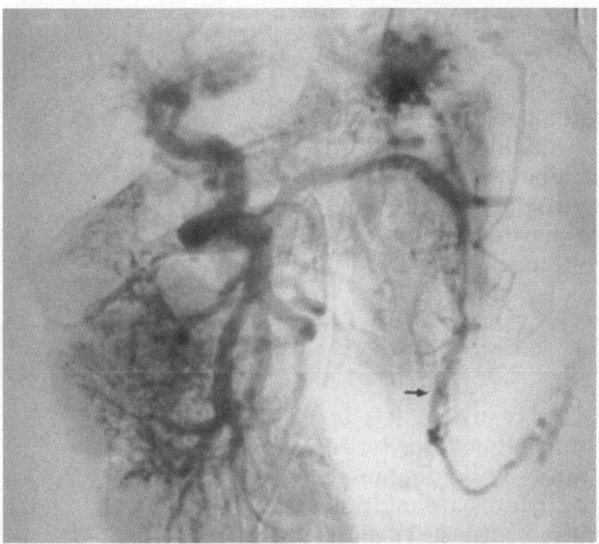

Fig. 3.7. Portal vein thrombosis: 4 years of age. Venous return of a superior mesenteric artery injection. The thrombosis includes the portal trunk. The superior mesenteric vein and the splenic vein are normal. The liver is opacified through pancreaticoduodenal veins. There is opacification of the oesophageal varices through the posterior gastric vein. There is a subcapsular splenic vein collateral (*arrow*).

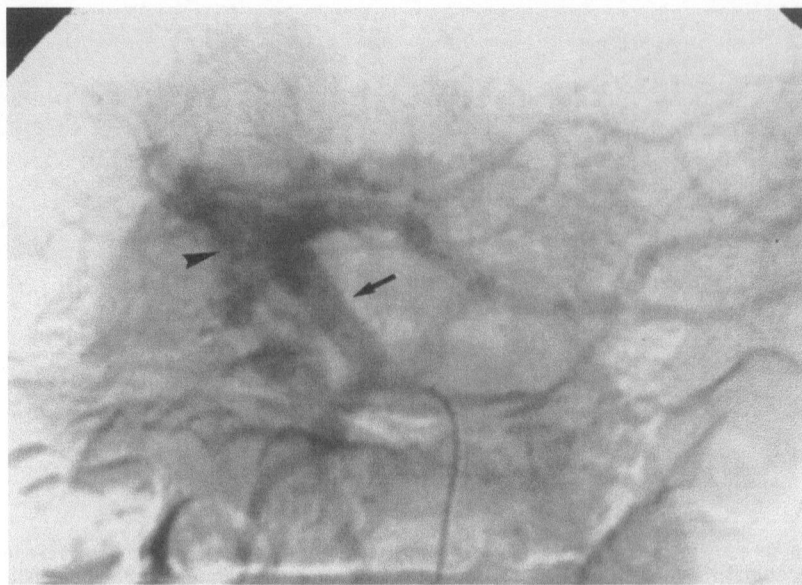

Fig. 3.8. Right portal vein thrombosis: 4-year-old boy with haematemesis and hypertrophy of the left lobe of the liver. Venous return of a superior mesenteric artery injection. The portal trunk (*arrow*) and the left portal vein are patent. The right portal vein is occluded (*arrowhead*).

Clinical Findings

Splenomegaly and hepatomegaly are usually present. There are variable modifications of liver volume and right or left lobe atrophy may be prominent. Upper gastrointestinal haemorrhage and liver failure may be the first signs of the disease, but they usually occur in the evolution of a previously diagnosed disease.

Diagnosis (Table 3.1)

The diagnosis of cirrhosis is easily made clinically or by ultrasound in macronodular types. The micronodular type can only be diagnosed by liver biopsy. Causes of cirrhosis are multiple in children and different from those encountered in adult patients. The most common cause is biliary cirrhosis.

Angiography

Angiography is nowadays only performed when a surgical porto-systemic shunt or a liver transplantation are considered.

Technique

There is progressive decrease of the portal vein flow toward the liver and, in the late evolution,

Table 3.1. Causes of cirrhosis in our series of angiographies

Biliary cirrhosis	
Biliary atresia	72
Idiopathic biliary cirrhosis	32
Choledochal cysts	5
Biliary ductular hypoplasia	9
Byler's disease	16
Other causes of cirrhosis	
Idiopathic	34
Posthepatitis	15
Alpha-1-antitrypsin deficiency	16
Rendu Osler disease	2
Active chronic hepatitis	3
Wilson disease	6
Cystic fibrosis	3

there may be partial or complete inversion of the portal flow. Simutaneously there is evident increase of the hepatic artery flow.

When the portal vein is not opacified in the late phase of superior mesenteric arteriography, the inverted portal flow can usually be demonstrated by hepatic arteriography with slow and prolonged injection of contrast medium.

Thin-needle transhepatic portography is also a good method of visualising the portal vein when there is no contraindication (ascites, coagulation disorder).

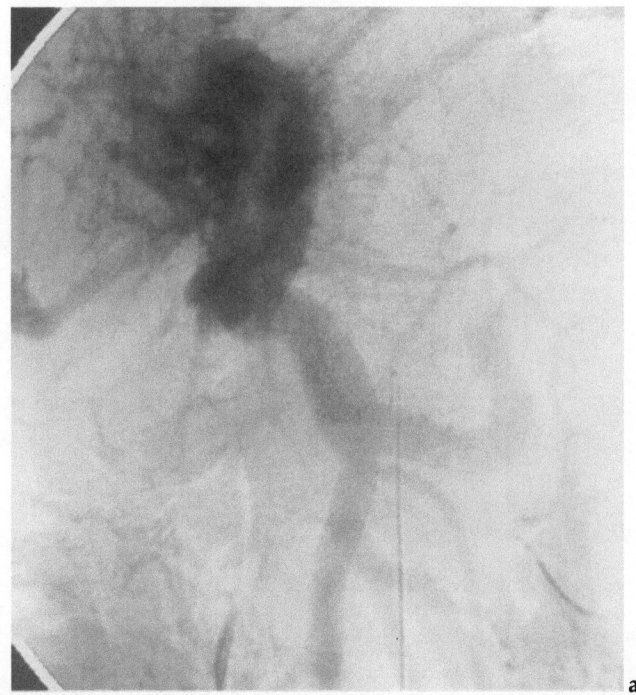

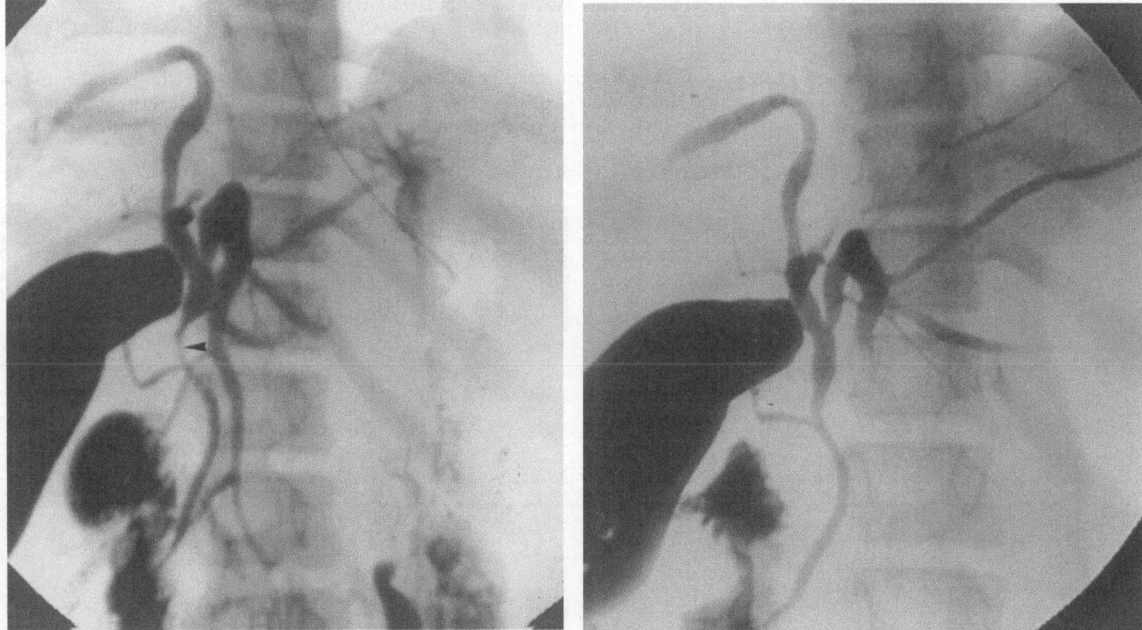

Fig. 3.9. Age: 11 years. Portal vein thrombosis and biliary cirrhosis with bile duct dilatation. Right lung hypoplasia. Atrophy of the right lobe of the liver. Hypertrophy of the left lobe. **a** Venous return of a superior mesenteric artery in-jection. The portal vein bifurcation is thrombosed. There is a very large collateral in the hilum of the liver. The proximal portal trunk is patent. **b** Percutaneous cholecystography. On the biliary opacification, there is a compression effect at the level of the cystic and common bile duct junction due to the dilatation of the portal vein collateral (*arrowhead*). **c** After portocaval shunt: diminution of the bile duct dilatation.

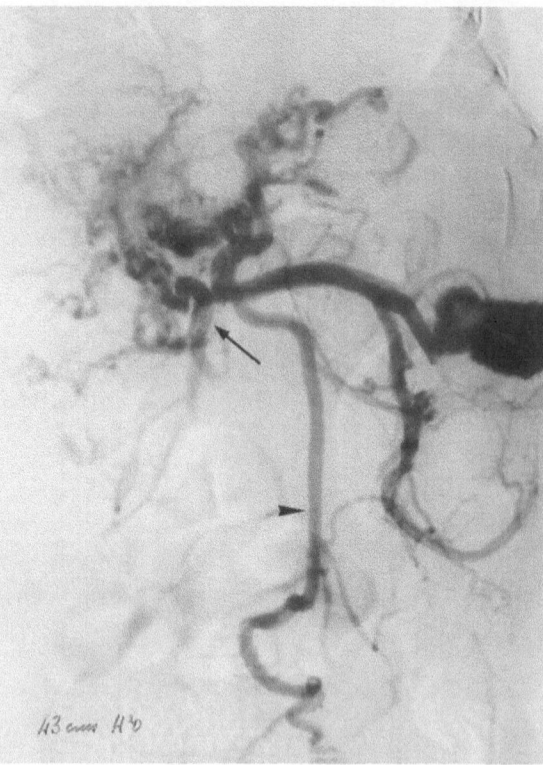

Fig. 3.10. Portal vein thrombosis: 4 years of age. Spleno-portography (splenic pressure 43 cm H₂O). The portal trunk is thrombosed. There are multiple collaterals around the common bile duct and the gallbladder. The superior mesenteric vein is normal (*arrow*). There is a reflux in the inferior mesenteric vein (*arrowhead*) and subcapsular splenic vein. The left gastric vein opacifies oesophageal varices.

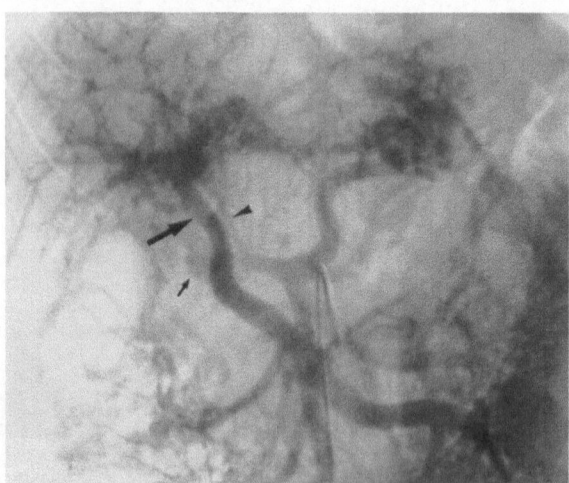

Fig. 3.11. Portal vein thrombosis. Umbilical vein catheterisation at birth. Pseudo-duplication of the portal trunk. Venous return of a superior mesenteric artery injection. There is small atretic remnant of the portal trunk (*arrowhead*) opacified through the superior mesenteric vein. A large pancreaticoduodenal collateral (*large arrow*) opacifies the liver and gives this pseudo duplication of the portal trunk. Note a large left gastric vein and oesophageal varices. Note (*small arrow*) posterior pancreaticoduodenal vein coming from the initial portal trunk (stereography).

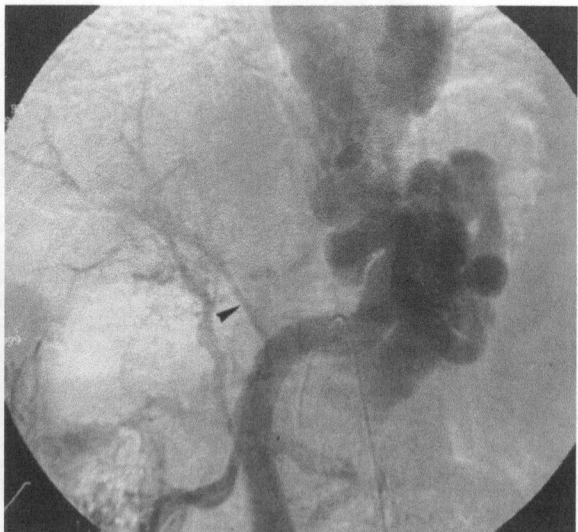

Fig. 3.12. Portal vein thrombosis with cirrhosis on histology: 14 years of age. Venous return of a superior mesenteric artery injection. The portal trunk is atretic (*arrowhead*). There is a small pancreaticoduodenal collateral. The hepatic portal perfusion is poor. The splenic vein is dilated and there is a spontaneous splenorenal shunt and massive opacification of the oesophageal varices through a posterior gastric vein.

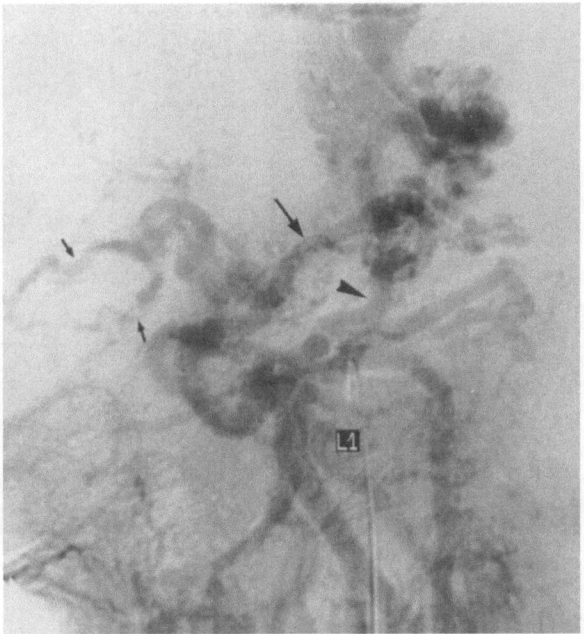

Fig. 3.13. Extensive portal vein thrombosis: 5 years of age. Venous return of a superior mesenteric artery injection. There is no recognisable vein. The liver is opacified through multiple pancreaticoduodenal collaterals. Note reflux in cystic veins (*small arrows*). The inferior mesenteric vein is opacified. The oesophageal varices are opacified through the left gastric vein (*arrowhead*) and the right gastric vein (*large arrow*).

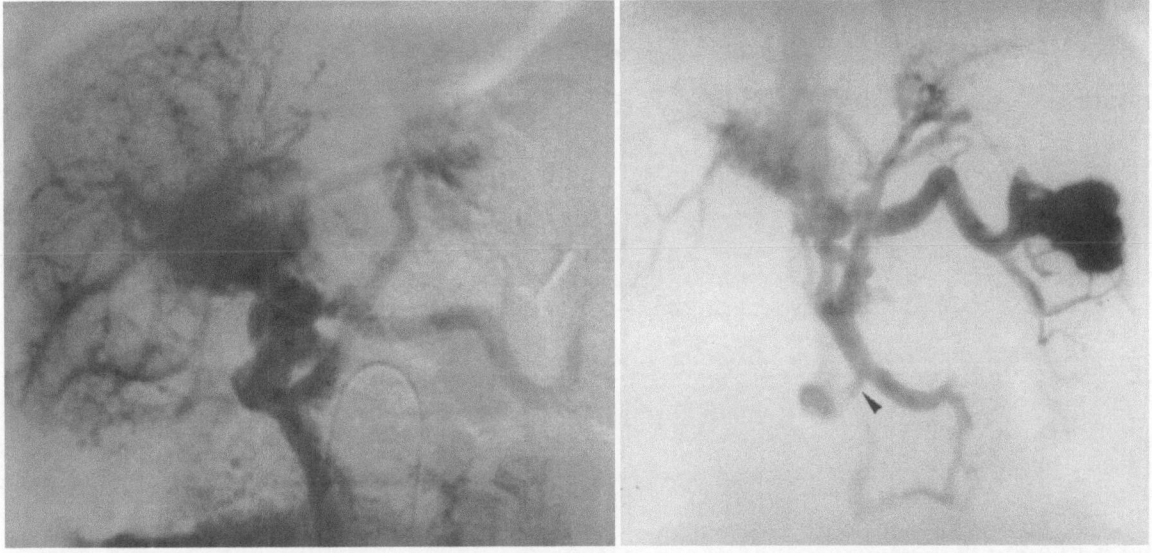

a   b

Fig. 3.14. Sickle cell disease, no umbilical catheterisation. **a** Venous return of a superior mesenteric artery injection. The portal vein is thrombosed. Multiple collaterals perfuse the liver. Opacification of oesophageal varices through left gastric vein. **b** Splenoportography after construction of a mesenterico-caval-anastomosis. Note opacification of the mesenterico-caval anastomosis (*arrowhead*). The oesophageal varices and the pancreaticoduodenal veins are smaller.

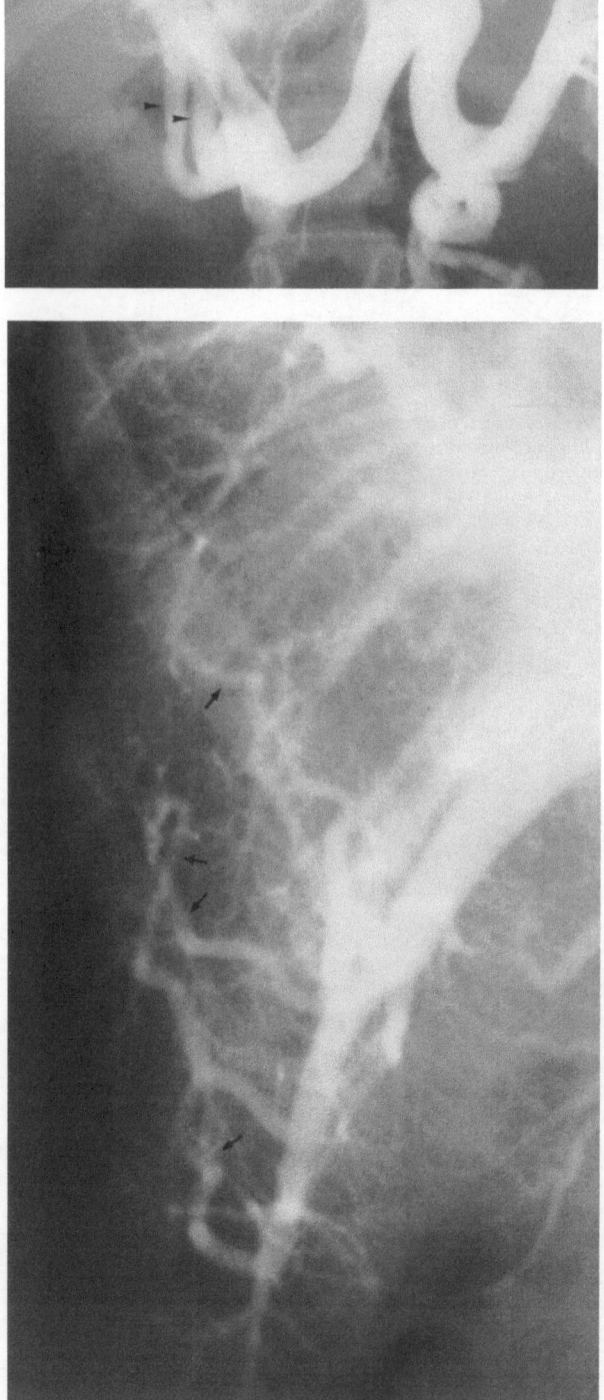

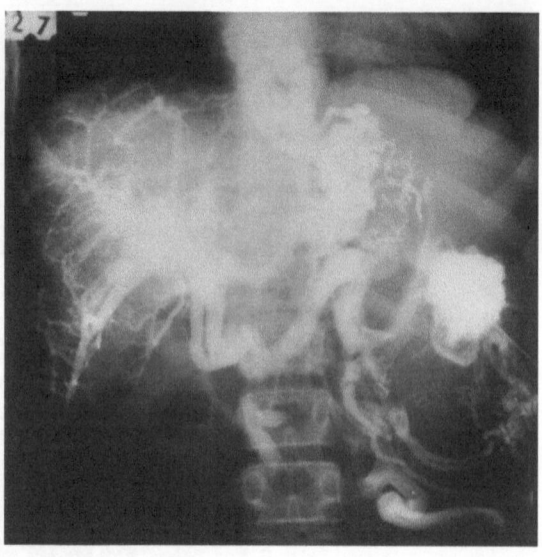

Fig. 3.15. Intrahepatic thrombosis: 14 years of age.
a, b Splenoportography; **c** Close-up view of the right
lobe of the liver. The portal trunk is patent (*large
arrows*), the hilum is thrombosed. The liver is perfused
by choledochal veins with a double appearance
(*arrowheads*). The oesophageal varices are opacified
through a posterior gastric vein. On the close-up view,
there is opacification of porto-portal anastomoses at the
periphery of the liver (*small arrows*).

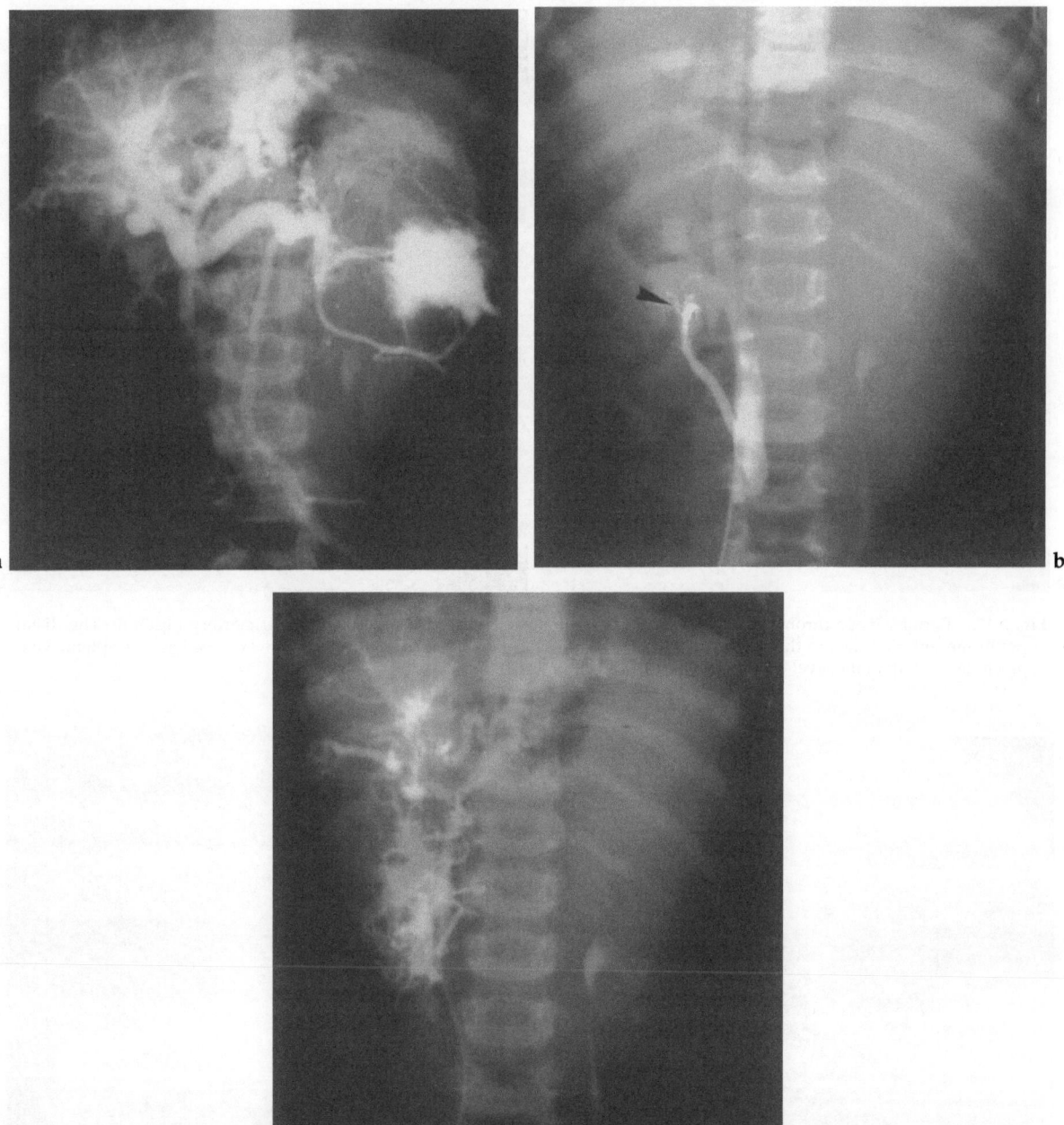

Fig. 3.16. Portal vein thrombosis: 6 years of age. **a** Splenoportography. The thrombosis is located at the level of the hilum. There are some oesophageal varices opacified by a right gastric vein. Reflux in the inferior mesenteric vein. **b** Mesenterico-caval anastomosis. Persistence of portal hypertension. Control of patency of the anastomosis. A catheter is placed in the anastomosis which is thrombosed (*arrowhead*). **c** Opacification with a ballon catheter. The cavernoma is opacified through small channels.

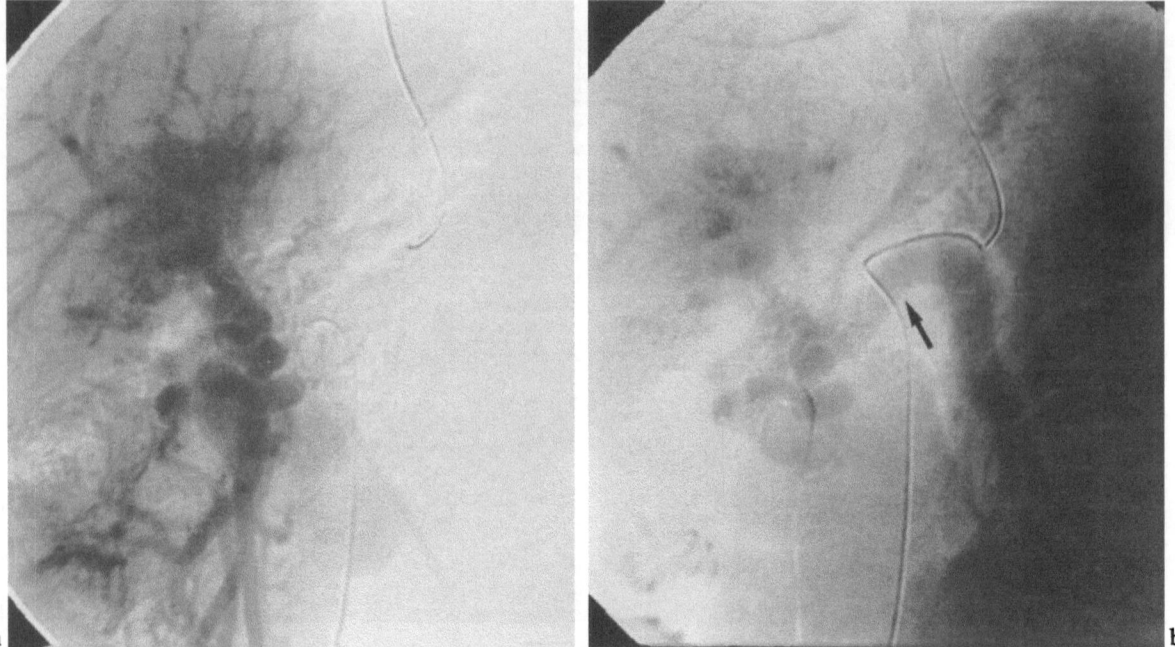

Fig. 3.17. Portal venous thrombosis: 11 years of age. **a** Venous return of a superior mesentric artery injection. The distal superior mesenteric vein and the portal trunk are thrombosed. **b** Venous return of a splenic artery injection. The splenic vein is patent (*arrow*) up to the level of the mesenteric vein.

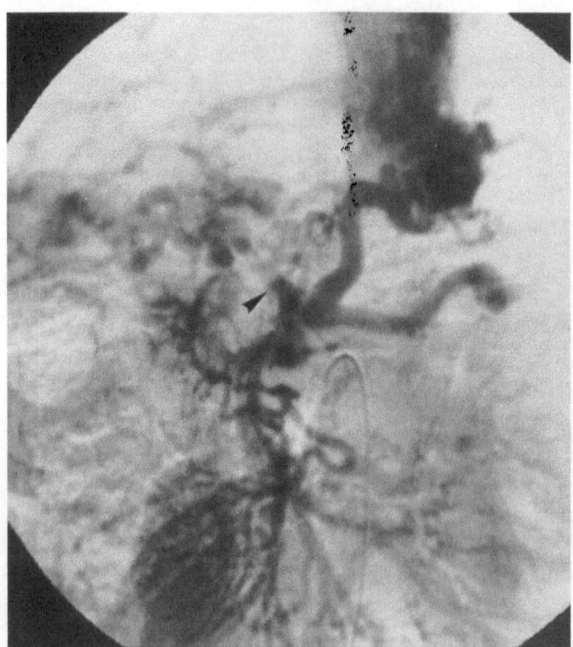

Fig. 3.18. Portal vein thrombosis, involving the distal superior mesenteric vein. Venous return of a superior mesenteric artery injection. Multiple pancreaticoduodenal collaterals are well seen. There is a reflux in the splenic vein. A portal vein stump is seen (*arrowhead*). The oesophageal varices are opacified by the left gastric vein.

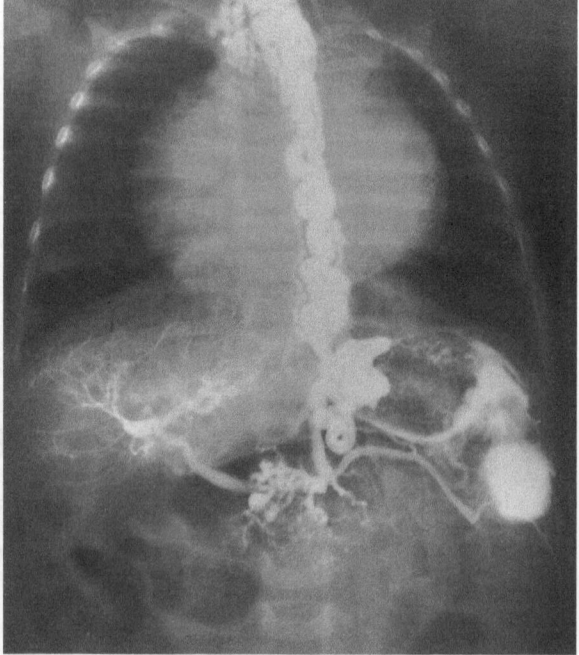

Fig. 3.19. Trisomy 21 plus cardiac malformation. Unusual case of segmental portal vein thrombosis. Splenoportogram (splenic pressure 35 cm H_2O). There is an obstruction of the splenomesenteric junction. The portal trunk and the intrahepatic branches are normal. Note large oesophageal varices fed by a posterior gastric vein. Note opacification of intrapancreatic collaterals.

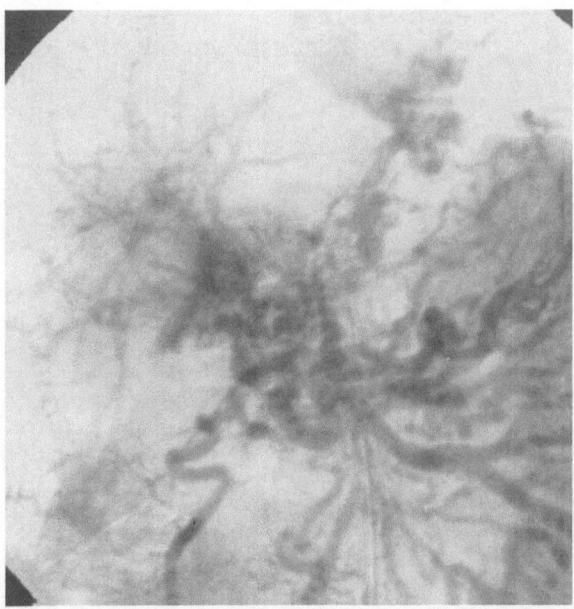

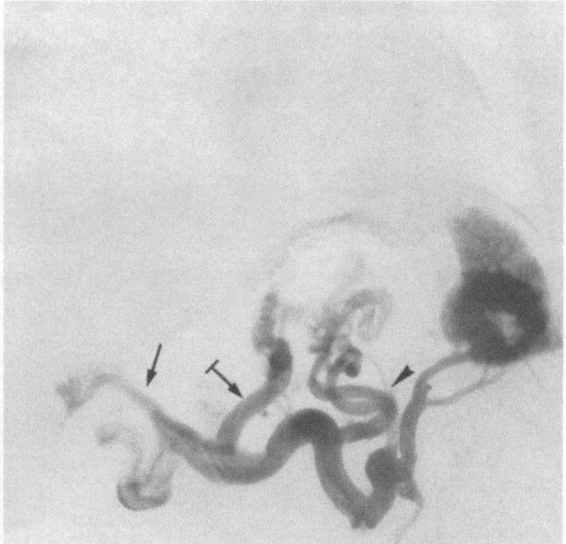

Fig. 3.20. Sickle cell disease and thalassaemia. Extensive portal vein thrombosis: 12 years of age. Superior mesenteric artery injection. Venous return. No single veins are recognisable. The liver is opacified through multiple collaterals.

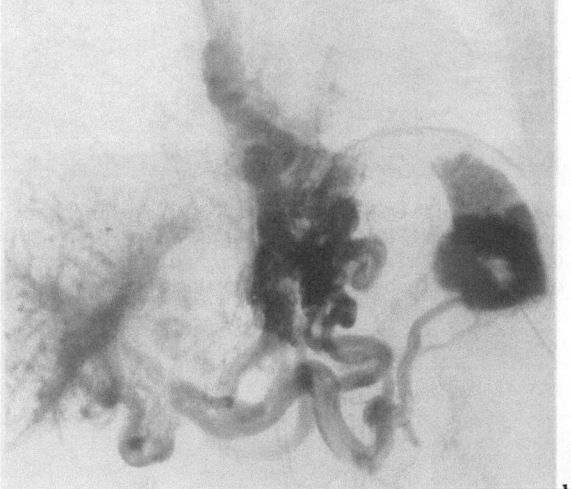

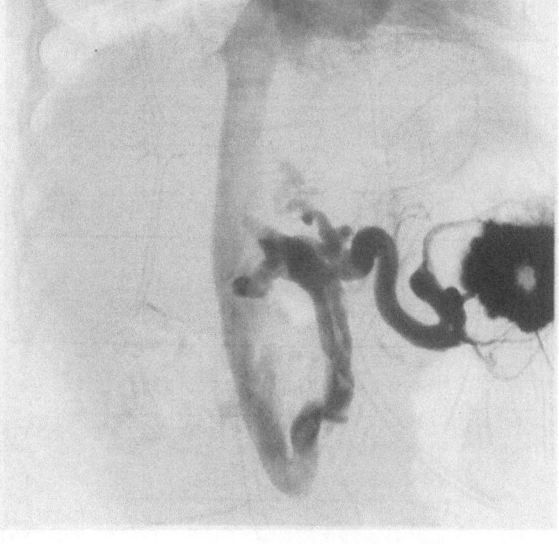

Fig. 3.21. Portal vein thrombosis: 5 years of age. **a, b** Splenoportogram. There is an atretic remnant of the portal vein (*arrow*). The liver is opacified through peribiliary veins. Large oesophageal varices, opacified by posterior gastric veins (*arrowhead*) and the left gastric vein (*arrow with bar*). **c** Same patient after ilio-mesenterico-caval anastomosis. Splenoportogram. Most of the blood is diverted toward the inferior vena cava through the shunt.

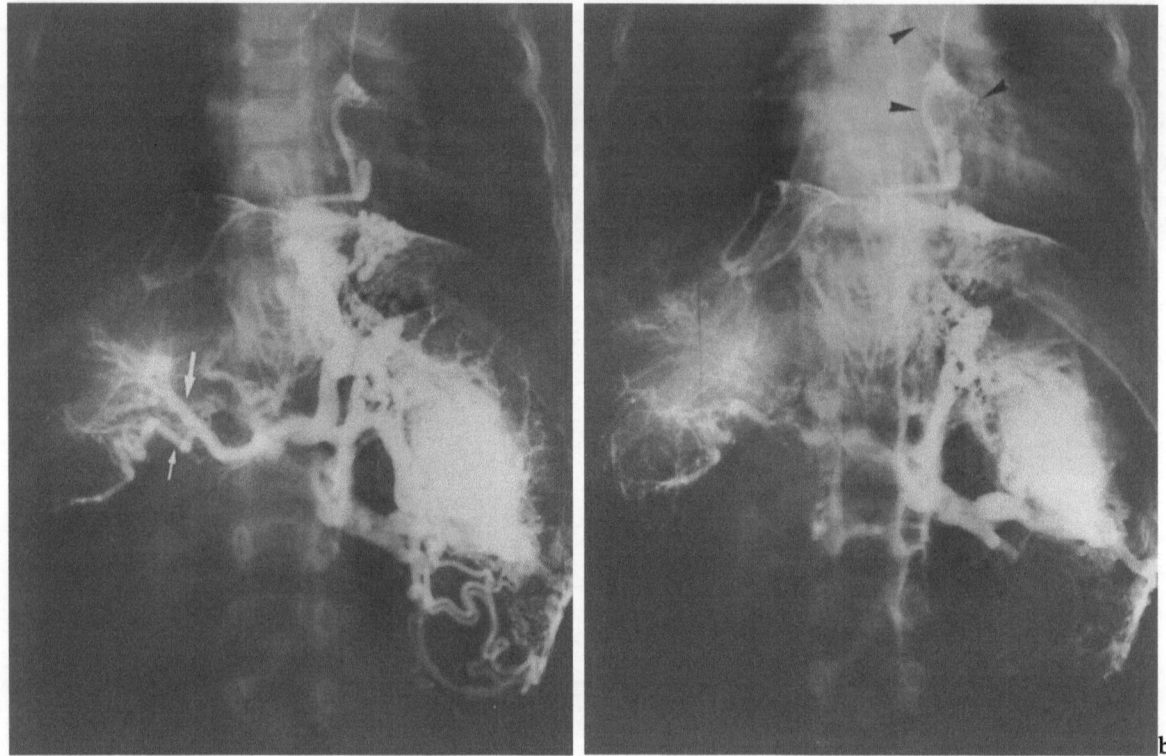

a   b

Fig. 3.22. Six-year-old boy with portal vein thrombosis secondary to a neonatal umbilical venous catheter. Spleno-portography. **a** Hilar thrombosis but the portal vein is patent (*large arrow*). Collateral veins are multiple: a large cystic vein (*small arrow*); a small left gastric vein; a large short gastric vein; diaphragmatic veins. **b** On the later film, there is also opacification of: a mediastinal vein joining a peribronchial vein (*arrowheads*); a splenorenal shunt; perivertebral veins.

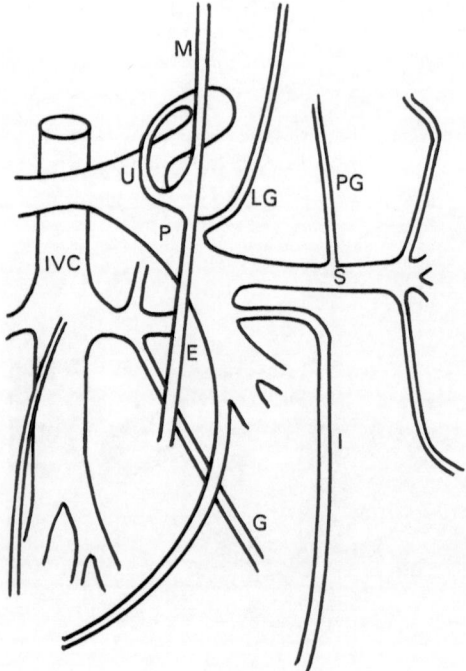

Fig. 3.23. Portosystemic Shunts.
Abbreviations: IVC, inferior vena cava; E, epigastric vein; I, inferior mesenteric; M, internal mammary; U, umbilical; P, portal; LG, left gastric; S, splenic; PG, posterior gastric; G, gonadal.

Findings (Figs. 3.24–3.35)

The hepatic artery is enlarged. Distal intra-hepatic branches are distorted by nodules of regeneration or have a corkscrew appearance in zones of atrophy.

The portal vein is of small size with poor branching. Inversion of flow can be partial, limited to one lobe or massive. Duplication of the intrahepatic portal veins has been observed, more frequently in biliary cirrhosis.

Portosystemic collaterals. In our experience no hepatopetal collateral vein has been observed in cirrhosis, probably because of the resistance due to the postsinusoïdal block.

Hepatofugal collaterals include, in addition to the usual gastro-oesophageal vein, the para-umbilical vein (20%) which anastomoses to the epigastric vein or to the internal mammary vein. Presence of a paraumbilical vein maintains hepatopetal flow in the left portal vein branch.

Portosystemic shunt may also be seen around surgical scars such as jejunostomies which were previously performed with the Kasai procedure in biliary atresia.

The inferior vena cava can be distorted due to atrophy of the liver or to compression by nodules of regeneration. One case of IVC thrombosis has been seen.

Biliary Atresia With Additional Malformations

In 10%–20% of cases, biliary atresia is associated with the so-called non-cardiac polysplenia syndrome.

Besides polysplenia, thoracic or abdominal situs inversus, small bowel malrotation, the syndrome may include various vascular anomalies.

In a series of 17 children explored by ultrasound and angiography, correlation was established with the surgical findings during Kasai or transplantation procedure. Type and frequency of anomalies were as follows (Figs. 3.36–3.42)

- Sex ratio: 12 girls, 5 boys
- Polysplenia: 16/17
- Heterotaxia: 6
    Abdominal situs inversus: 4
    Thoracic situs inversus: 1
    Thoraco-abdominal situs inversus: 1
- Abnormal IVC: 17
    Azygous continuation: 13
    Left IVC: 3
    Left hemiazygous continuation: 1

In these cases the hepatic veins drain directly into the right atrium.
- Portal vein:
    Thrombosis: 1
    Preduodenal portal vein: 13
The location of the portal vein is at best identified by ultrasound on its anteriorly convex course in front of the bright echoes of the duodenum. On angiogram the pre-duodenal portal vein may be incurved toward one or the other side, but it may be perfectly straight and overlooked. In one case there was a very unusual appearance of the portal vein, suggesting persistence of both embryonic vitelline veins.
- Hepatic artery: aberrant in all cases; there was no case of regular common hepatic artery.
    7 cases: 2 hepatic arteries.
    4 cases: a replaced right hepatic artery arising from the superior mesenteric artery.
    6 cases: a replaced left hepatic artery arising from the left gastric artery. In these cases the hepatic artery has a vertical ascending course parallel to the hepatofugal left gastric vein.

Congenital Hepatic Fibrosis

Definition

Congenital hepatic fibrosis (CHF) is a recessive autosomal disease characterised by enlarged fibrotic portal spaces containing numerous bile ductules more or less ectatic communicating with the biliary tree.

The liver disease is associated in virtually all cases with renal abnormalities consisting of polycystic kidney disease of variable severity. A child may have a predominent renal involvement, leading to renal insufficiency or a predominant liver disease.

Clinical Symptoms

Hepatomegaly is always present but liver function tests are normal. The possible complications are portal hypertension, cholangitis more rarely, renal failure and exceptionally in the late outcome cholangiocarcinoma.

The diagnosis may be strongly suggested by ultrasound of the liver and kidneys. It is unequivocally made by surgical liver biopsy but needle biopsy may miss the fibrotic areas.

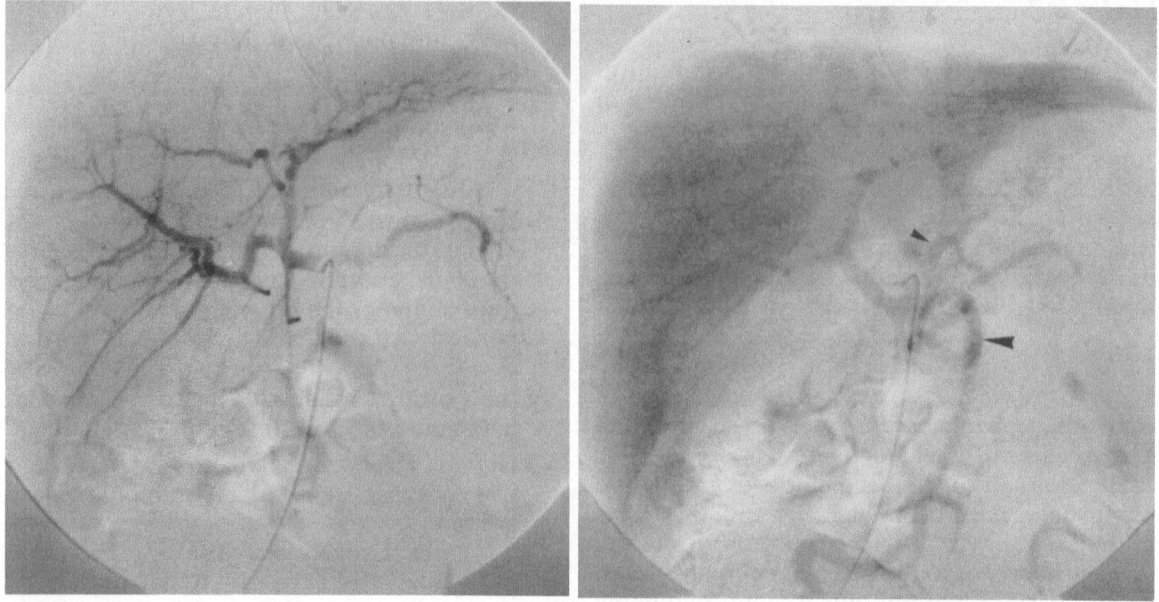

a   b

Fig. 3.24. Byler's disease and cirrhosis. Pretransplantation work-up. **a** Hepatic angiogram: the hepatic artery is dilated but the gross anatomy is normal. **b** Late phase: Inversion of flow in the portal system with opacification of the portal trunk, splenic vein and inferior mesenteric vein (*large arrowhead*). Left gastric vein and oesophageal varices are opacified (*small arrowhead*).

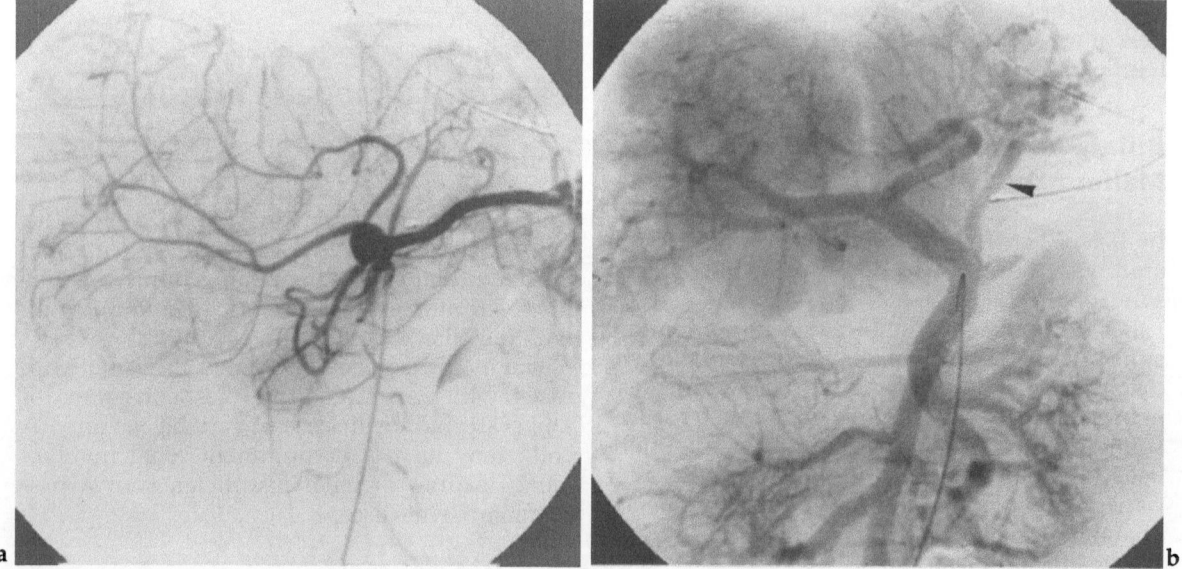

a   b

Fig. 3.25. Idiopathic macronodular cirrhosis. **a** Hepatic angiogram. There is marked distortion of the intrahepatic anatomy due to the multinodular liver. **b** Venous return of a mesenteric artery injection. There is marked distortion of the intrahepatic portal branches. The multinodular architecture of the liver is well seen, segments II and III are atrophic. Left gastric vein is opacified (*arrowhead*).

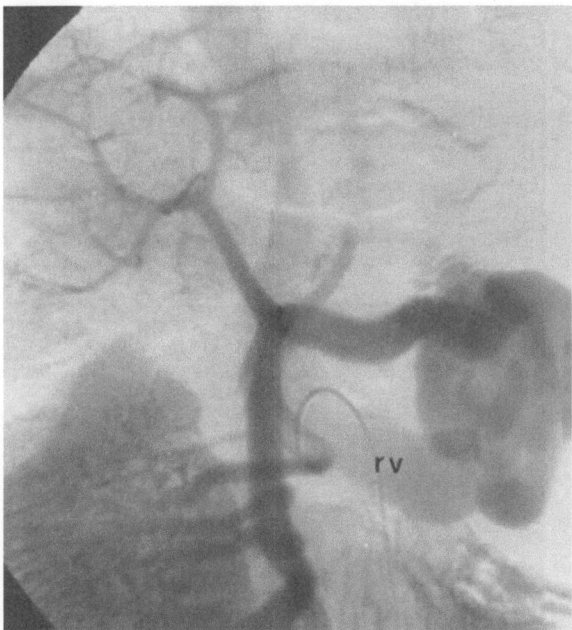

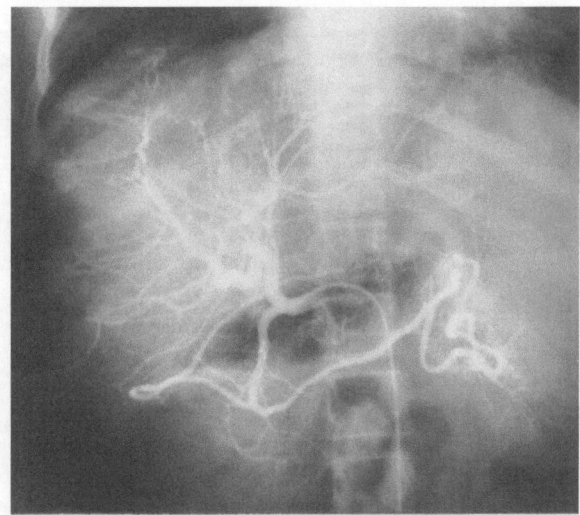

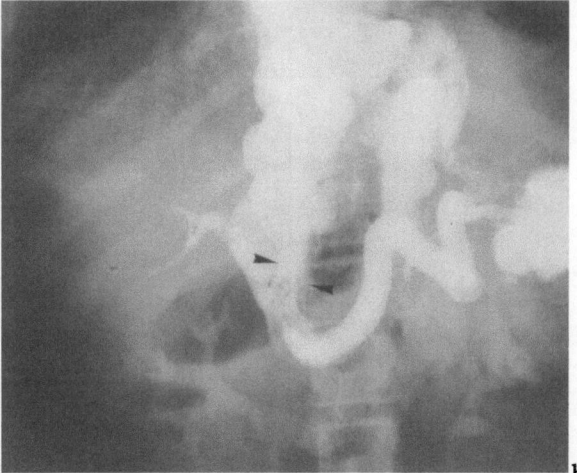

Fig. 3.26. Alpha 1 antitrypsin deficiency. Pretransplantation work-up. Venous return of a superior mesenteric artery injection. The superior mesenteric vein is opacified. The portal vein trunk is hypoplastic as well as the intrahepatic branches. The anatomy is distorted. There is an inversion of the flow in the splenic vein with an opacification of a spontaneous splenorenal shunt with opacification of the left renal vein (rv) and inferior vena cava. The left gastric vein is partialy opacified.

Fig. 3.27. Alpha 1 antitrypsin deficiency. **a** Hepatic artery ▶ injection. Moderate hypervascularisation. Slightly distorted intrahepatic anatomy. In the late phase (not shown) there was an inversion of the portal flow. **b** Splenoportography (splenic pressure: 25 cm H_2O). The intrahepatic branches of the portal vein are not opacified due to the inversion of flow. Large left gastric vein (*arrowheads*) opacifies the large oesophageal varices. **c** Same injection late phase. The splenorenal shunt is well seen with opacification of the left renal vein (rv) and inferior vena cava.

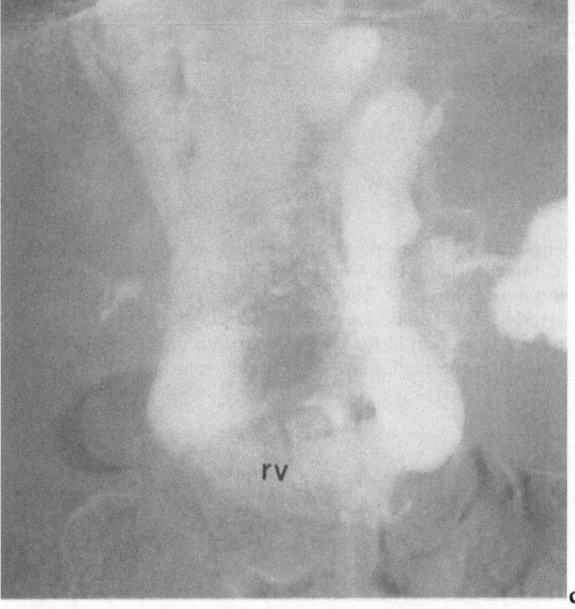

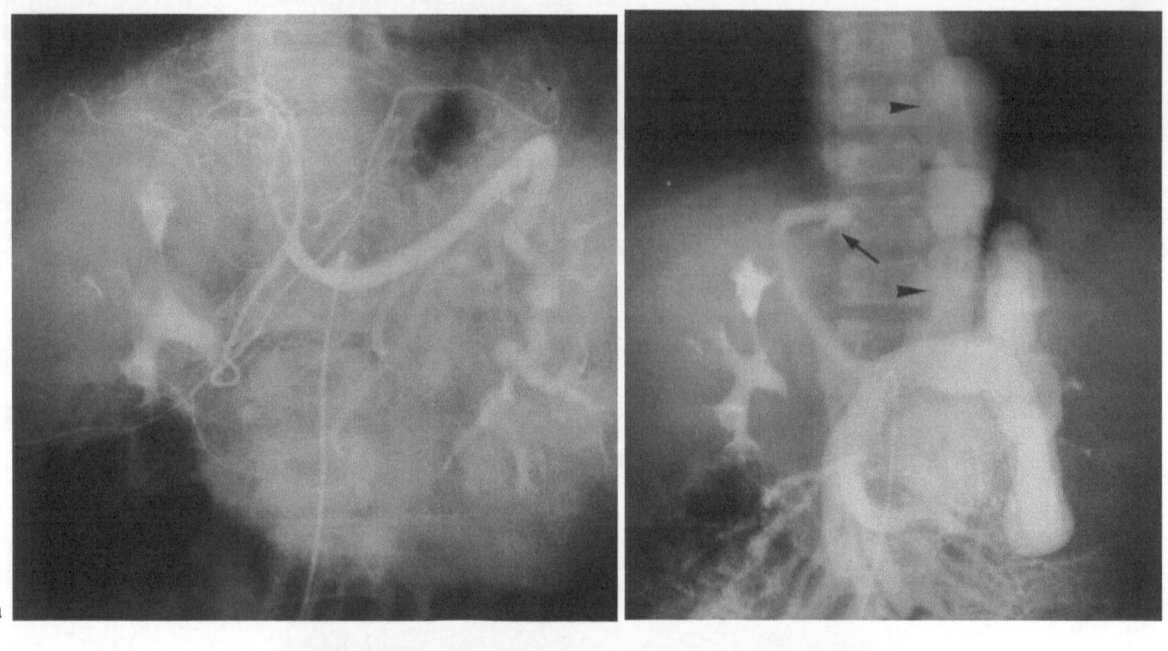

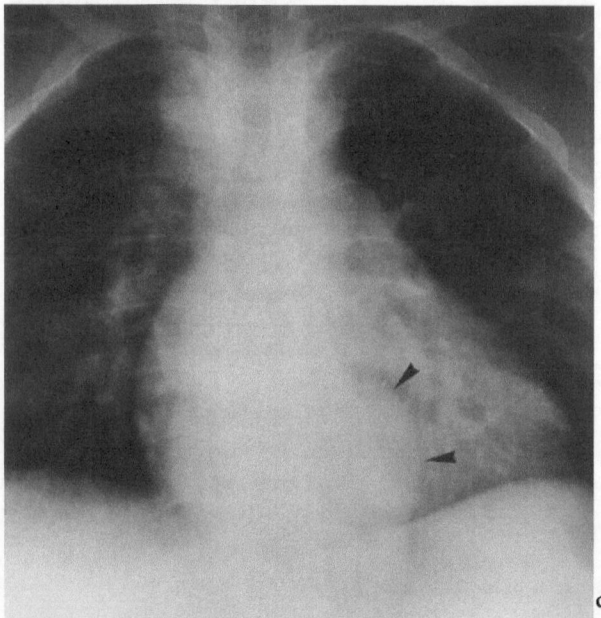

Fig. 3.28. 14-year-old girl presenting with biliary cirrhosis secondary to sclerosing cholangitis associated with histiocytosis X. Pretransplantation work-up. **a** Celiac trunk opacification: there is a large hypovascular nodule in the right lobe. The rest of the liver is atrophic. The splenic artery is enlarged with aneurysmal dilatations. **b** Venous phase of the superior mesenteric arteriogram. The portal vein is hypoplastic. There is a large indirect splenorenal spontaneous anastomosis draining into the hemiazygos vein (*arrowheads*). A paraumbilical vein is also seen (*arrow*). The right portal branch is not opacified. **c** On the chest film the displacement of the left paravertebral mediastinal line (*arrowheads*) corresponds to the enlarged hemiazygos vein.

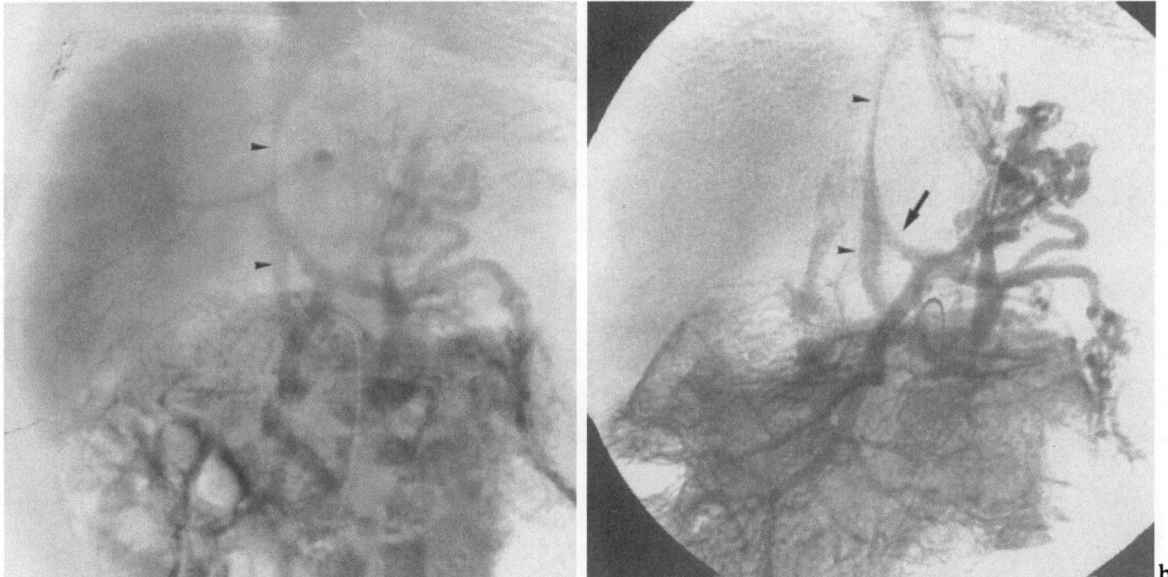

a   b

Fig. 3.29. Biliary atresia. Hepato-porto-enterostomy. Failure. Pretransplantation work-up. **a** 9 months of age. Venous return of superior mesenteric artery injection. The portal trunk and the intrahepatic portal branches are small but patent. There is retrograde opacification of the splenic vein and of a splenorenal shunt with opacification of the inferior vena cava (*arrowheads*). **b** Same patient: 20 months of age. Venous return of a superior mesenteric artery injection. There is no more opacification of the intrahepatic portal system because of inversion of the portal blood flow (*arrow*). Most of the mesenteric blood is diverted through oesophageal varices and splenorenal shunt.

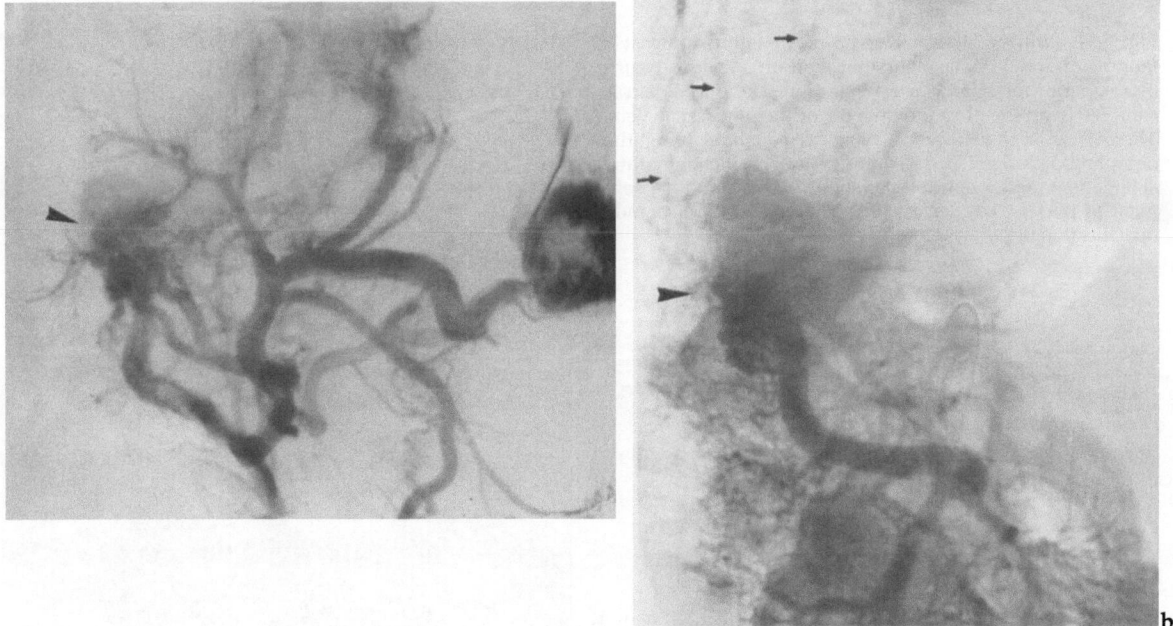

a   b

Fig. 3.30. Biliary atresia, portal hypertension. **a** Splenoportography. There is a large collateral coming from the first three jejunal veins towards the mouth of the jejunostomy (*arrowhead*). **b** Late phase of a superior mesenteric artery injection. Most of the mesenteric blood is draining into parietal veins (*small arrows*) around the mouth of the jejunostomy (*arrowhead*).

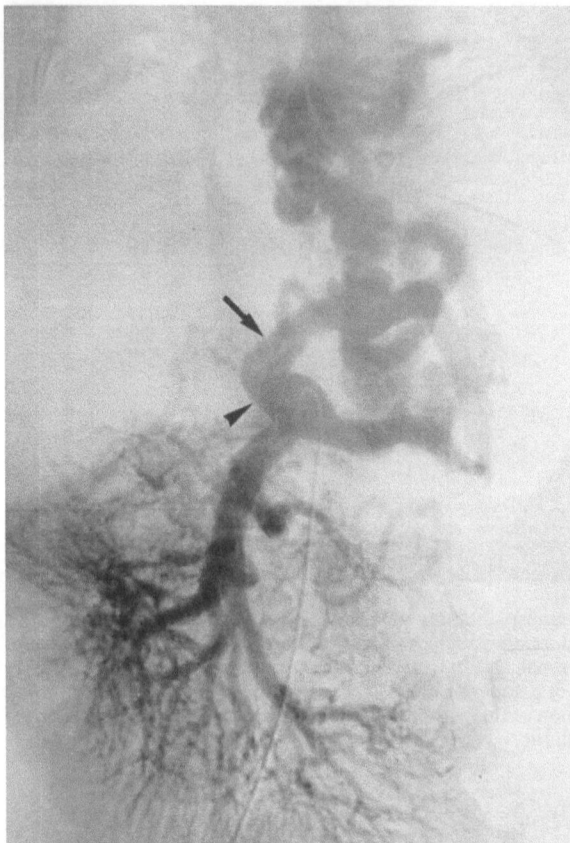

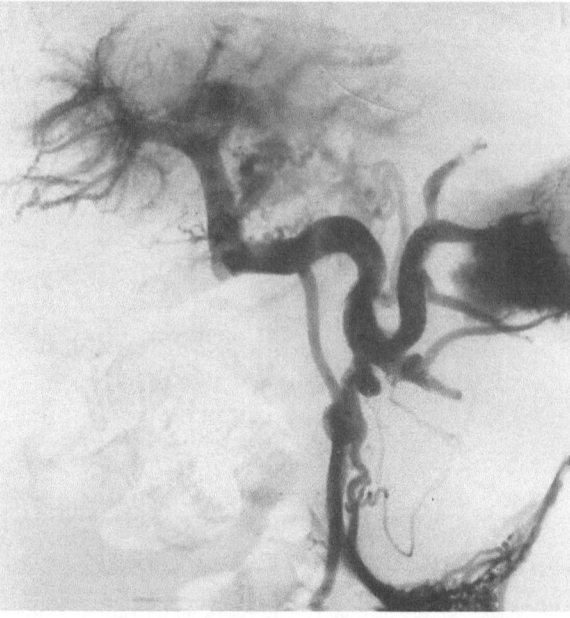

Fig. 3.32. Biliary atresia. Hepato-porto-enterostomy. Spleno-portography at 8 years of age (splenic pressure 38 cm H$_2$O). Opacification of the inferior mesenteric vein and perisplenic collaterals. Note some intrahepatic portal vein duplications.

Fig. 3.31. Biliary atresia. Hepato-porto-enterostomy at 3 months of age. Pretransplantation work-up. Venous return of a superior mesenteric artery injection. The portal vein is completely atretic after the take off of the left gastric vein. There is a large left gastric vein (*arrow*) opacifying the oesophageal varices. There is retrograde opacification of the splenic vein and a splenorenal shunt. Large proximal segment of portal trunk (*arrowhead*). There was no retrograde opacification of portal vein on hepatic angiogram.

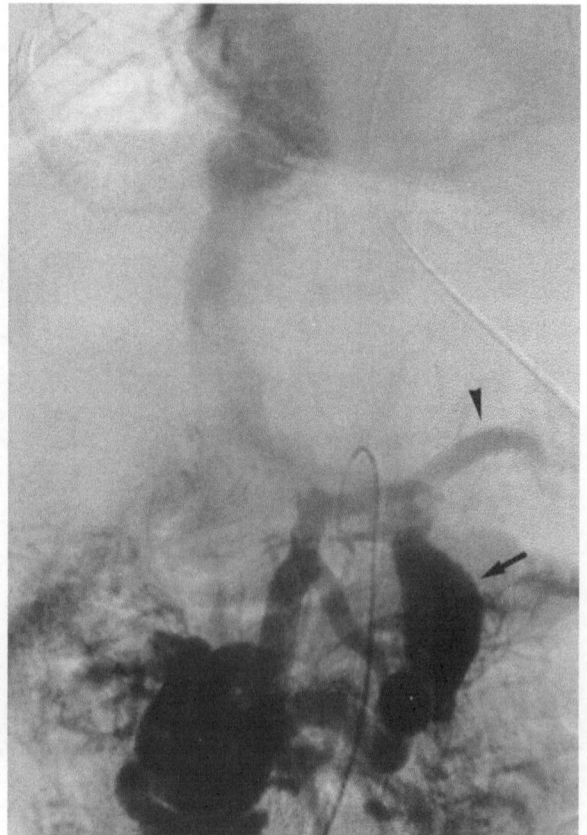

Fig. 3.33. Biliary atresia. Hepato-porto-enterostomy with ▶ jejunostomy. Failure at 8 years of age. Pretransplantation work-up. Venous return of the superior mesenteric artery injection. The superior mesenteric vein drains into multiple collaterals around the jejunostomy and into a left gonadic (*arrow*) vein draining into the left renal vein and the inferior vena cava. There is a reflux in the splenic vein (*arrowhead*). There is no opacification of the portal vein.

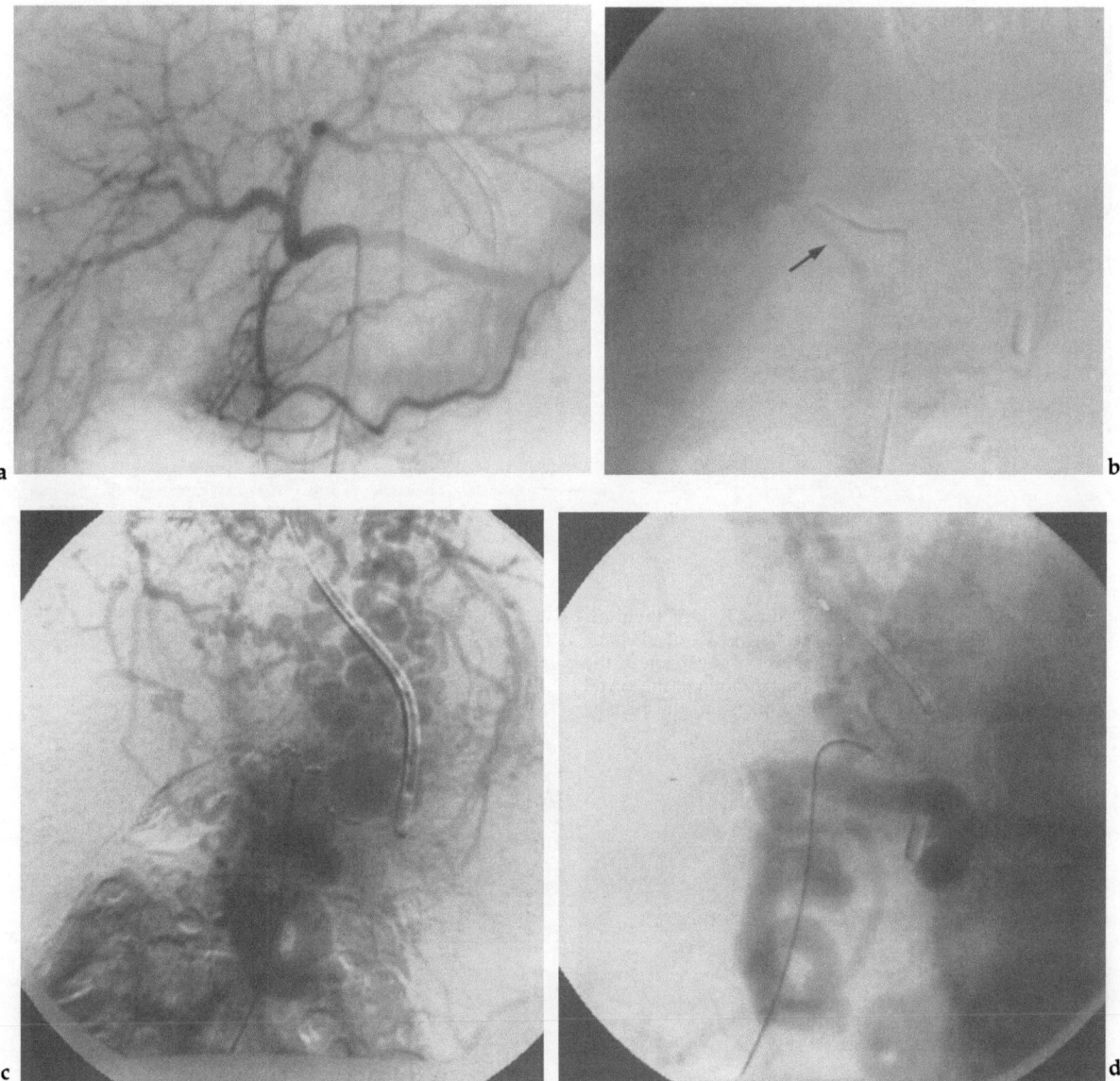

Fig. 3.34. Biliary atresia. Hepato-porto-enterostomy (D 71) with jejunostomy. Persistance of jaundice. Pretransplantation work-up. 13 months of age. **a** Hepatic angiogram. The hepatic artery is dilated but the anatomy is normal. **b** Late phase. The portal vein is opacified because of reversion of flow. The portal trunk is small (*arrow*). **c** Venous phase of the superior mesenteric artery injection. Most of the mesenteric blood flow opacifies parietal veins, which are anterior and secondary to the jejunostomy. **d** Same patient. Venous return of the splenic artery injection. There is an inversion of flow in the superior mesenteric vein and parietal veins.

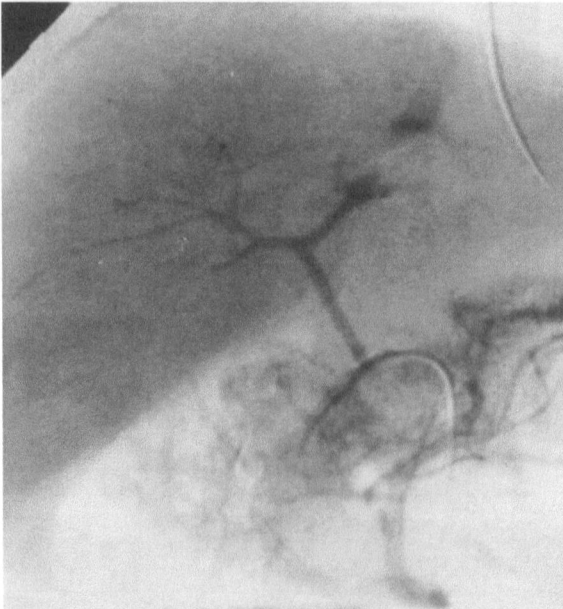

Fig. 3.35. Biliary atresia. Kasaï procedure. Failure. Pretransplantation work-up. 8 months of age. Late phase of a hepatic artery injection. This is a typical aspect of inversion of the portal blood flow with retrograde opacification of the portal system and portal trunk on the late phase of the hepatic artery injection.

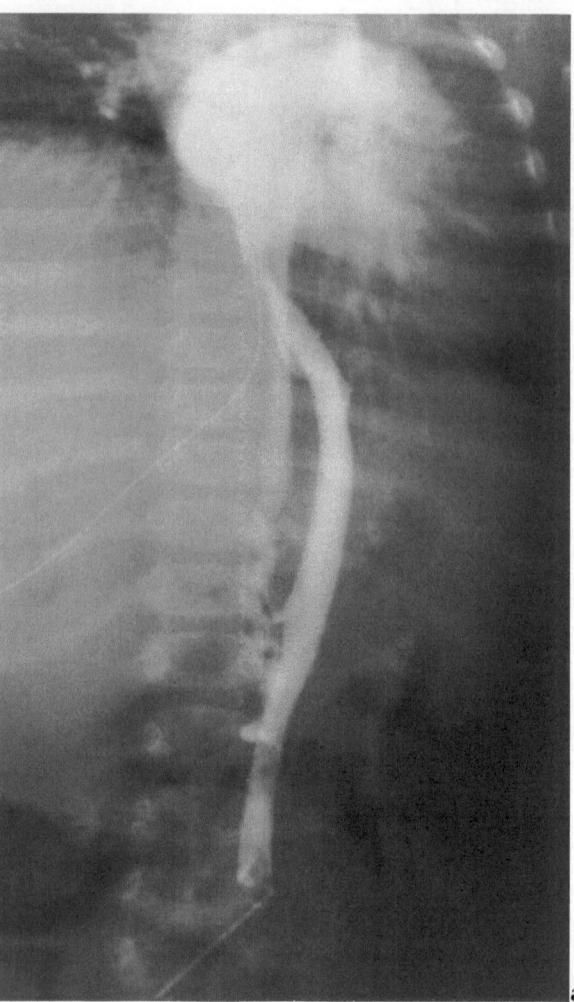

a

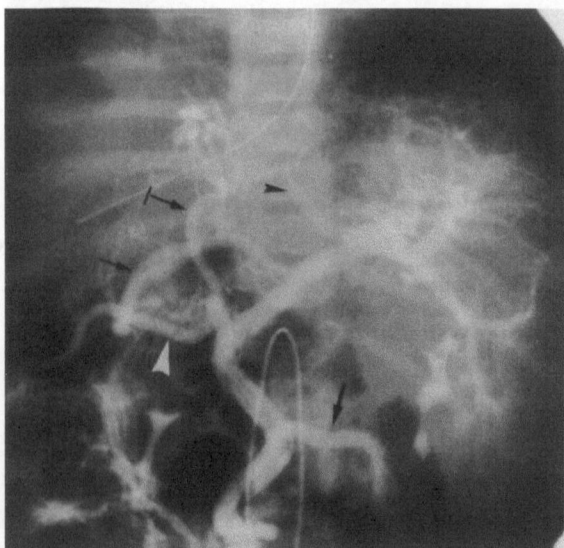

Fig. 3.36. Thoracic and abdominal situs inversus. The portal vein has an inverted course toward the liver which is in the left side of the abdomen. It was preduodenal on ultrasound and at surgery. There is partial inversion of flow in the right portal branch (*small arrowhead*). There is opacification of the splenic vein (*large arrowhead*), the left gastric vein (*arrow with bar*), the right gastric vein (pyloric vein) (*small arrow*), the inferior mesenteric vein (*large arrow*).

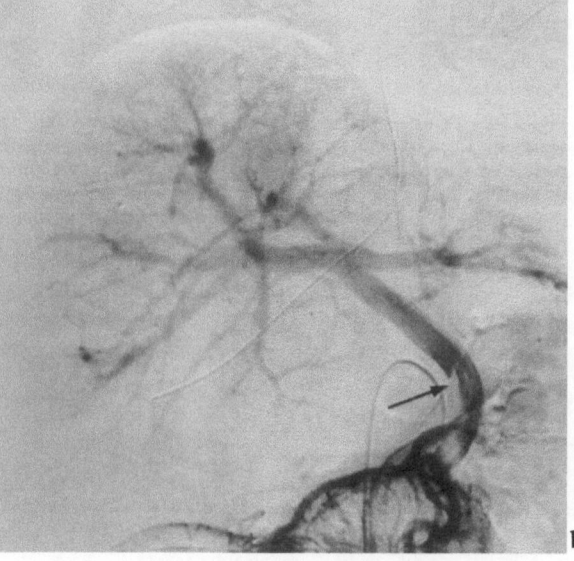

b

Fig. 3.37. Abdominal situs inversus. *Caption opposite*

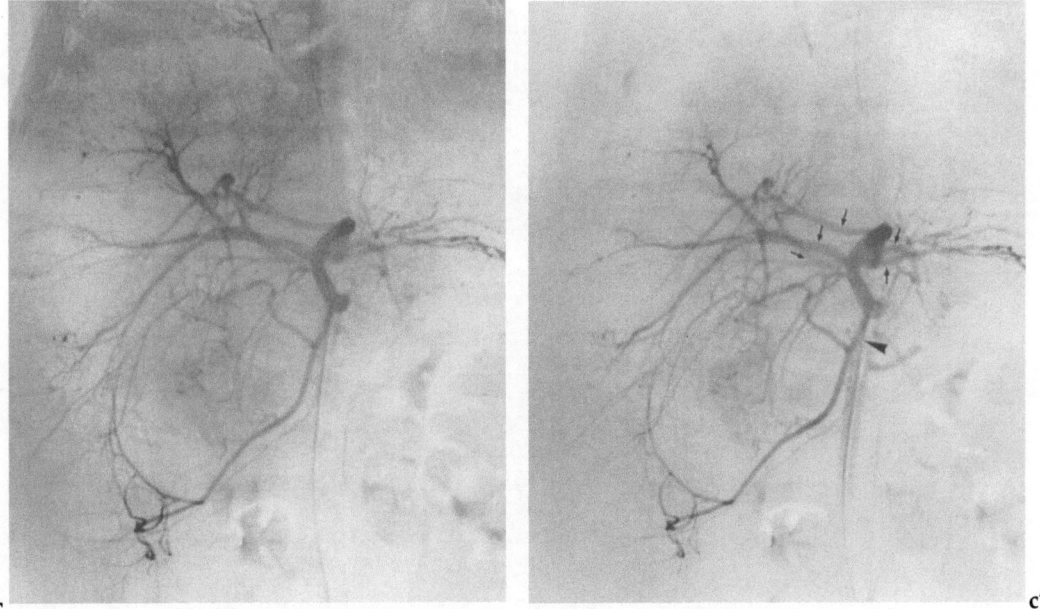

c   c′

Fig. 3.37. Abdominal situs inversus (*continued*). **a** The inferior vena cava is left-sided and crosses the midline to join the right atrium. There is also opacification of a left hemiazygous vein. **b** Venous phase of the superior mesenteric arteriogram. The liver is mainly located in the right upper quadrant. The superior mesenteric vein is on the left of the superior mesenteric artery, but the portal vein has an usual course. There is no opacification of the splenic vein (*arrow*). **c** Hepatic arteriogram with stereographic technique. The hepatic artery has a vertical ascending course and gives three branches to the right and two to the left (*small arrows*). The left gastric artery arises (*arrowhead*) just at the origin of the hepatic artery.

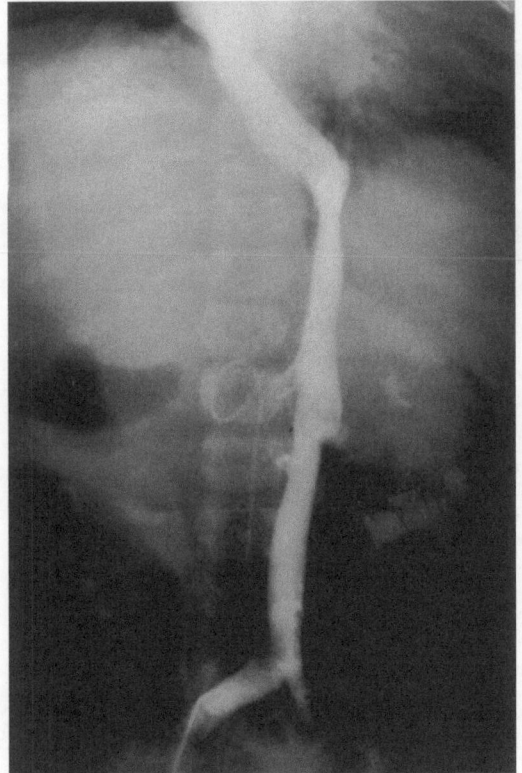

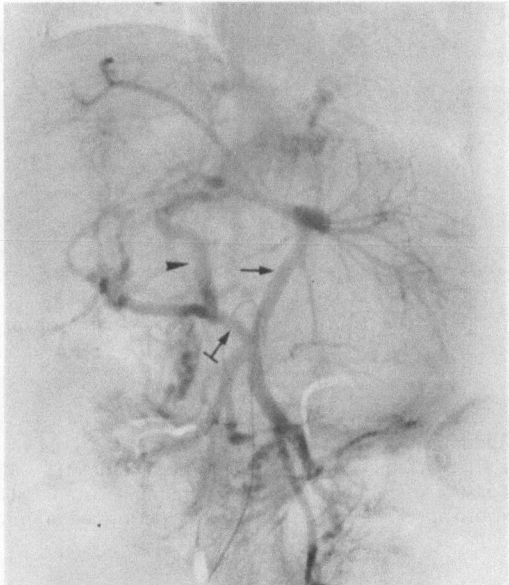

b

Fig. 3.38. Abdominal situs inversus. **a** The inferior vena cava is left-sided and crosses the midline at the level of the diaphragm to join the right atrium. **b** Venous phase of the superior mesenteric arteriogram. The liver is mainly located into the left upper quadrant and the portal vein has an inverted course (*arrow*). It was preduodenal on ultrasound. There is opacification of the splenic vein (*arrow with bar*) and of the left gastric vein (*arrowhead*) which supplies gastric varices. *Continued overleaf.*

a

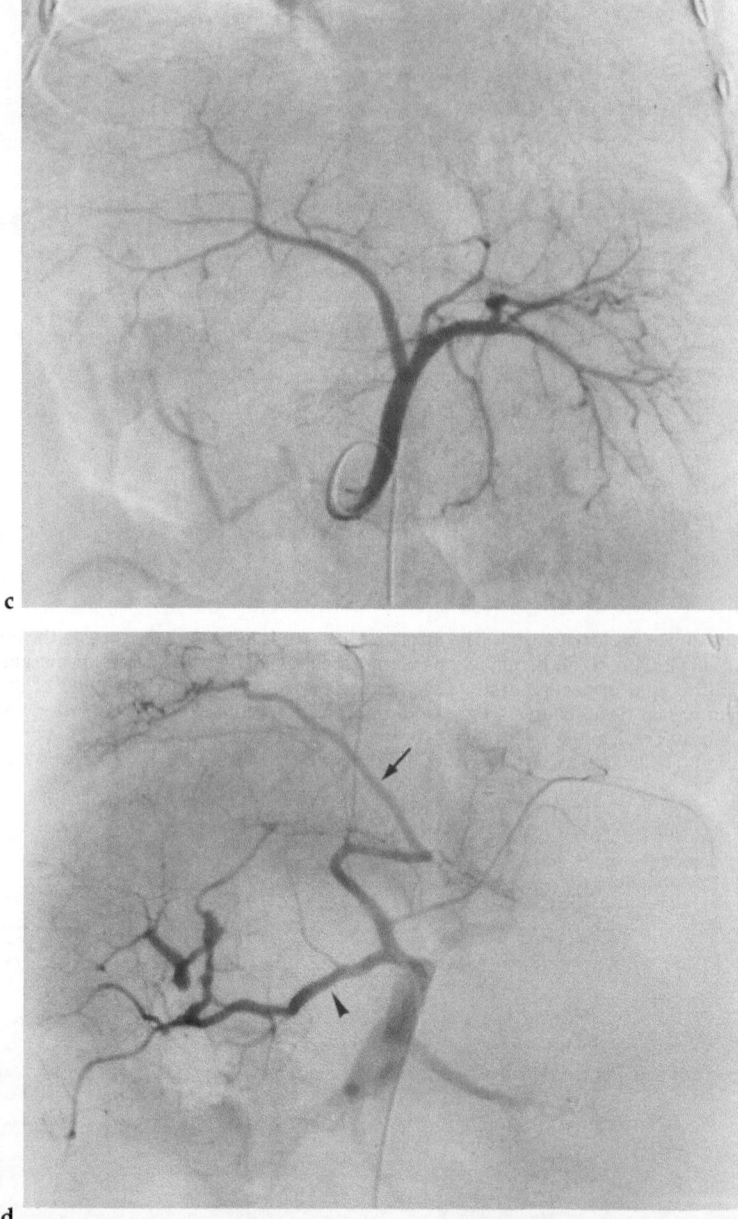

Fig. 3.38. Abdominal situs inversus (*continued*). **c** The arterial vascularisation of the liver is mainly supplied by a replaced right hepatic artery arising from the superior mesenteric artery. **d** There is also an accessory hepatic artery (*arrow*) arising from the left gastric artery. Both inferior diaphragmatic arteries also originate from the left gastric artery. The splenic artery (*arrowhead*) is also opacified. The arterial study is performed in stereoangiography.

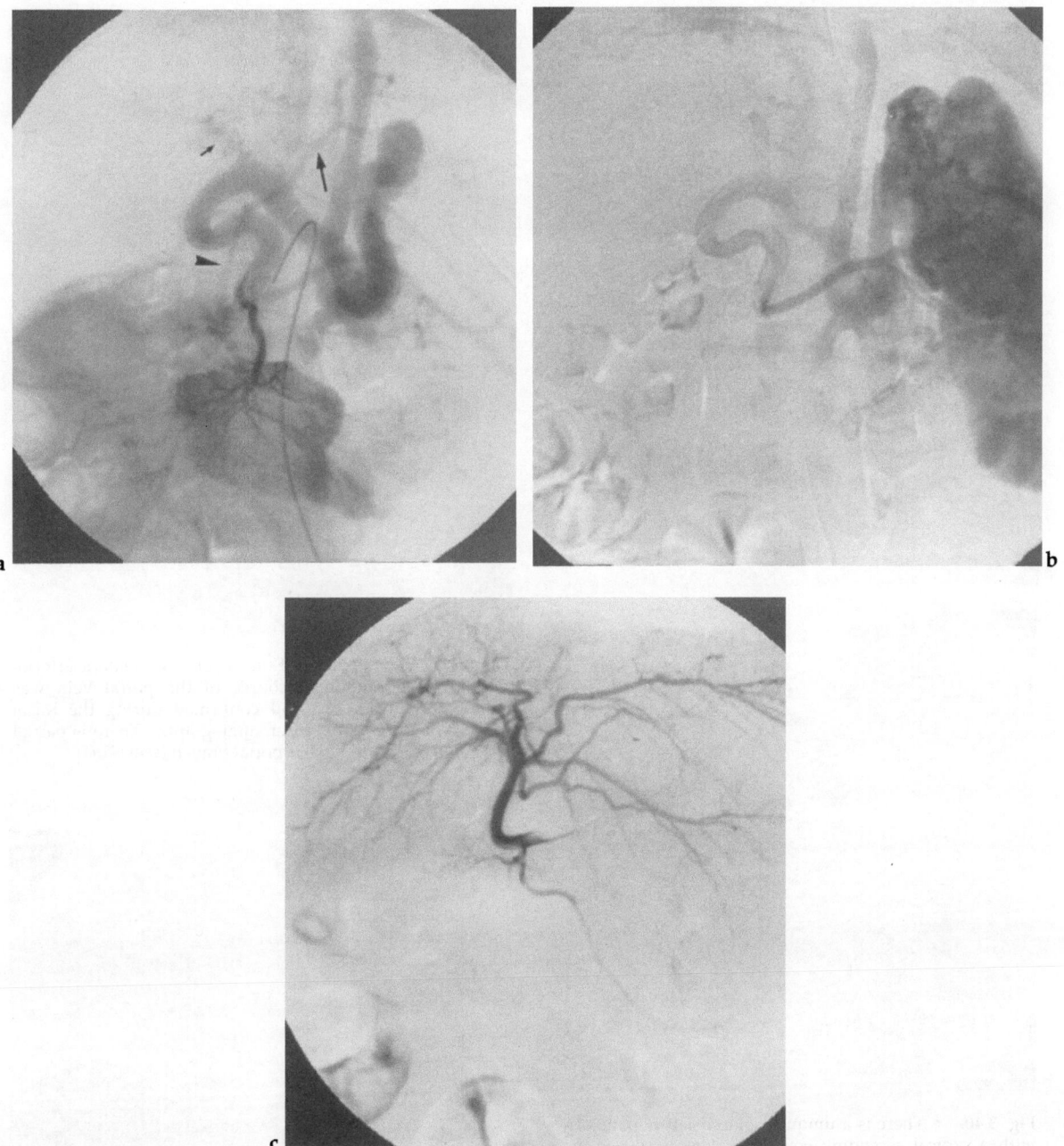

Fig. 3.39. Complex anatomy. **a** Venous phase of the superior mesenteric arteriogram. Left (*large arrow*) and tortuous right portal (*small arrow*) branches arise from a small portal vein (*arrowhead*). There is also opacification of a large vein going toward the hepatic hilum but then joining an indirect spontaneous splenorenal shunt, which drains into a left hemiazygos vein. **b** This splenorenal shunt is well opacified on the venous phase of the splenic artery injection. **c** The liver is in a middle position. There is a unique replaced left hepatic artery with a vertical ascending course.

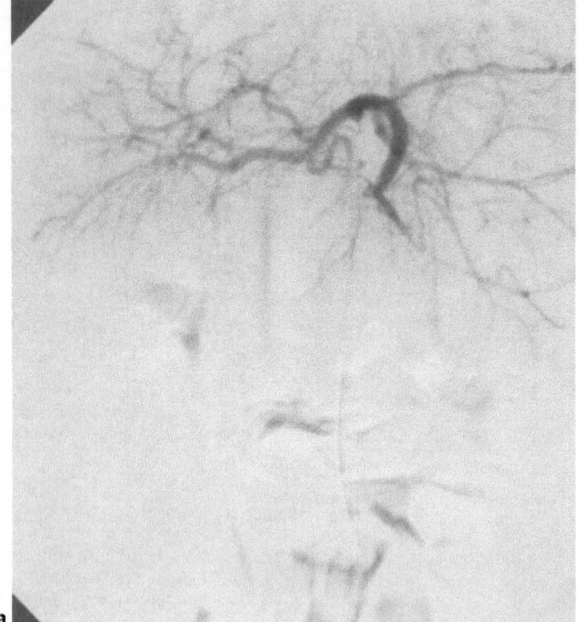

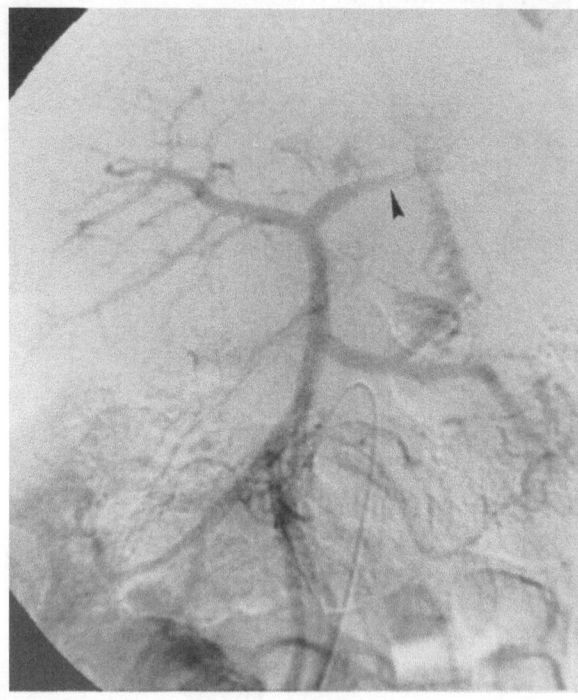

Fig. 3.41. Venous phase of the superior mesenteric arteriogram. The preduodenal course of the portal vein was evident on ultrasound and confirmed during the Kasaï procedure but is not seen on angiography. There is partial inversion of flow in the left portal branch (*arrowhead*).

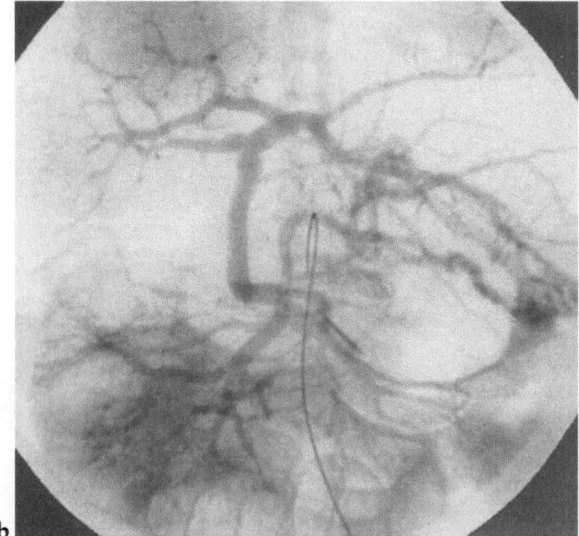

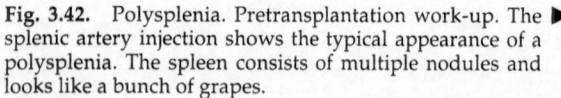

Fig. 3.40. a There is a unique replaced left hepatic artery with a typical ascending course. **b** Venous phase of the superior mesenteric arteriogram. The portal vein is preduodenal and has an unusual course incurvated toward the right side.

Fig. 3.42. Polysplenia. Pretransplantation work-up. The ▶ splenic artery injection shows the typical appearance of a polysplenia. The spleen consists of multiple nodules and looks like a bunch of grapes.

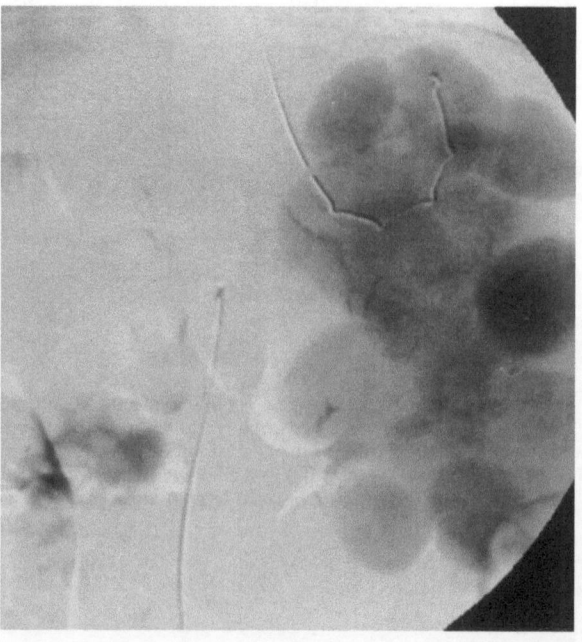

Angiography (Figs. 3.43–3.52)

Among 74 cases of CHF seen in our institution, 30 were studied by angiography as a pre-operative work-up before a surgical porto-systemic shunt.

Duplication of the intrahepatic portal veins are well described. They now are known not to be specific of the disease as they may also be encountered in other diseases, mainly in biliary cirrhosis. They probably represent intrahepatic peribiliary collaterals, secondary to either thrombosis or hypoplasia of the portal venules as shown in the portal tracts on liver biopsy. Such duplications were seen in all cases with portal hypertension.

In 10 cases (66% of cases) hepatopetal collateral veins were also seen, doubling the patent portal vein and proximal branches. This hepatopetal network was extensive in three cases, mimicking a portal cavernoma. It probably corresponds to peribiliary veins which shunt the presinusoïdal block present in congenital hepatic fibrosis.

The association of hepatofugal and hepatopetal collateral veins contrasting with a patent portal trunk and proximal branches is unusual and should suggest the diagnosis of congenital hepatic fibrosis.

In one case aneurysmal dilatation of the left portal vein branch was found. Opacification of the Arantius duct was also seen in another case.

Arterial hypervascularity was also seen probably compensating the portal hypoperfusion.

Cholangiography

Although cholangiography is liable to cause complications in CHF, it was performed three times to assess the diffusion of the disease. In two cases typical ectasias such as described in Caroli's disease were found. In one case, slight biliary dysplasia was present. We think that in a child with Caroli's disease the kidneys should be checked for recessive polycystic kidney disease.

Budd–Chiari Syndrome

Definition

Budd–Chiari syndrome is present when there is a block at the level of the main hepatic veins and/or the suprahepatic inferior vena cava. It should be differentiated from veno-occlusive disease and liver involvement in cardiac disease. It is a rare occurrence in children. In most cases no cause is found.

Clinical Findings

Hepatomegaly is always present. It may be fortuitously discovered or associated with ascites, splenomegaly, collateral venous circulation, abdominal pain or unexplained fever.

Liver function tests are usually normal or minimally abnormal. In two of our cases a tumoral aetiology was present (epithelioïd haemangioendothelioma and amoebic abcess). Familial Budd–Chiari syndrome was seen with two sisters involved.

Diagnosis

It is usually suggested by ultrasonography with Doppler which shows abnormal anatomy or flow of the IVC or the hepatic veins.

Liver biopsy shows sinusoïdal dilatation with centrolobular haemorrhagic infiltration and portal fibrosis. In rare cases cirrhosis is evident.

Angiography confirms the diagnosis, shows the level and the extent of the obstacle and is critical to planning surgical treatment.

Treatment consists in portocaval anastomosis to relieve the venous congestion of the liver.

Angiography

Technique

General anaesthesia must be avoided because of the poor haemodynamic status of these children. A pressure recording of the pulmonary capillary and artery, right ventricle, atrium and IVC should be taken. The pressure of the IVC must be measured and compared to the portal vein pressure.

The radiological work-up includes cavography, opacification of the hepatic veins, and of the portal vein system. Opacification of the hepatic veins can be obtained by a retrograde catheterisation via a femoral vein or a jugular vein approach. When there is no ascites or coagulation disorder, a transhepatic approach is possible, allowing opacification and pressure recording of the hepatic and portal veins.

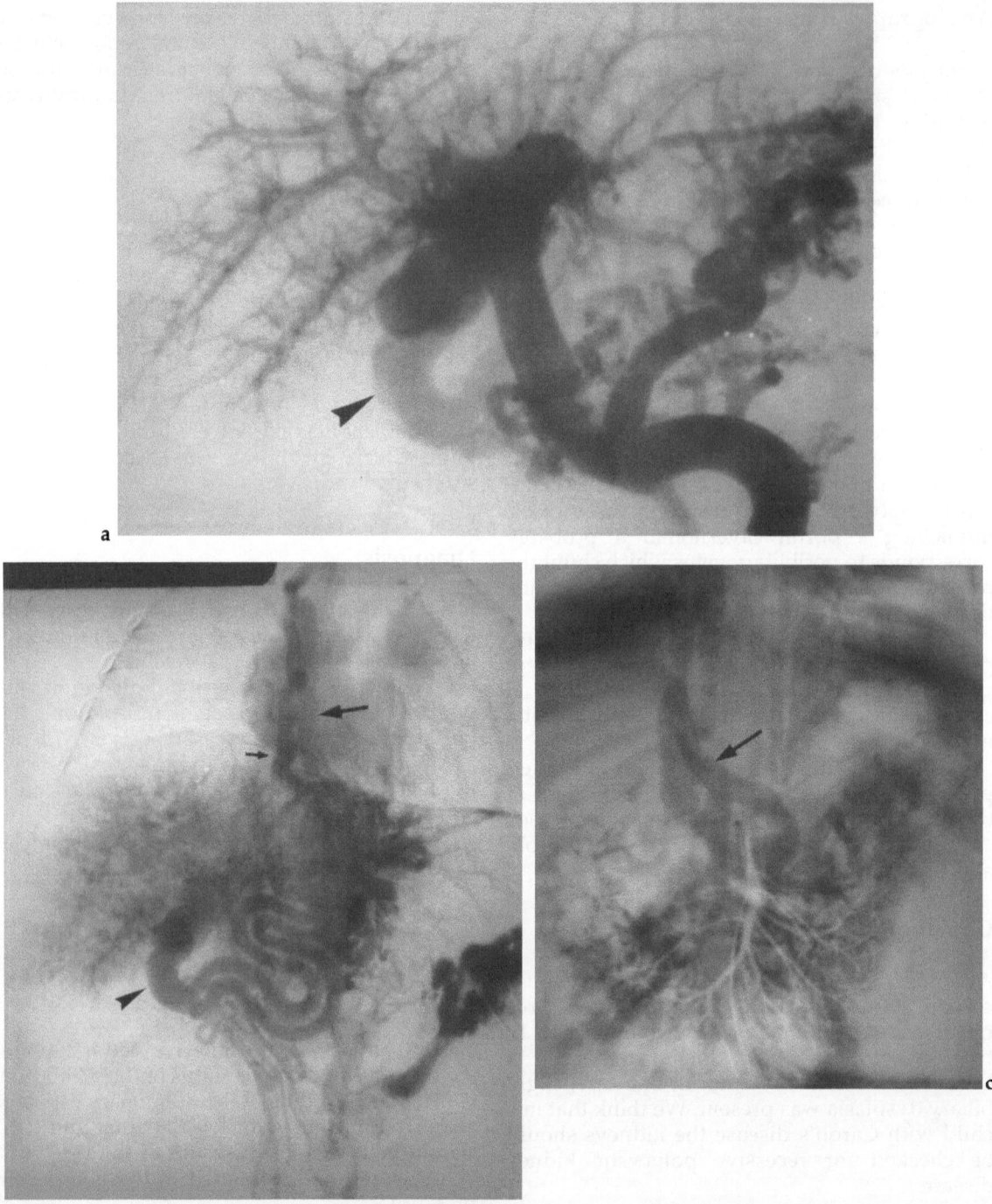

Fig. 3.43. **a** Splenoportography. The classic finding of duplication of the intrahepatic portal veins is seen. The large left gastric vein is opacified (*arrowhead*). **b** There is a large duplicated umbilical vein (*arrowhead*) draining into the right internal mammary vein (*small arrow*). The right azygos vein (*large arrow*) is opacified through oesophageal varices. Portal pressure: 34 cm H$_2$O. **c** Same patient after surgical spleno-renal shunt. Venous phase of superior mesenteric artery injection. The portal trunk (*arrow*) is partialy opacified, the splenic vein is entering the left renal and opacifies the inferior vena cava.

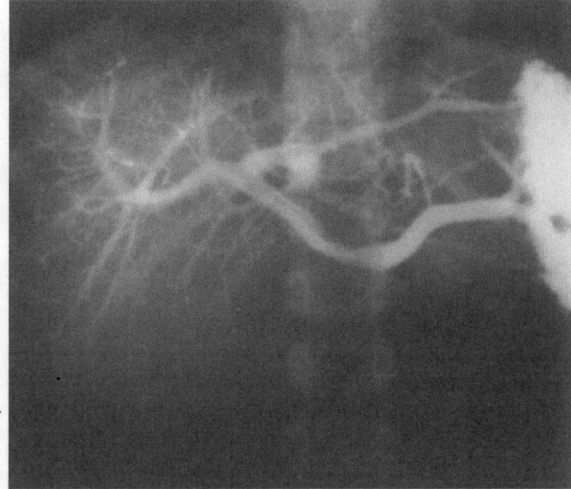

Fig. 3.44. Congenital hepatic fibrosis. Splenoportography. The intrahepatic portal arborisation is normal. There is an opacification of a posterior gastric vein. Splenic pressure 16cm of H$_2$O, normal.

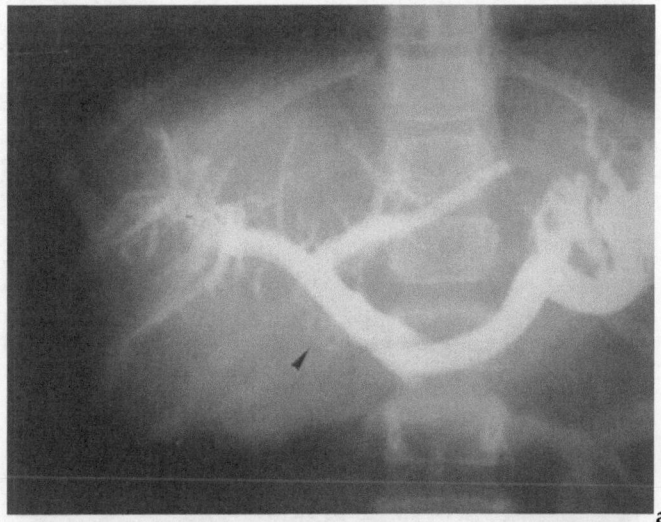

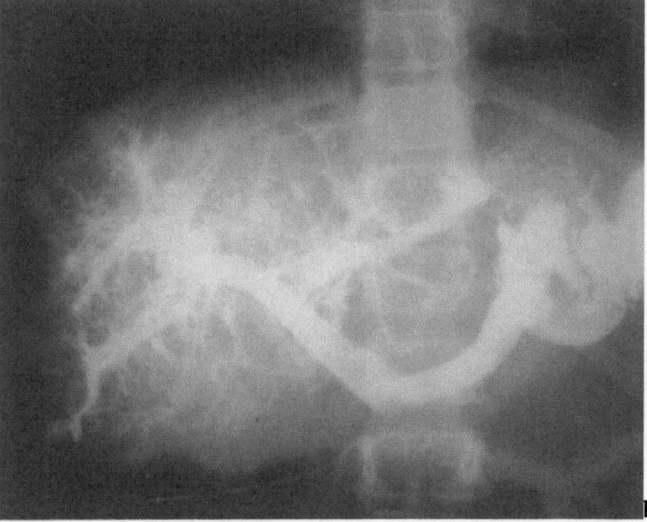

Fig. 3.45. 9 years of age. Splenic pressure 21 cm H$_2$O. **a, b** Splenoportogram. Some small portal vein branches are lacking probably due to segmental thrombosis. Portal vein branch duplications well seen. There is opacification of some posterior gastric veins. And an opacification of a hepatopetal (peribiliary) vein (*arrowhead*).

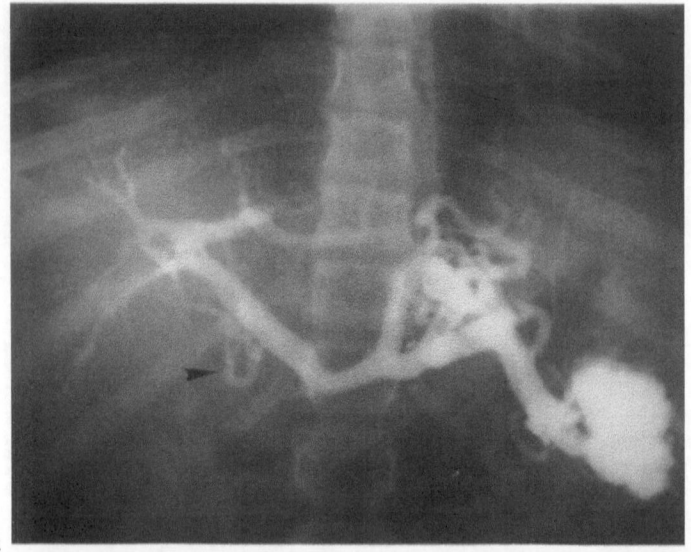

a

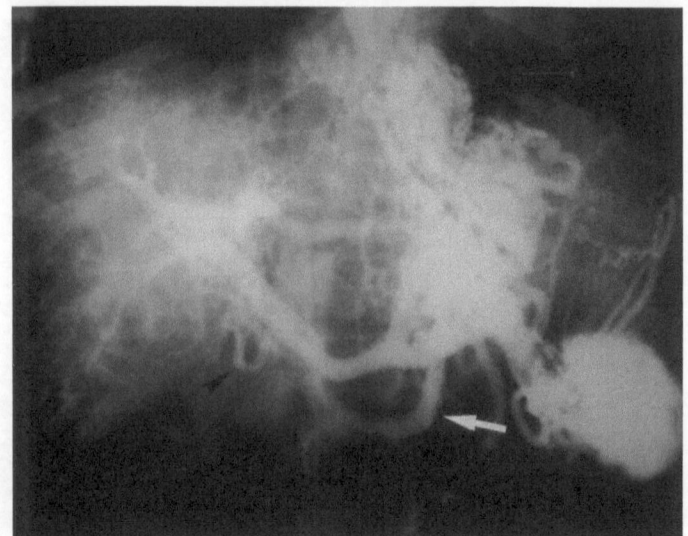

b

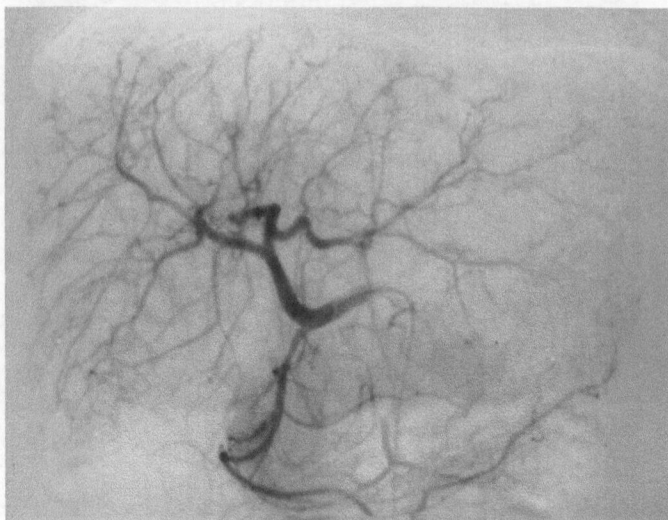

c

Fig. 3.46. 11 years of age. **a, b** Splenoportogram. The intrahepatic anatomy is distorted with some segmental thrombosis. Some intrahepatic veins are duplicated. There is opacification of a hepatopetal peribiliary vein (*arrowhead*) (choledochal vein). The left gastric and posterior gastric veins are opacified. Large oesophageal varices are seen. Splenorenal shunt (*arrow*). Portal pressure: 24 cm H_2O. **c** Same patient. Hepatic angiogram. Moderate hypervascularisation, mainly at the periphery of the liver.

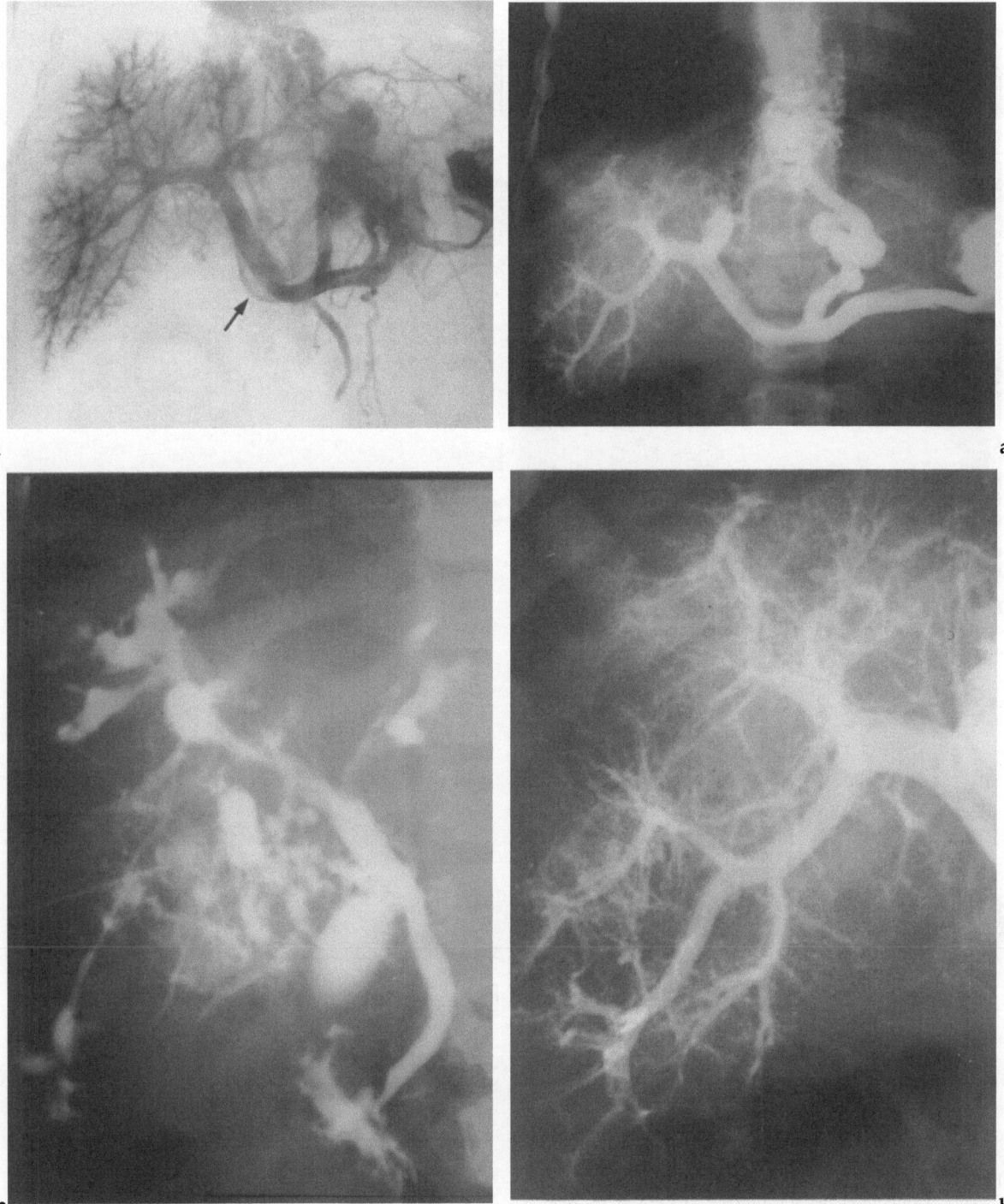

Fig. 3.47. Congenital hepatic fibrosis. Recessive polycystic kidney disease, portal hypertension, moderate renal insufficiency. **a** Splenoportography. Duplication of the intrahepatic portal branches. Opacification of the oesophageal varices through the left gastric vein and posterior gastric veins. Splenorenal shunt (*arrow*). **b** Percutaneous transhepatic cholangiography. Multiple communicating cysts are seen through out the liver.

Fig. 3.48. Congenital hepatic fibrosis: 13 years of age. **a** Splenoportogram. Portal pressure: 27 cm H$_2$O. A large left gastric vein is seen. **b** Close-up view demonstrates clearly the intrahepatic duplication, sometimes triplication of the intrahepatic portal vein branches.

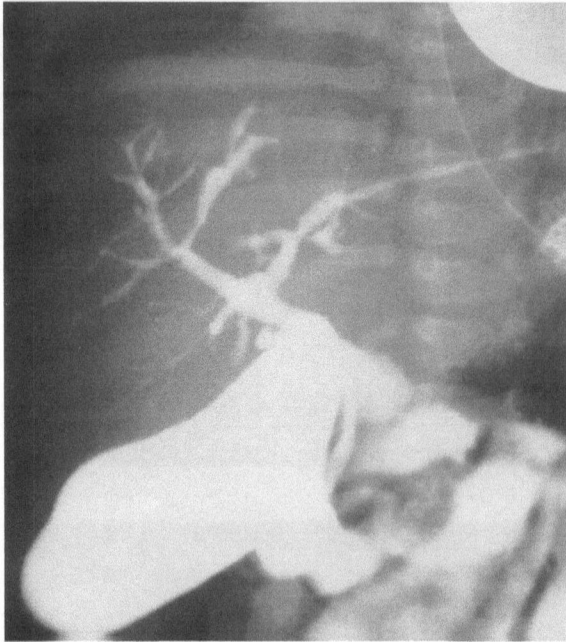

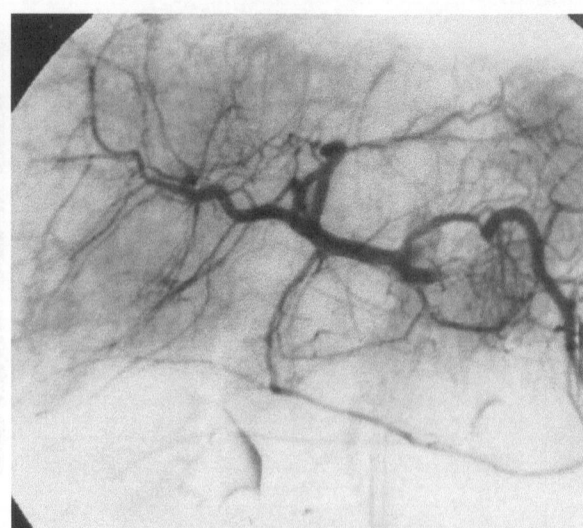

Fig. 3.49. 17 months of age. Percutaneous transhepatic cholecystography. The intrahepatic biliary ducts are moderately dilated, with some ectasias.

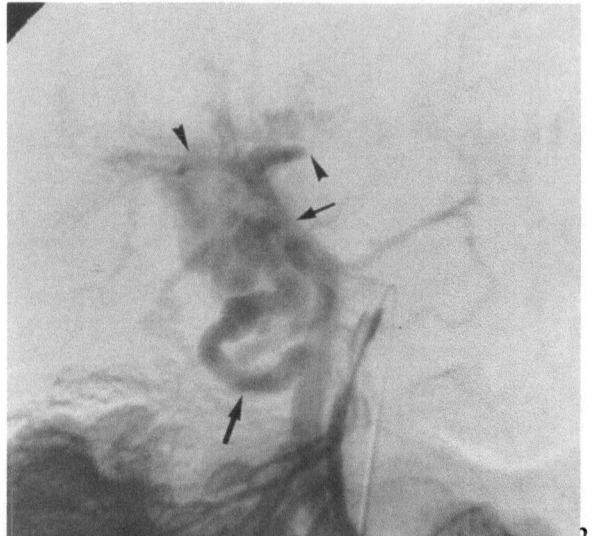

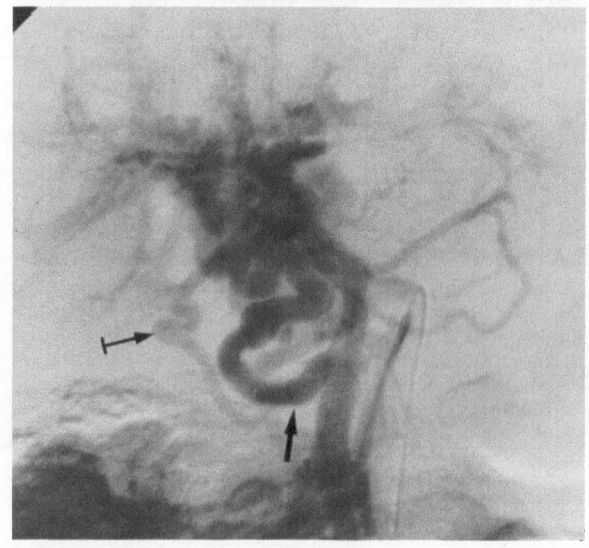

Fig. 3.50. A 4-year-old girl presenting with hepatosplenomegaly. Congenital hepatic fibrosis diagnosed by liver biopsy. **a** Hepatic angiogram. The hepatic arteries are dilated. Some segmental arteries are duplicated or triplicated. **b, c** Venous return of superior mesenteric artery. The portal vein is patent (*small arrow*). There is abrupt tapering of both the left and right portal vein branches (*arrowheads*). There is a large pancreaticoduodenal collateral (*large arrow*) arising from the superior mesenteric vein, and doubling the portal vein. There are also multiple duplicating intrahepatic veins. A paraumbilical vein is opacified (*arrow with bar*). There is only a slight reflux in the left gastric vein.

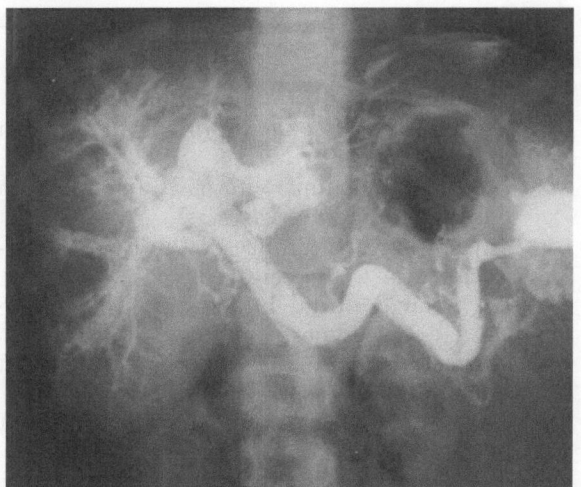

a

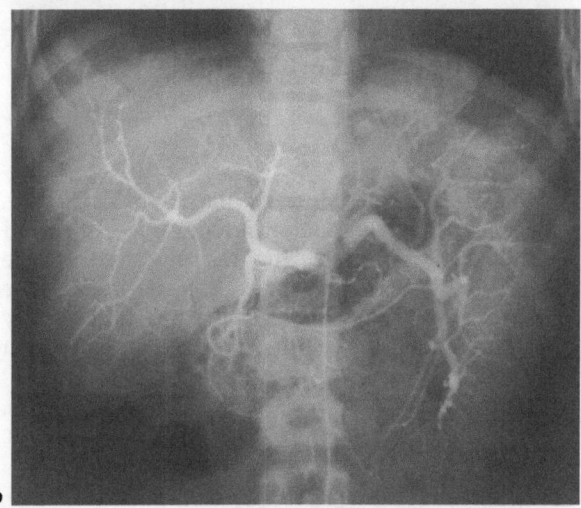

b

◀ **Fig. 3.51.** 10 years of age. **a** Splenoportogram. Multiple duplications are seen in the liver. A large varix of the left portal vein is seen. Portal pressure: 35 cm H_2O. **b** Same patient, hepatic angiogram: slight distortion of the arterial pattern in the periphery of the liver.

Fig. 3.52. Cholestasis of unknown aetiology: an 11-year-old boy presenting with microcephaly, mental retardation, cholestasis, splenomegaly and severe portal hypertension. Splenoportography: the portal pressure is measured at 37 cm H_2O. All the veins opacified are markedly enlarged (diameter of the splenic vein: 2 cm). There is a very large left gastric vein. The portal vein (*arrows*) is patent but there is a tortuous hepatopetal vein doubling it. The right portal vein branch presents with abrupt tapering and duplicating veins are evident. These features were suggestive of congenital hepatic fibrosis but this was not confirmed on the surgical biopsy performed during the splenorenal anastomosis.

▼

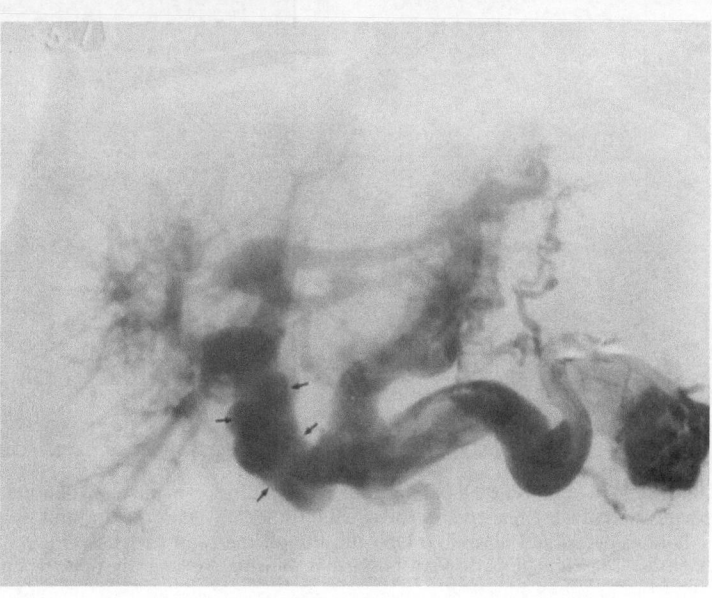

Findings (27 children) (Figs. 3.53–3.64)

Inferior vena cava. The following features were identified:

- Obstruction of the IVC was present in five cases, and in three of these the obstacle was consistent with a membranous web.
- In four cases, there was severe narrowing of the IVC with reflux opacification of the renal vein and the perivertebral veins.
- In 18 cases the IVC was normal or only compressed.

Hepatic veins. Abnormalities of the hepatic veins can be summarised in three schematic patterns:

1. Abnormal ostium in seven cases,
2. Extensive stenosis of the hepatic vein in 14 cases,
3. No hepatic vein identified in four cases.

In the first two patterns numerous intrahepatic collaterals are opacified giving a spider's web appearance to the angiogram. These collaterals represent dilated intrahepatic anastomoses. (The presence of this sign should suggest the diagnosis even if the opacified hepatic vein is normal.) Extrahepatic venous drainage can join the diaphragmatic, epigastric or other parietal veins. In the third pattern it represents the only drainage of the liver which is opacified.

Portal vein. Anomalies revealed by portal angiography included:

- Thrombosis of the portal vein in two cases
- Spontaneous congenital portacaval shunt in one case
- Portohepatic shunt with early hepatic vein opacification in two cases
- A granular appearance of the liver parenchyma, due to uneven stasis
- An opened portal bifurcation due to the caudate lobe hypertrophy
- A partial inversion of the portal vein branches flow in some cases
- Gastro-oesophageal veins may be opacified, but usually are not prominent.

Veno-occlusive Disease
(six cases)

Clinically similar to Budd–Chiari syndrome, this disease associates hepatomegaly, ascites and sometimes jaundice. The lesions involve the intrahepatic radicles of the hepatic veins. The main trunks are normal. The diagnosis is usually based on histology, but may be suggested on ultrasonography.

Angiography shows normal hepatic veins, which may be very thin, due to low blood flow.

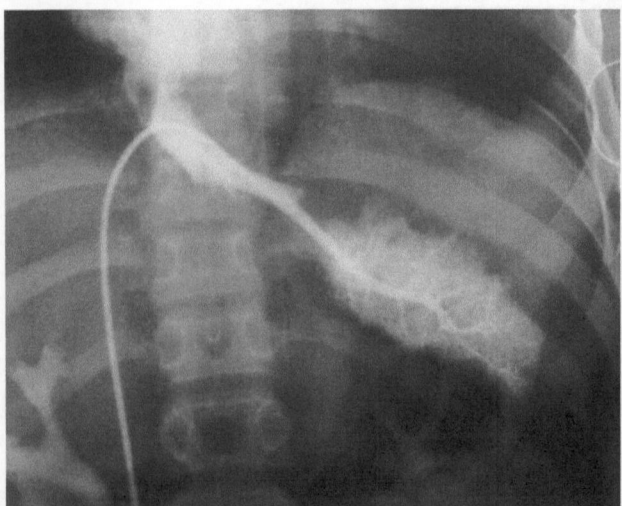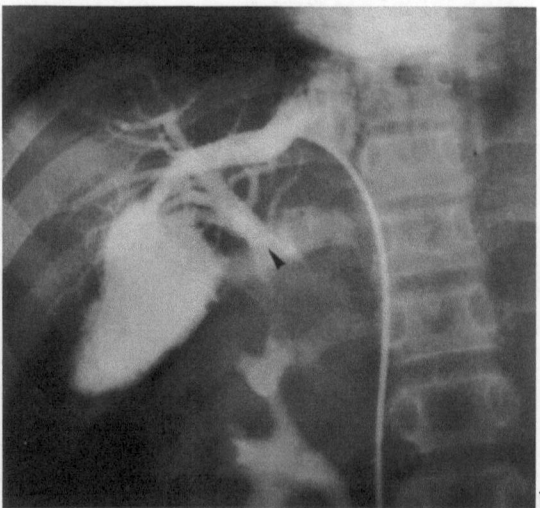

Fig. 3.53 Suspician of Budd–Chiari syndrome. Hepatomegaly; portal fibrosis; suspicion of abnormal centrolobular veins on biopsy. **a** Retrograde opacification of left hepatic vein. The small intrahepatic veins are fine and normal. The opacification of the liver parenchyma is homogeneous and normal. **b** Opacification of the right hepatic vein. Wedged injection. The liver parenchyma is homogeneuos. The right hepatic vein is normal. Normal retrograde opacification of the portal system (*arrowhead*).

When a portography is obtained, the parenchymatous phase is similar to Budd–Chiari syndrome, granular and heterogeneous.

The causes are various: toxic ("wild" teas), chemotherapy, radiotherapy, bone marrow graft.

Cardiac Causes of Post-hepatic Blocks

These include constrictive pericarditis, congestive cardiac failure, and also the exceptional cor triatriatum dextrum which may present as Budd–Chiari syndrome. It is due to a membranous web dividing the right atrium and two cases have been seen in our hospital recently.

Postradiotherapy Liver Disease

Radiotherapy is no longer performed for nephroblastoma, but in five of our cases, it was used to treat angiomas of the liver.

Angiography shows a cork-screw appearance of the distal branches of the hepatic artery. Portal hypertension may be present.

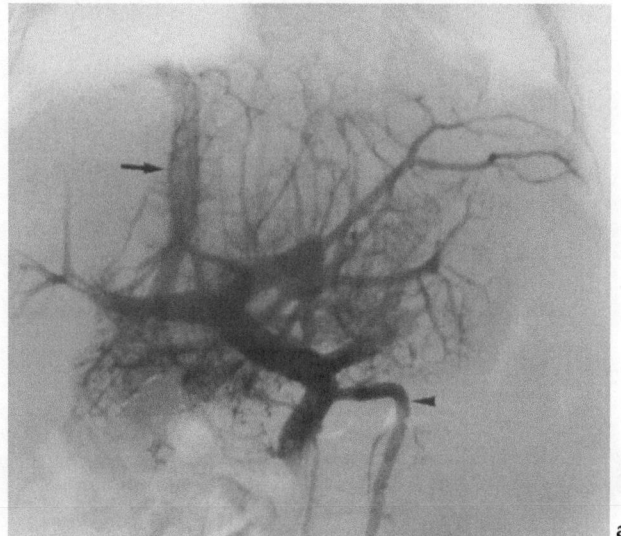

a

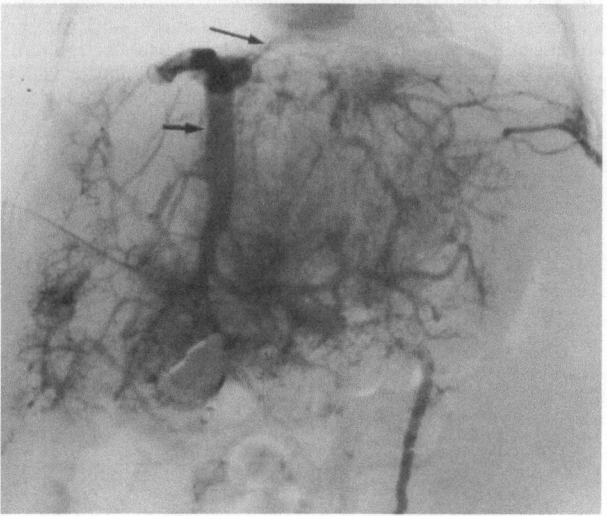

b

Fig. 3.54. Budd–Chiari syndrome. **a** Transhepatic opacification of the portal system (3 s). Hepatomegaly of mainly the left lobe. Massive opacification of the medial hepatic vein (*arrow*). Opacification of the inferior mesenteric vein (*arrowhead*). **b** Late phase (6 s). The medial vein is obstructed. There is a narrow communication toward the right atrium (*arrow*). Opacification of multiple abnormal small hepatic veins.

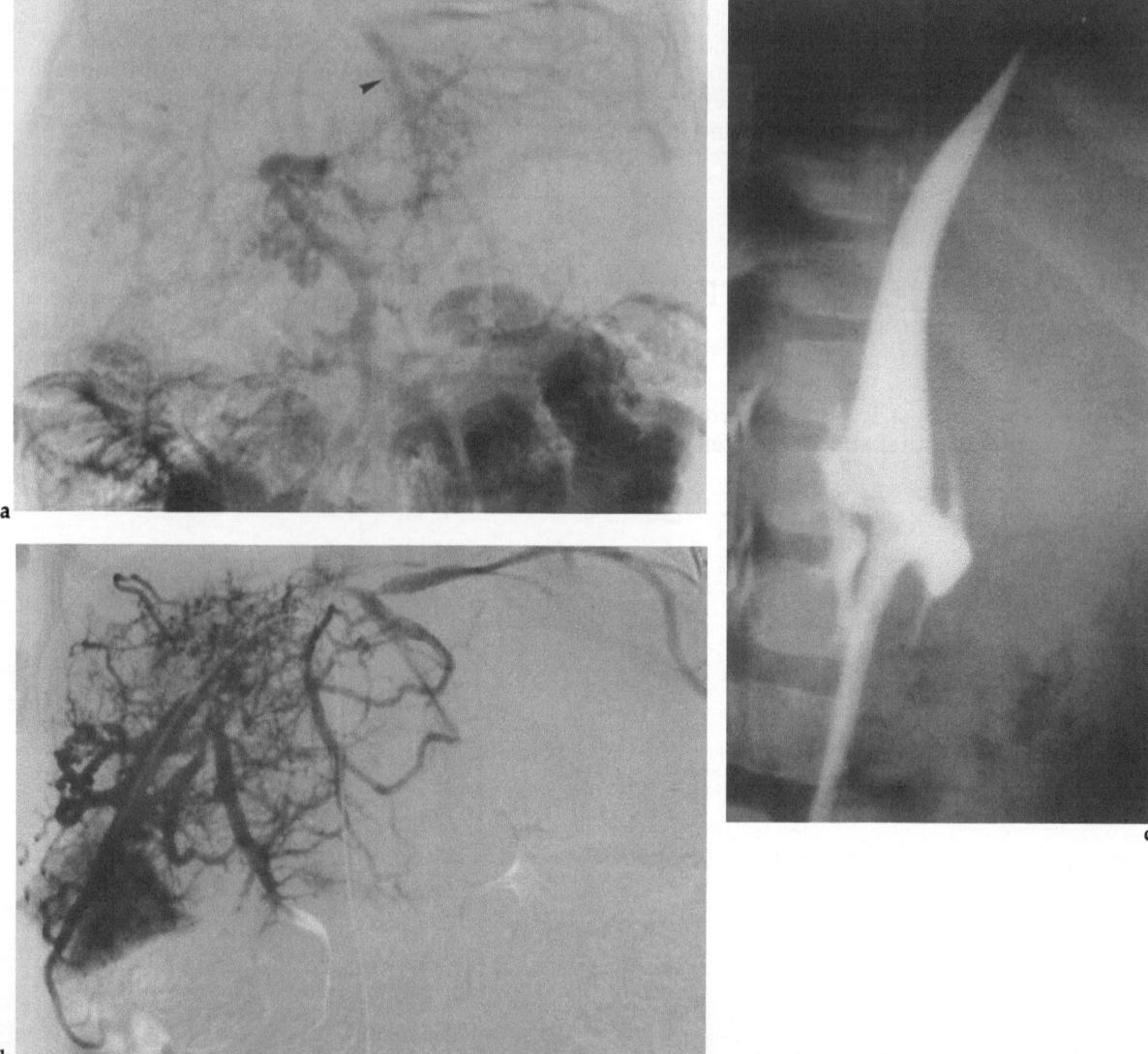

Fig. 3.55. Familial Budd–Chiari syndrome: 2 years of age, hepatomegaly. **a** Venous phase of the superior mesenteric artery injection (10 s after the beginning of arterial injection). The right portal vein is not opacified (thrombosis?). There is a rapid opacification of the left hepatic vein due to a portohepatic shunt (*arrowhead*). **b** Retrograde opacification of the right hepatic vein. There is a stenosis of the right, medial and left hepatic vein ostium. The entire vein system is opacified through the right hepatic vein injection. **c** Lateral view of the inferior vena cava, which is compressed by the hepatomegaly.

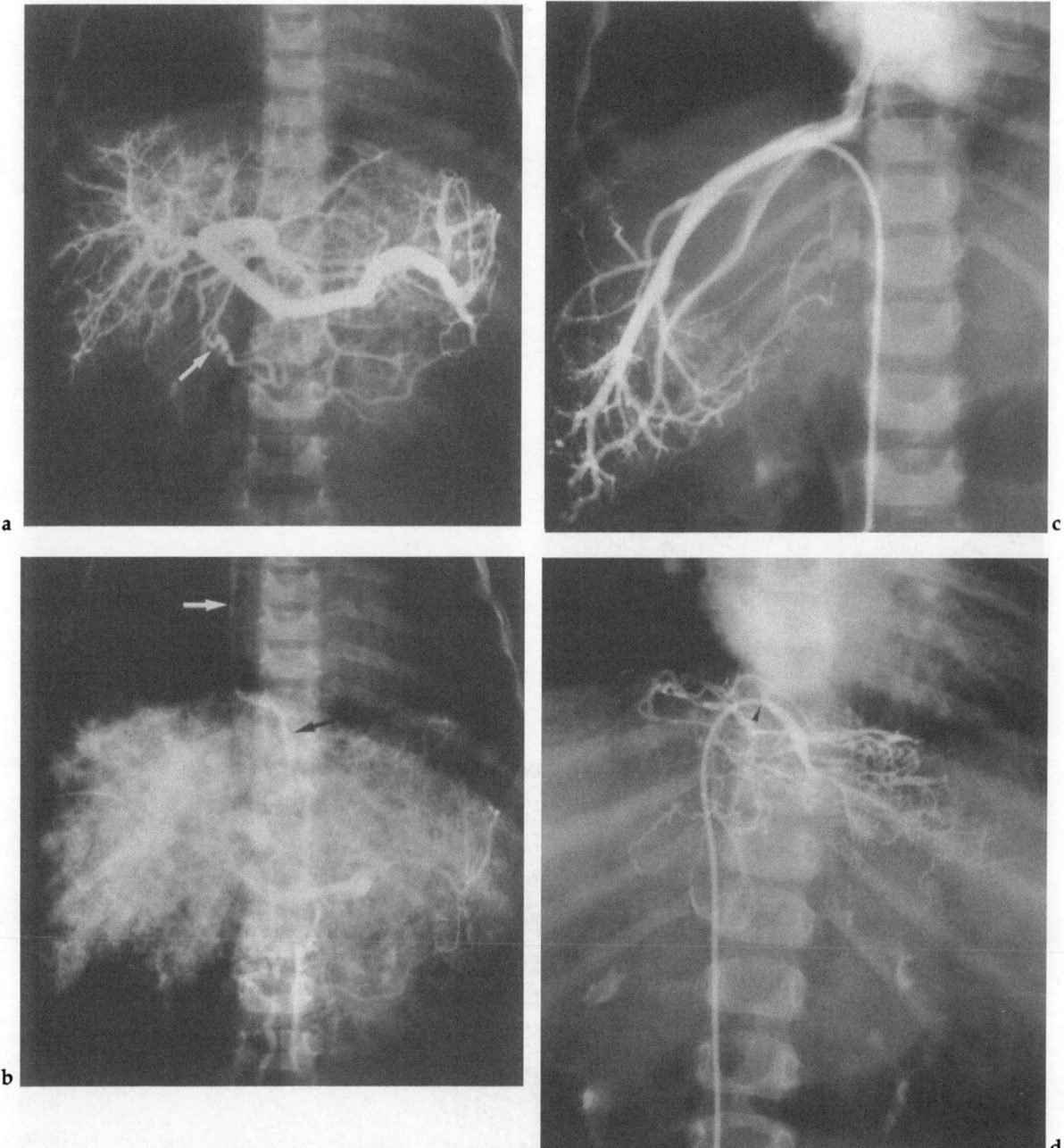

Fig. 3.56. Familial Budd–Chiari syndrome: 2 years of age, (sister of patient in Fig. 3.55). **a** Transphepatic portography. Hepatomegaly (mainly left lobe). Recanalisation of the umbilical vein (*arrow*). **b** Late phase, macronodular appearance of the parenchymography. The epigastric and internal mammary veins are opacified by the umbilical vein (*arrow*). **c** Retrograde opacification of the right hepatic vein. No stenosis is seen but there are numerous intrahepatic collaterals with opacification of the hepatic vein of the spiegel lobe. **d** Left hepatic vein opacification. Tight stenosis of the left hepatic vein (*arrowhead*).

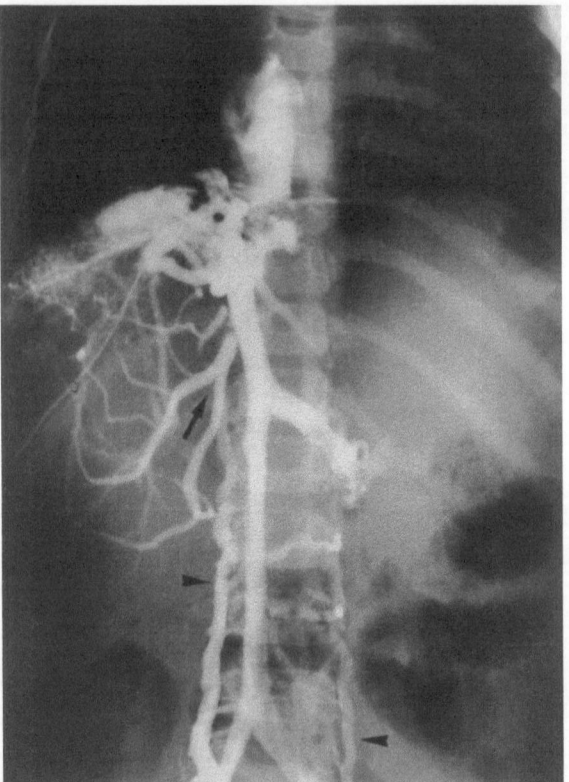

◀ **Fig. 3.57.** Budd–Chiari, syndrome: 7 years of age. Transhepatic opacification of the right vein. The terminal segment of the inferior vena cava is obstructed. The right atrium is opacified through multiple narrow collaterals. The flow is inverted in the inferior vena cava with opacification of the left renal and right and left ascending lumbar veins (*arrowheads*). There is opacification of multiple intrahepatic vein collaterals with opacification of the hepatic vein of the spiegel lobe (*arrow*). Infrahepatic vena cava pressure: 10 mm Hg.

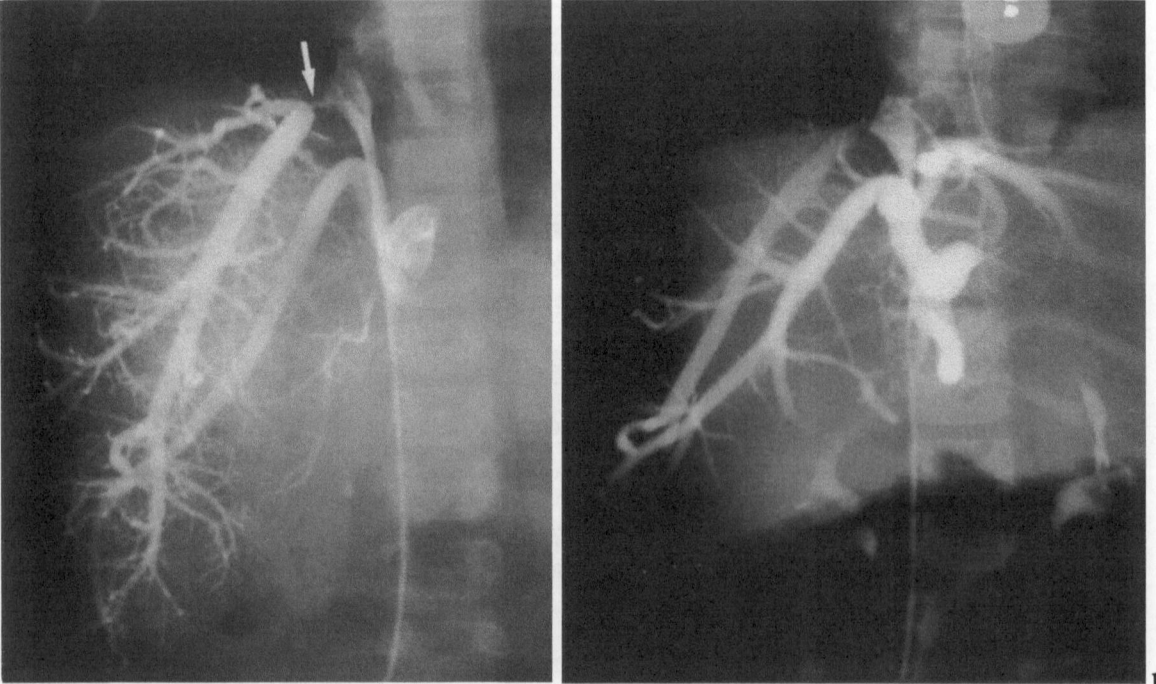

Fig. 3.58. Budd–Chiari syndrome. **a** Retrograde opacification of the right hepatic vein. There is a tight (*arrow*) stenosis of the ostium. There is opacification of an accessory right hepatic vein and spiegel vein through collaterals. **b** Selective opacification of a large spiegel vein. This opacification drains into the two right hepatic veins. The left hepatic vein is also opacified.

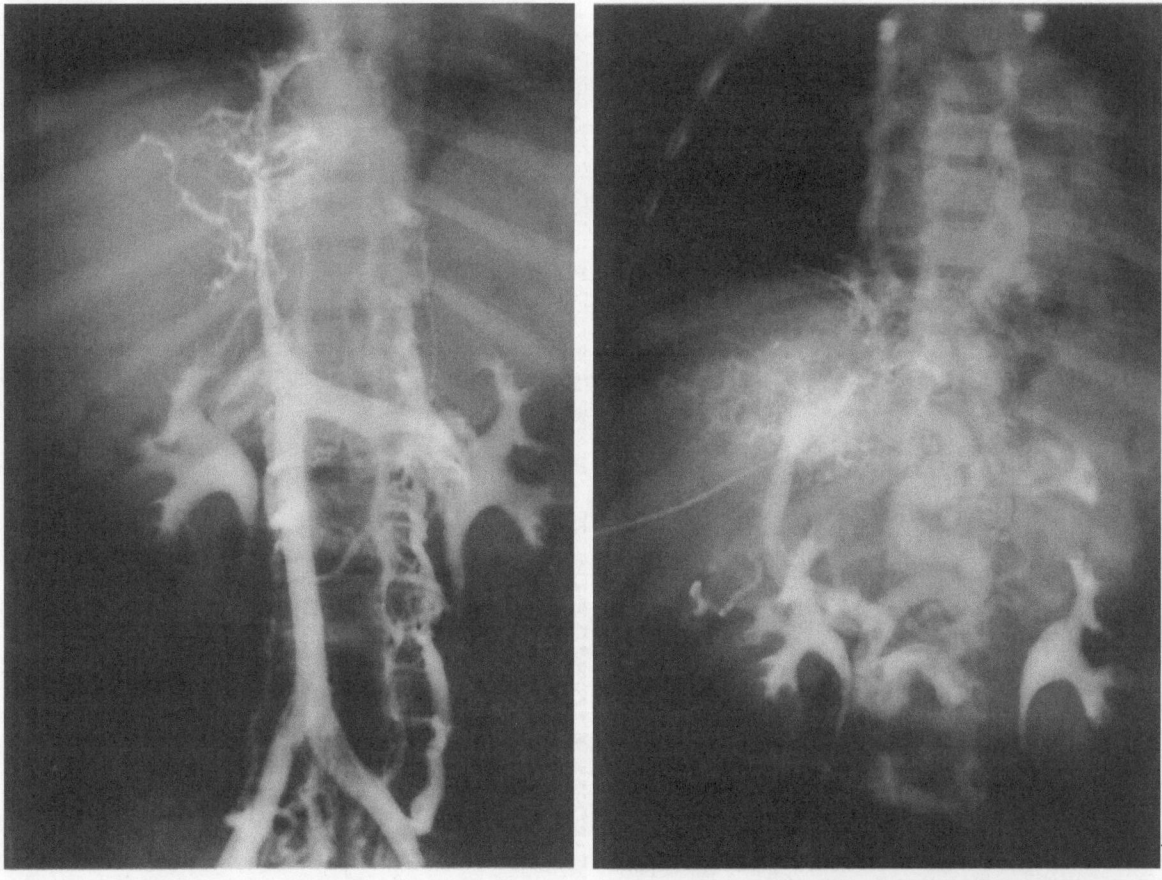

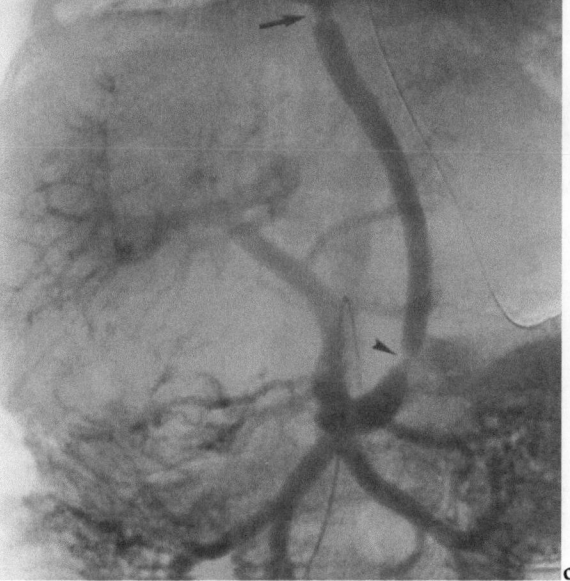

Fig. 3.59. Budd–Chiari syndrome: 4 years of age. **a** Cavography: the retrohepatic portion of the inferior vena cava is nearly thrombosed. Small collaterals are seen. The inferior vena cava drains into the left renal vein and perivertebral plexus. **b** Transhepatic opacification: no intrahepatic hepatic veins are seen. There is one large vein draining toward the umbilical vein with massive opacification of the internal mammary veins (hepatico-ombilical shunt). **c** Mesentericoatrial Dacron shunt. The shunt has been constructed because of the thrombosis of the inferior vena cava. Venous phase of the superior mesenteric artery injection. There is a stenosis between the jugular graft (*arrowhead*) and the Dacron graft and a moderate stenosis between the right atrium and the Dacron graft (*arrow*). Angioplasty was performed through a right jugular vein approach.

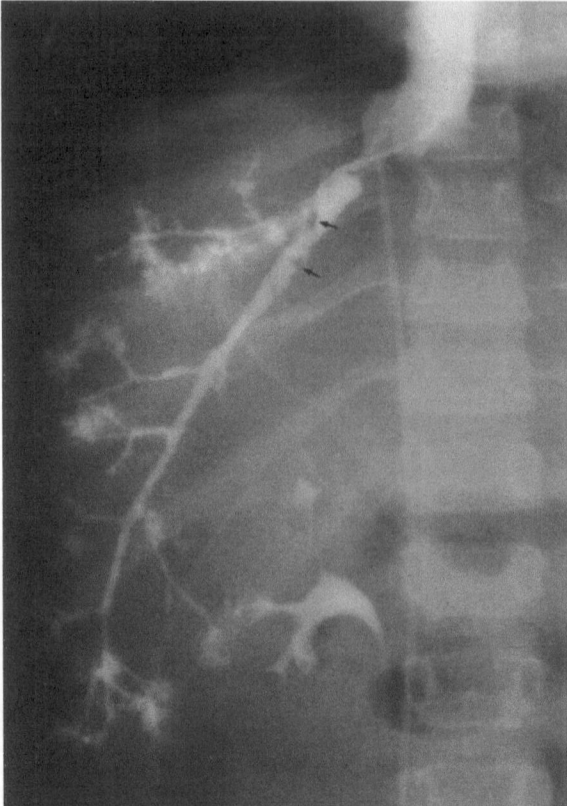

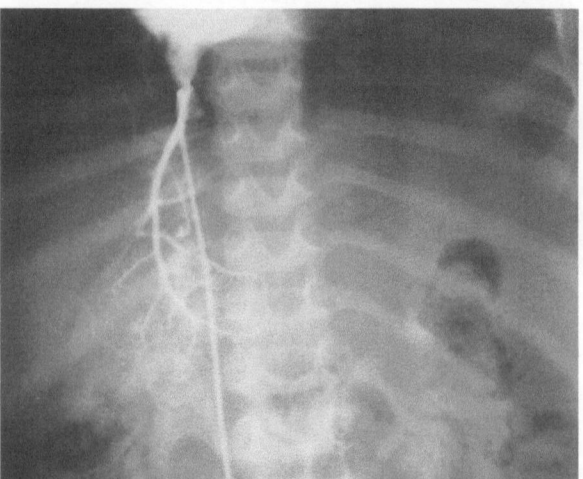

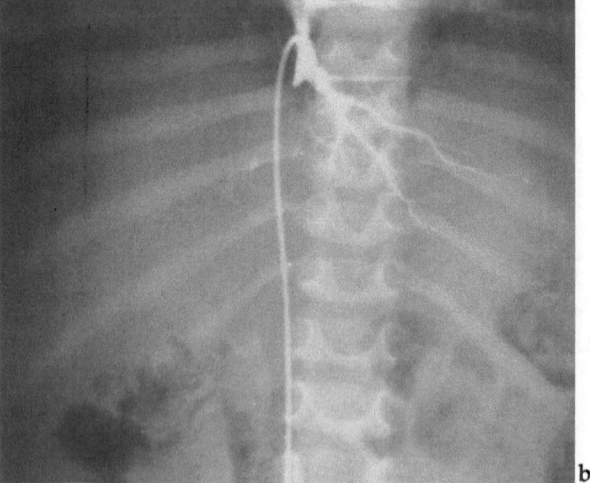

Fig. 3.60. Acute Budd–Chiari syndrome. Right hepatic vein opacification shows a tight ostial stenosis. The right hepatic vein is narrow with multiple mobile filling defects (clots) (*arrows*). (Radiocinema) No hepatic vein collaterals are seen.

Fig. 3.61. Veno-occlusive disease, hepatomegaly, ascites ▶ (bush tea intoxication) (pyrrolizidine alkaloid). 2.5 years of age. **a** and **b** Opacification of the medial and left hepatic veins. The hepatic veins are gracile. There are some collaterals, but there is no stenosis of the ostium. Wedged hepatic pressure: 14 mm Hg. Free hepatic vein pressure: 5 mm Hg. **c** Venous phase of superior mesenteric artery injection. Irregular aspect of portal system? hypoperfusion of the right lobe of the liver. Multiple subdiaphragmatic derivations in the left lobe.

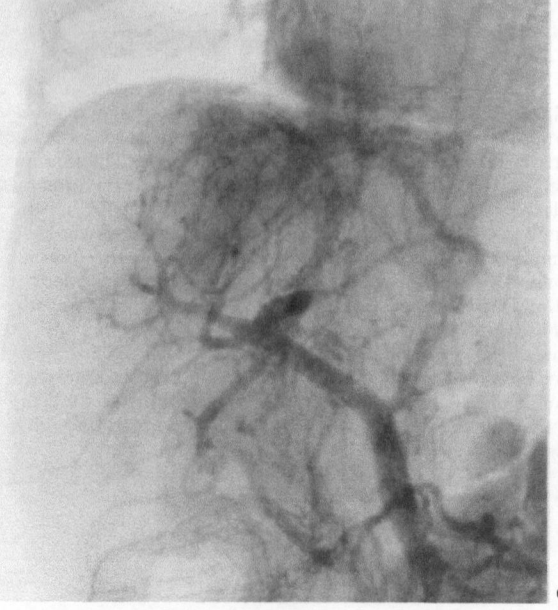

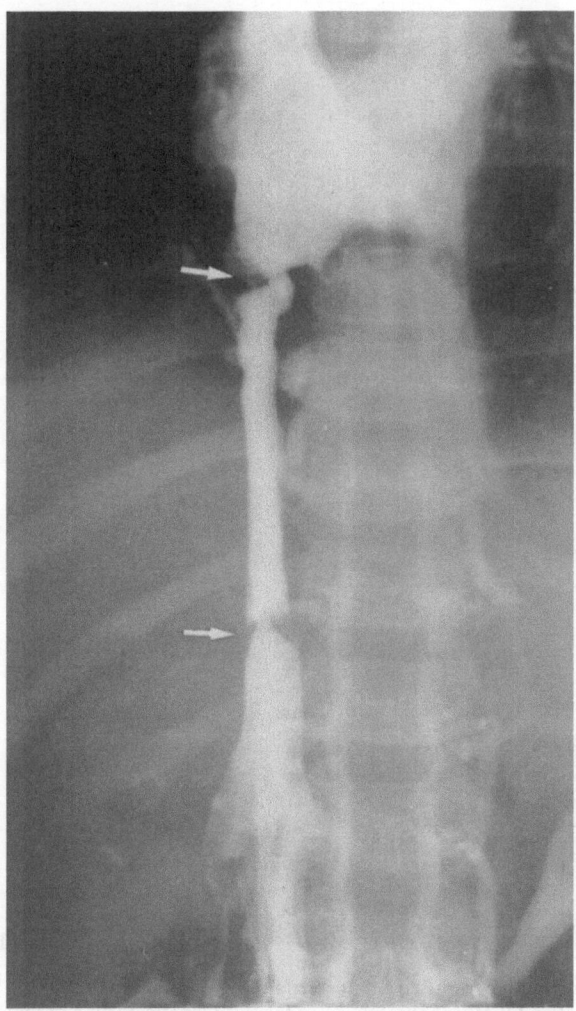

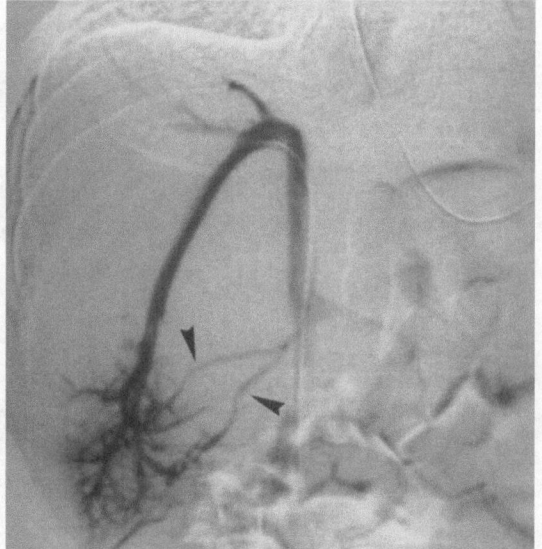

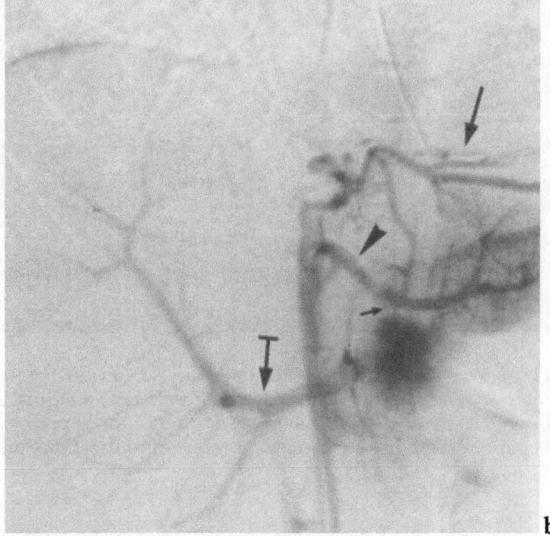

Fig. 3.62. Budd–Chiari syndrome: 9-year-old boy. Cavography shows one stenosis above the ending of the renal vein (*arrow*) and one stenosis just below the right atrium (*arrow*). These stenosis are consistent with membranous webs.

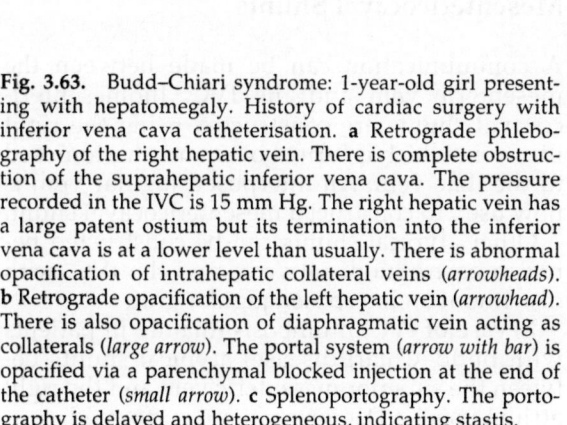

Fig. 3.63. Budd–Chiari syndrome: 1-year-old girl presenting with hepatomegaly. History of cardiac surgery with inferior vena cava catheterisation. **a** Retrograde phlebography of the right hepatic vein. There is complete obstruction of the suprahepatic inferior vena cava. The pressure recorded in the IVC is 15 mm Hg. The right hepatic vein has a large patent ostium but its termination into the inferior vena cava is at a lower level than usually. There is abnormal opacification of intrahepatic collateral veins (*arrowheads*). **b** Retrograde opacification of the left hepatic vein (*arrowhead*). There is also opacification of diaphragmatic vein acting as collaterals (*large arrow*). The portal system (*arrow with bar*) is opacified via a parenchymal blocked injection at the end of the catheter (*small arrow*). **c** Splenoportography. The portography is delayed and heterogeneous, indicating stastis.

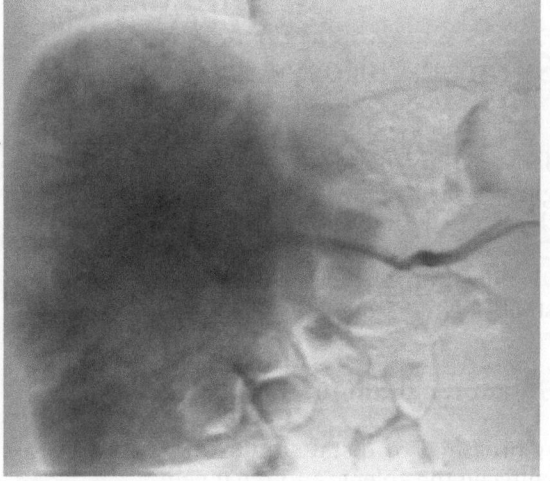

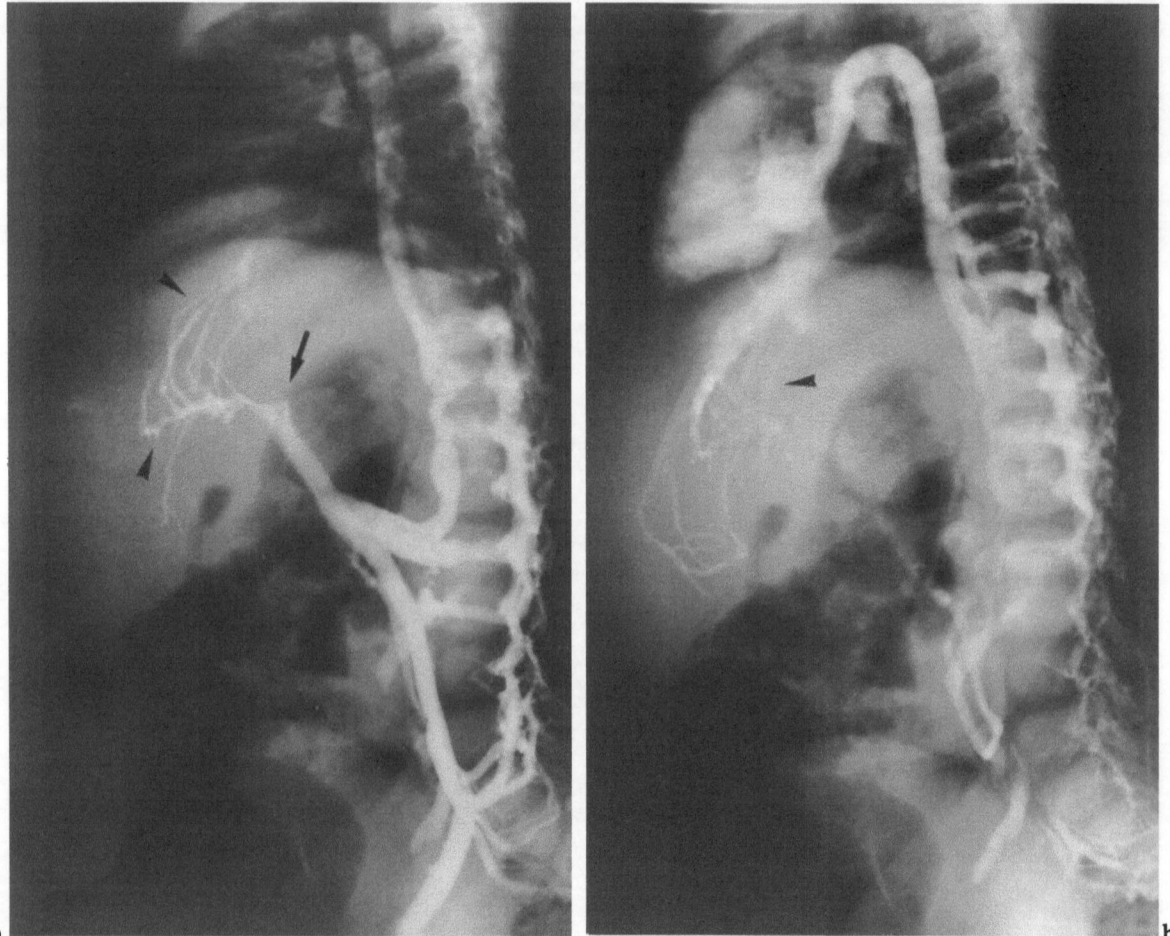

a   b

Fig. 3.64. Budd–Chiari syndrome: 15-year-old boy presenting with a right corticosurenaloma. Preoperative work-up. Inferior vena cava opacification lateral projection. **a** Displacement and localised thrombosis of the retrohepatic portion of the inferior vena cava (*arrow*). **b** Opacification of the suprahepatic portion of the inferior vena cava by a network of collateral hepatic veins (*arrowheads*). There is reflux of contrast medium in the renal veins and in the azygos system.

Surgical Portosystemic Shunts

Treatment of portal hypertension includes surgical portosystemic shunts (Fig. 3.65). Patency of the shunt is monitored by ultrasound. Colour Doppler is also useful. A complete angiographic visualisation of the shunts is useful to understand their anatomy.

Splenorenal Shunts

A proximal or distal shunt can be constructed between the splenic and renal vein.

Mesentericocaval Shunts

A communication can be made between the mesenteric vein and the IVC. Iliomesentericocaval shunts are constructed using the right iliac vein which is turned over and anastomosed to the iliac vein. An interposed jugular vein is now used to construct a mesentericocaval shunt.

Other atypical shunts can be constructed between gastroduodenal veins and the IVC, with or without an interposed jugular graft.

In case of IVC thrombosis (mainly in patients with Budd–Chiari disease) atypical shunts between the superior mesenteric vein and the right atrium using a Dacron graft are performed.

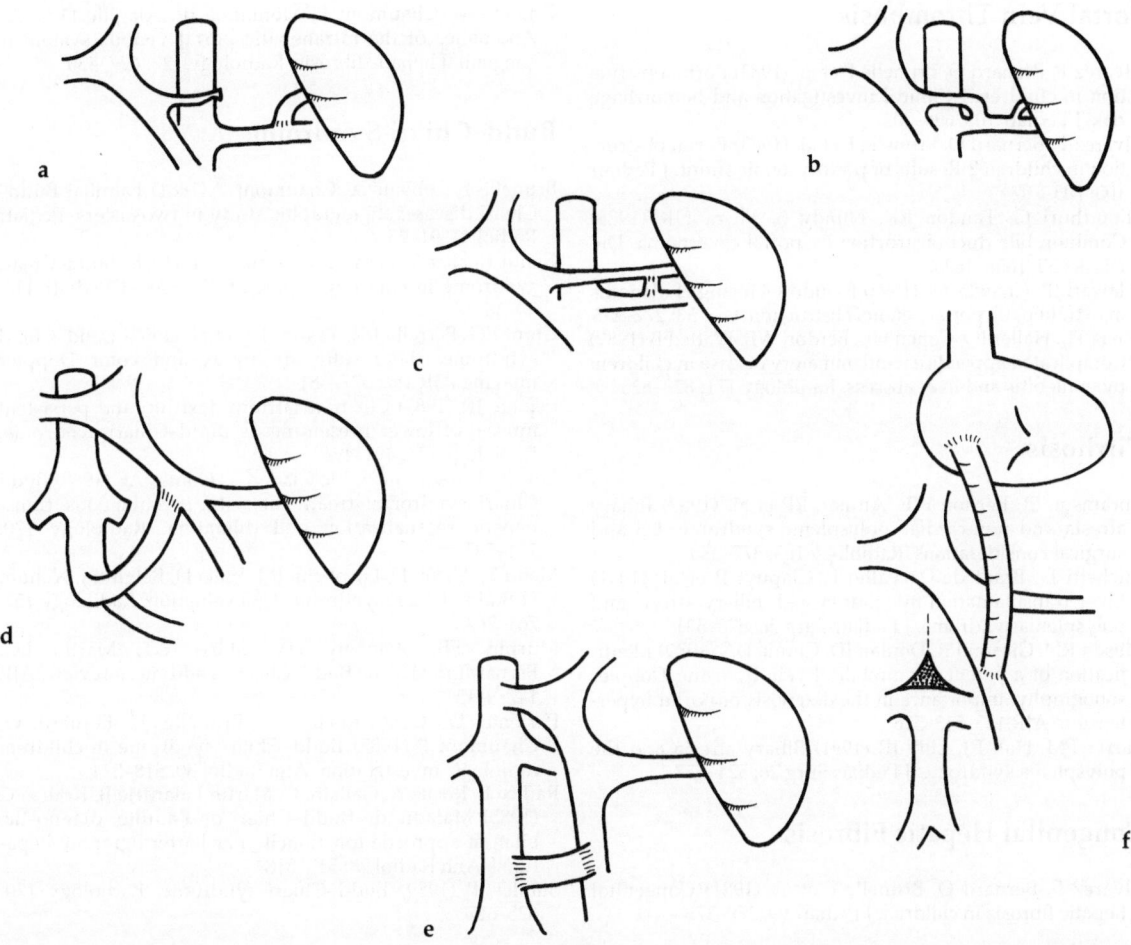

Fig. 3.65. Portosystemic shunts. **a** Distal splenorenal shunt. **b** Proximal splenorenal shunt. **c** Proximal splenorenal shunt with a jugular graft. **d** Iliomesentericocaval shunt. **e** Mesentericocaval shunt with a jugular graft. **f** Mesenterico-atrial shunt.

Portocaval Shunt

Recently, distal portocaval shunts with interposed jugular graft have been placed in those cases of cirrhosis, in which liver transplantation may be considered later. This procedure allows the proximal portal vein to remain of sufficient calibre.

Bibliography

General

Balkanci F, Farid N, Guran S, Senaati S, Atique MH, Yuce A (1991) A high incidence of spontaneous splenorenal shunting shown by digital splenoportography. Pediatr Radiol 21: 145–147

Bernard O, Alavarez F, Brunelle F, Hadchouel P, Alagille D (1985) Portal hypertension in children. Clin Gastroenterol 14: 33–35

Boucher D, Brunelle F, Bernard O et al. (1985) Ultrasonic demonstration of portocaval anastomosis in portal hypertension in children, Pediatr Radiol 15: 307–310

Brunelle F, Alagille D, Pariente D, Chaumont P (1981) An ultrasound study of portal hypertension in children. Ann Radiol 24: 121–130

Nunez D, Russell E, Yrizarry J, Pereiras R, Viamonte M Portosystemic communications studied by transhepatic portography. Radiology 127: 75–79

Patriquin H, Tessier G, Grignou, A Boisvert J (1985) Lesser omental thickness in normal children: baseline for detection of portal hypertension. AJR 145: 693–696

Patriquin H, Lafortune M, Burns P et al. (1987) The duplex Doppler examination of children and adults with portal hypertension. Technique and anatomy AJR 149: 71–76

Patriquin H, Lafortune M, Weber A et al. (1987) Surgical portosystemic shunts in children: assessment with duplex Doppler US. Radiology 165: 25–28

Portal Vein Thrombosis

Alvarez F, Bernard O, Brunelle F et al. (1983) Portal obstruction in children 1-Clinical investigation and hemorrhage risk. J Pediatr 103: 696–702

Alvarez F, Bernard O, Brunelle F et al. (1983) Portal obstruction in children 2-Results of portosystemic shunt. J Pediatr 103: 703–707

Choudhuri G, Tandon RK, Nundy S, Misra NK (1988) Common bile duct obstruction by portal cavernoma. Dig Dis Sci 33: 1626–1628

Dilawari JB, Chawla YK (1992) Pseudosclerosing cholangitis in extrahepatic portal venous obstruction. Gut 33: 272–276

Slovis TL, Haller JO, Cohen HL, Berdon WE, Watts FB (1989) Complicated appendiceal inflammatory disease in children: pylephlebitis and liver abscess. Radiology 171: 823–825

Cirrhosis

Abramson SJ, Berdon WE, Altman RP et al. (1987) Biliary atresia and non-cardiac polysplenic syndrome: US and surgical considerations. Radiology 163: 377–380

Falchetti D, Brant de Carvalho F, Clapuyt P et al. (1991) Liver transplantation in children with biliary atresia and polysplenia syndrome. J Pediatr Surg 26: 528–531

Gibson RN, Gibson PR, Doulan JD, Clunie DA (1989) Identification of a patent paraumbilical vein by using Doppler sonography: importance in the diagnosis of portal hypertension. AJR 153: 513–516

Karrer FM, Hall RJ, Lilly JR (1991) Biliary atresia and the polysplenia syndrome. J Pediatr Surg 26: 524–527

Congenital Hepatic Fibrosis

Alvarez F, Bernard O, Brunelle F et al. (1981) Congenital hepatic fibrosis in children. J Pediatr 99: 370–375

Odièvre M, Chaumont P, Montagne JP, Alagille D (1977) Anomalies of the intrahepatic portal venous system in congenital hepatic fibrosis. Radiology 122: 427–430

Budd–Chiari Syndrome

Brunelle F, Leblanc A, Chaumont P (1981) Familial Budd–Chiari disease: angiographic study in two sisters. Pediatr Radiol 11: 91–95

Gentil-Kocher S, Bernard O, Brunelle F (1988) Budd–Chiari syndrome in children: report of 22 cases. J Pediatr 113: 30–38

Grant EG, Perrella RR, Tessler FN et al. (1989) Budd–Chiari syndrome: the results of duplex and color Doppler imaging AJR 152: 377–381

Lepage JR (1983) Cor triatriatrium dextrum and persistent muscle of lower presenting as Budd–Chiari syndrome. Radiology 134: 491–494

Lois JF, Hartzmann S, Mc Glade CT, Gomes AS (1989) Budd Chiari syndrome: treatment with percutaneous transhepatic recanalization and dilatation. Radiology 170: 791–793

Menu Y, Alison D, Lorphelin JM, Valla D, Belghiti J, Nahum H Budd–Chiari syndrome: US evaluation. Radiology 157: 761–764

Murphy FB, Steinberg HV, Shires GT, Martin LG, Bernardino ME The Budd–Chiari syndrome: a review. AJR 147: 9–15

Pariente D, Gentil-Kocher S, Brunelle F, Bernard O, Chaumont P (1987) Budd–Chiari syndrome in children: radiologic investigation. Ann Radiol 30: 518–524

Radice L, Roche A, Gallaire C, Martin Lalardrie B, Kraiem C (1985) Maladie de Budd–Chiari de l'adulte: diagnostic, bilan et approche fonctionelle par l'artériographie hépatique. Ann Radiol 28: 513–518

Stanley P (1989) Budd–Chiari syndrome. Radiology 170: 625–627

4 Hepatic Tumours

Angiomas

Clinical Findings

Hepatic angiomas are the most common benign hepatic tumours. They present in infancy usually with hepatomegaly. The female to male ratio is about 2 to 1. The possible complications are cardiac failure, thrombopenia (Kasabach–Merritt syndrome) and very rarely intraperitoneal haemorrhage. They have a natural tendency to regression, often after a period of rapid growth.

The diagnosis is strongly suspected in an infant with hepatomegaly, cardiac failure and cutaneous angiomas. In all cases the diagnosis can be made by ultrasonography, CT scan with bolus injection or MR T_1 with gadolinium, and T_2 weighted images.

Hepatic angiomas can be divided into two groups: multiple and solitary angiomas which roughly correspond to different clinical presentation and evolution.

Multiple hepatic angiomas in most cases present after a free interval after birth, whereas solitary angiomas are usually diagnosed at birth and can be discovered antenatally. In our series cutaneous angiomas were present in 13 of 14 cases of multiple angiomas whereas they were present in only one solitary angioma.

Cardiac failure is more frequent in multiple than in solitary angiomas whereas thrombopenia is more frequent in solitary forms.

Regression of solitary angiomas is more rapid, starting before the third month and calcifications are more frequent than in multiple forms.

Recurrence of multiple angiomas later in life has been reported and was observed in three of our cases, with a fatal issue in all cases. The overall prognosis of multiple angiomas is more pejorative than that of solitary ones.

Pathologically a distinction has been made between infantile haemangioendothelioma and cavernous haemangioma, but in fact there is no clear separation. They differ by the size of the vascular spaces but in both types there are endothelial cells, and areas of infarction, fibrosis and foci of calcification. Both types have been encountered in the same patient.

In multiple angiomas, the differential diagnosis mainly includes metastatic neuroblastoma (Pepper's syndrome) and in solitary forms hepatoblastomas. The α-fetoprotein level can be slightly increased in both types but less than in hepatoblastomas.

Angiography (Figs. 4.1–4.12)

Angiography is nowadays indicated when there is a complication and embolisation is considered.

In our institution 20 cases of hepatic angiomas have been explored by means of angiography in a series of about 70 angiomas seen and 12 out of them have been embolised. Three types of angiographic findings have been encountered. All cases had a dilated hepatic artery and a decrease of the diameter of the aorta below its origin.

"Capillary" Type of Angiomas

In 13 of 14 cases studied the involvement of the liver was diffuse. In all of them there was nodular capillary staining, homogeneous or with a dense peripheral rim. There was no rapid opacification of the hepatic veins. Extrahepatic arterial collateral vascularisation of the liver was observed in five cases, it arose from the mesenteric, diaphragmatic or parietal arteries.

The angioma filled via the portal vein in one case. In three cases there was also a portohepatic fistula and in one a localised arterioportal fistula.

"Cavernous" Type

Of the five cases observed four were solitary. In the fifth case there were multiple nodules, but localised to one lobe of the liver. In this type the small ectatic channels are rapidly opacified only in the periphery of the mass. There is stasis of contrast in these capillary-venous lakes and no visualisation of the hepatic veins.

In one case a portohepatic fistula was opacified via an umbilical vein catheter.

"Fistulous" Angiomas

Two similar cases presented with a mass in the liver. In both cases there was rapid opacification of a network of small tortuous veins and massive appearance of hepatic veins. In both cases arterial collateral supply was observed and cardiac failure was observed. One case was treated by embolisation and the other by radiotherapy.

Embolisation (n= 13 cases)

Embolisation was performed in 12 cases of multiple angiomas. Indications included cardiac insufficiency and thrombopenia. Embolisation uses the polymerising glue (cyanoacrylate) mixed with lipiodol.

Two patients died despite embolisation. In one, the death was the consequence of secondary lesions, appearing one year after embolisation. One embolisation was performed during a second haemorrhagic episode. No complication directly attributable to the embolisation was seen. Inadvertent splenic embolisation occurred in one patient with no detectable clinical effect. In two patients, angiographic control showed revascularisation of the lesions by intrahepatic peribiliary collaterals. Two angiographic controls showed an improvement of the portal perfusion after embolisation.

One persisting case of solitary angioma was embolised at 2 years of age, subsequent US and

CT were normal; there was no residual mass. Two patients were operated upon. One had a cardiac arrest during mobilisation of the liver. Surgery was postponed and the lesion regressed and calcified.

Malignant Hepatic Tumours (Table 4.1)

Introduction and Clinical Findings

These represent 60% of all hepatic tumours in children. Most of these are epithelial tumours including hepatoblastomas and hepatocarcinomas. The initial clinical finding is usually an abdominal mass. Very rarely, this mass is accompanied by jaundice (2% of the cases) and then usually is a rhabdomyosarcoma or a lymphoma. Hepatoblastoma has been described in association with hemihypertrophy (Beckwith–Wiedemann syndrome) and with a variety of paraneoplastic syndromes.

Table 4.1. Malignant Hepatic Tumour Pathology

Hepatoblastoma	46
Hepatocarcinoma	6
Sarcoma	9
Rhabdomyosarcoma	4
Lymphoma	1
Fibrolamellar	2
Nevocarcinoma	1
Epithelioid haemangioendothelioma	3
Unclassified	6
Malignant mesenchymoma	2
Metastasis	11

Epithelial Tumours

The α-fetoprotein serum level is elevated in almost all cases and thus the only differential diagnosis is teratoma with liver metastases.

Hepatoblastomas tend to occur in younger patients under 3 years of age, and have been reported antenatally. Treatment is surgical after chemotherapy. Prognosis is poor in multicentric tumours or when pulmonary metastases are present.

Hepatocarcinomas usually occur on underlying hepatic diseases such as virus B cirrhosis or hepatitis or even antigene carrier, tyrosinaemia, biliary atresia cirrhosis, glycogen storage disease with adenoma, Byler's disease and α_1-antitrypsin deficiency. Prognosis depends on the extent of the tumour and on the severity of the underlying disease. Liver transplantation is the treatment of choice when the disease is limited to the liver.

Other Tumours

The non-secreting tumours include sarcoma (rhabdomyosarcoma or undifferentiated sarcoma), lymphoma, fibrolamellar hepatocarcinoma, epithelioid haemangioendothelioma and metastases.

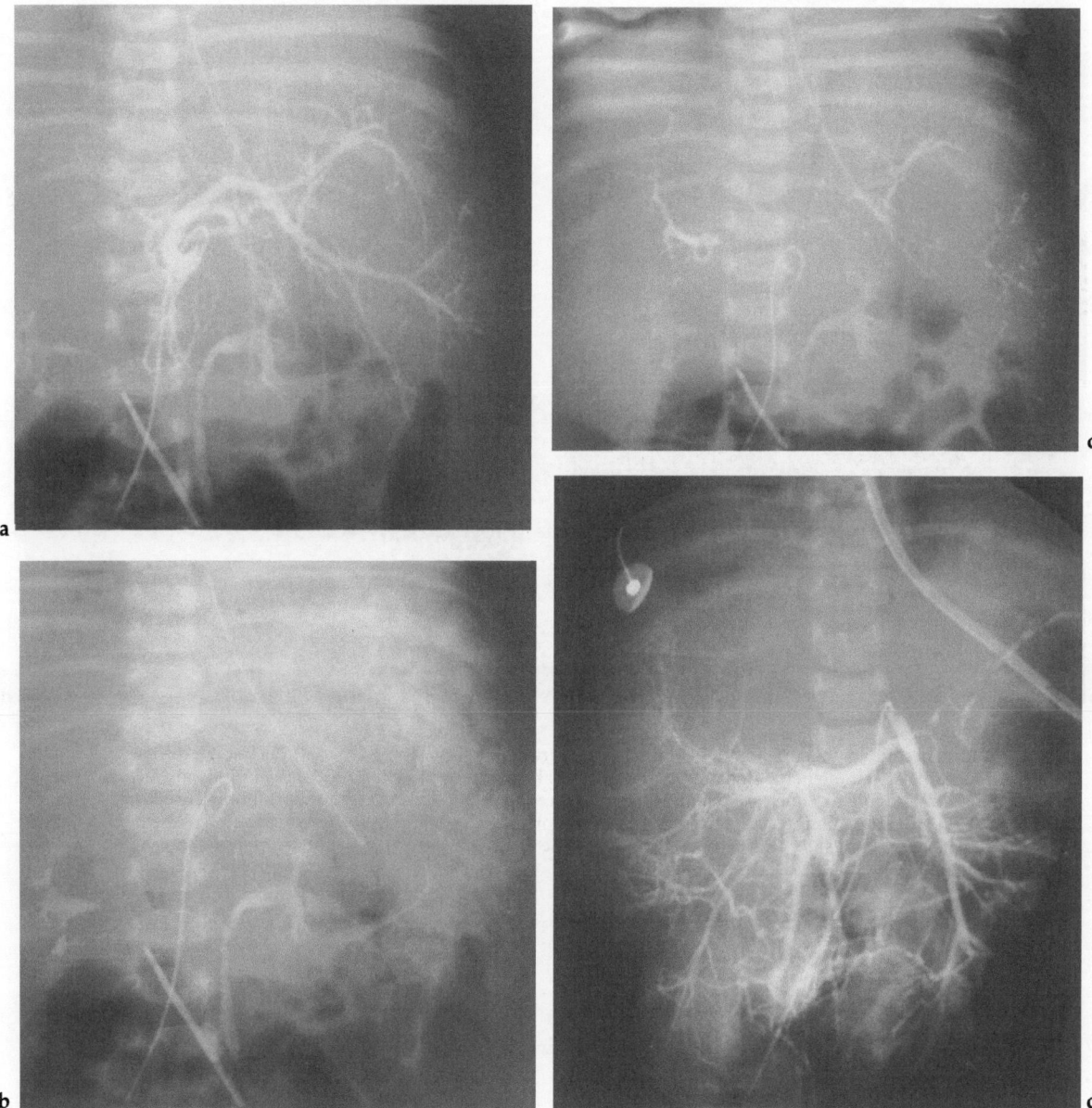

Fig. 4.1. Hepatic angioma, diffuse form: 2 months of age. **a** Selective injection of the left hepatic artery, early phase. **b** On the late phase, there is a diffuse hypervascularisation of the left lobe of the liver. **c** After embolisation of both hepatic arteries with cyanoacrylate and lipiodol. **d** Selective injection of the superior mesenteric artery 2 months later shows that there are some collaterals coming from the right hepatic artery revascularising the right lobe. The radio-opaque embolic material is seen in the left lobe of the liver.

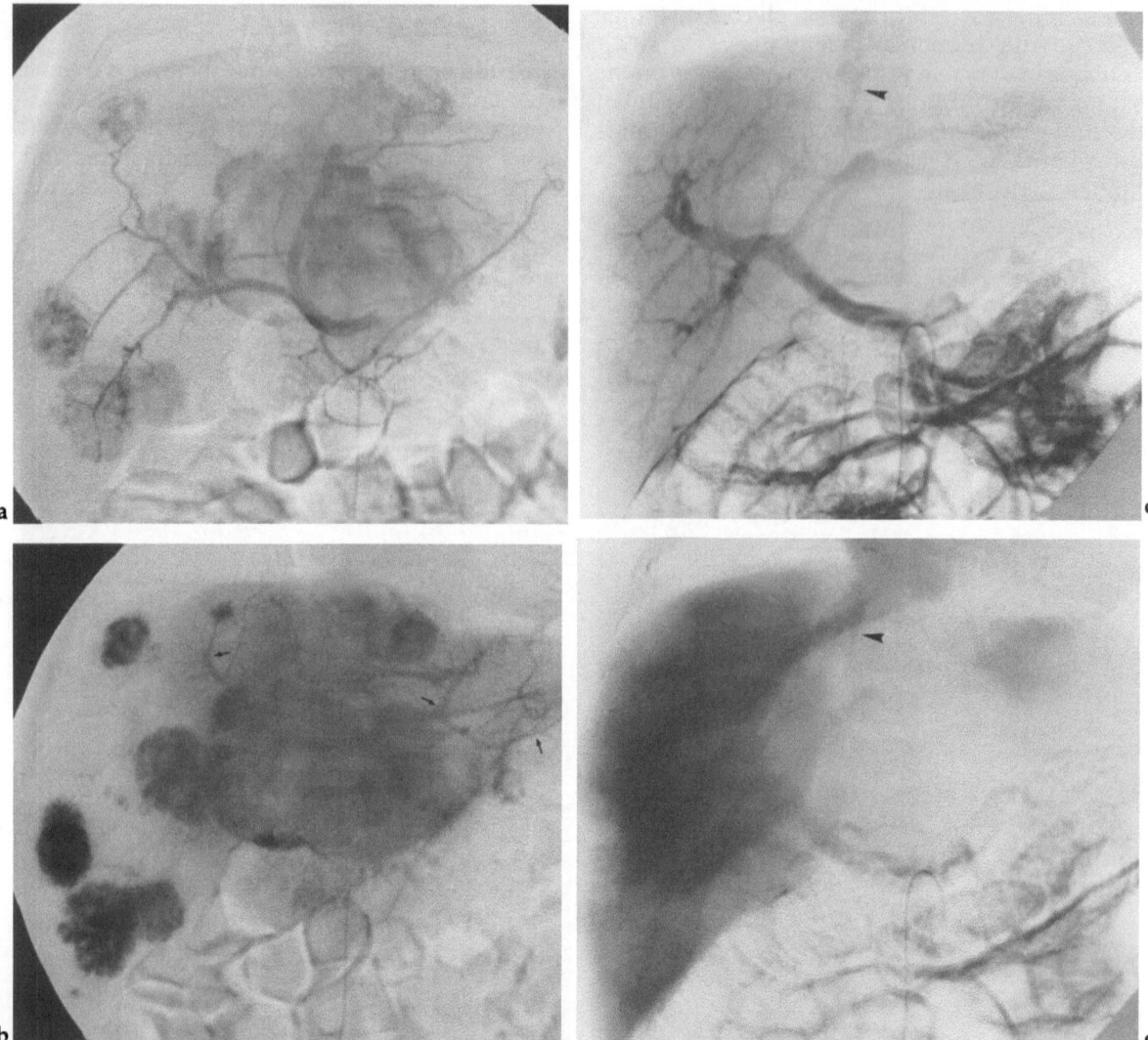

Fig. 4.2. Diffuse hepatic angioma: 6 months of age. **a** Hepatic artery injection. There are multiple but not diffuse well-limited nodules with capillary staining in the right and in the left lobe. **b** Late phase. The nodules of the right lobe are homogeneous whereas the central nodule has only peripheral staining. There is opacification of the left portal branches (*arrows*). **c** and **d** Late phase of superior mesenteric artery injection. There is a portohepatic fistula with the opacification of the medial hepatic vein (*arrowhead*). There is a large defect of portography in the left lobe because of the arterioportal shunt and also of the multiple angiomatous nodules.

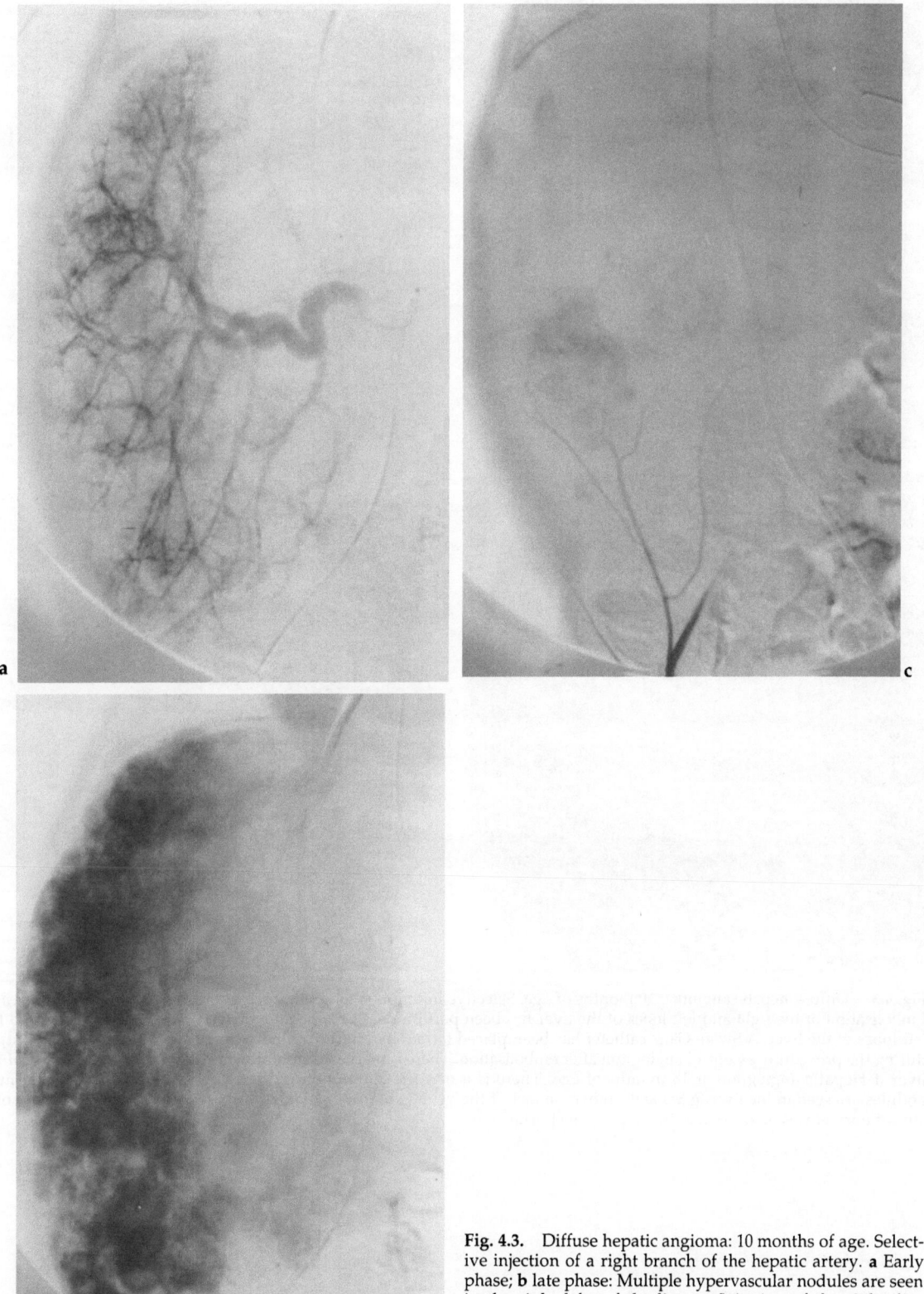

Fig. 4.3. Diffuse hepatic angioma: 10 months of age. Selective injection of a right branch of the hepatic artery. **a** Early
phase; **b** late phase: Multiple hypervascular nodules are seen
in the right lobe of the liver. **c** Injection of the right iliac
artery showing a dilated epigastric artery participating in the
angiomatous vascularisation of the right liver lobe.
Continued overleaf.

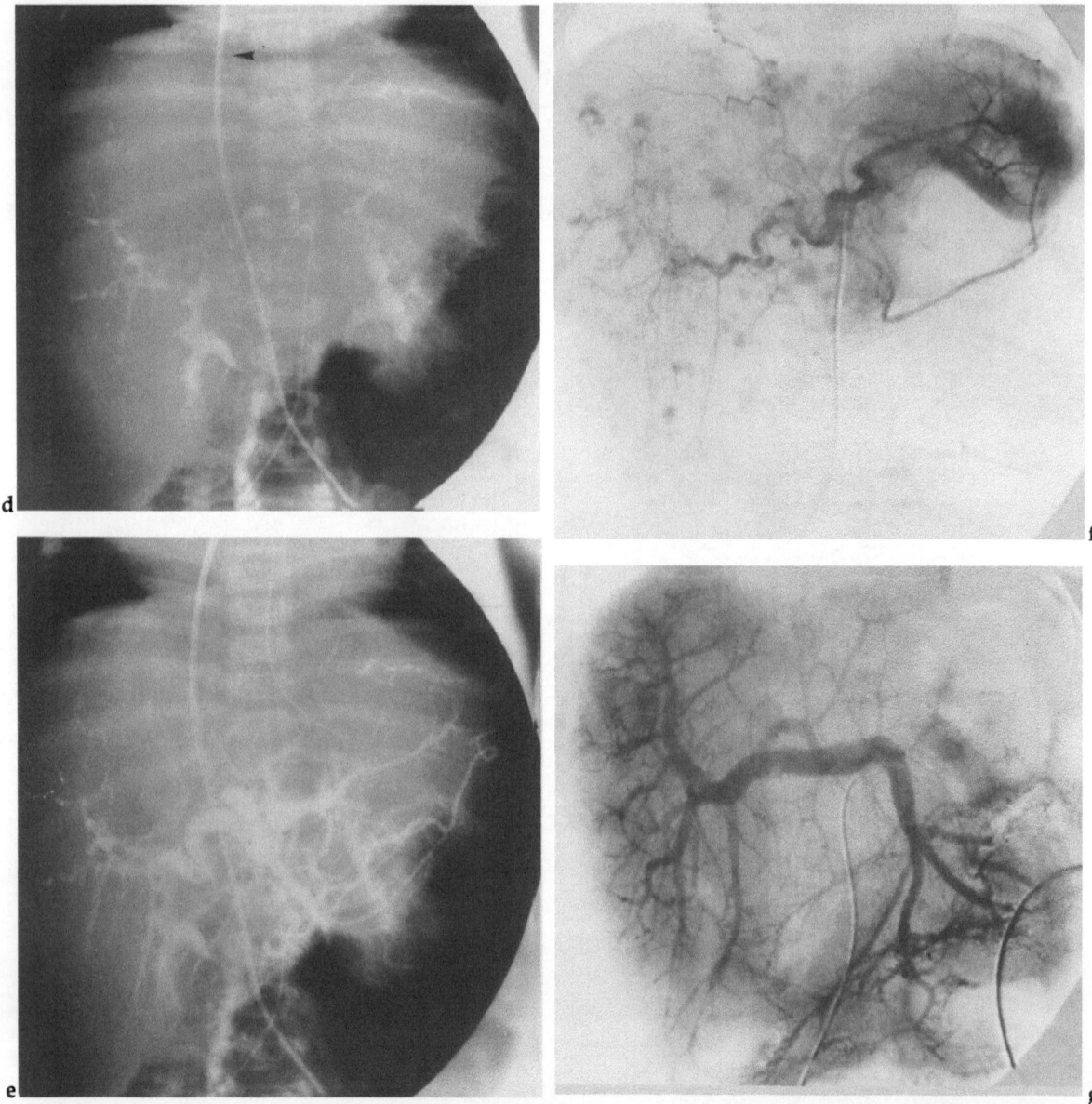

Fig. 4.3. Diffuse hepatic angioma: 10 months of age. Selective injection of a right branch of the hepatic artery. (*continued*) **d** Embolisation of the right and left lobes of the liver has been performed. Radio-opaque material is seen in the right and the left lobes of the liver. A Swan–Ganz catheter has been placed (*arrowhead*) in the pulmonary artery to control cardiac output during the procedure. **e** Control angiogram after embolisation. There is marked diminution of the hypervascularisation of the liver. **f** Hepatic angiogram at 18 months of age. There is a marked diminution of the hypervascularisation. Only small nodules are seen in the liver. **g** Same examination as in **f** the venous return of a superior mesenteric artery injection shows almost normal vascularisation of the liver by the portal vein.

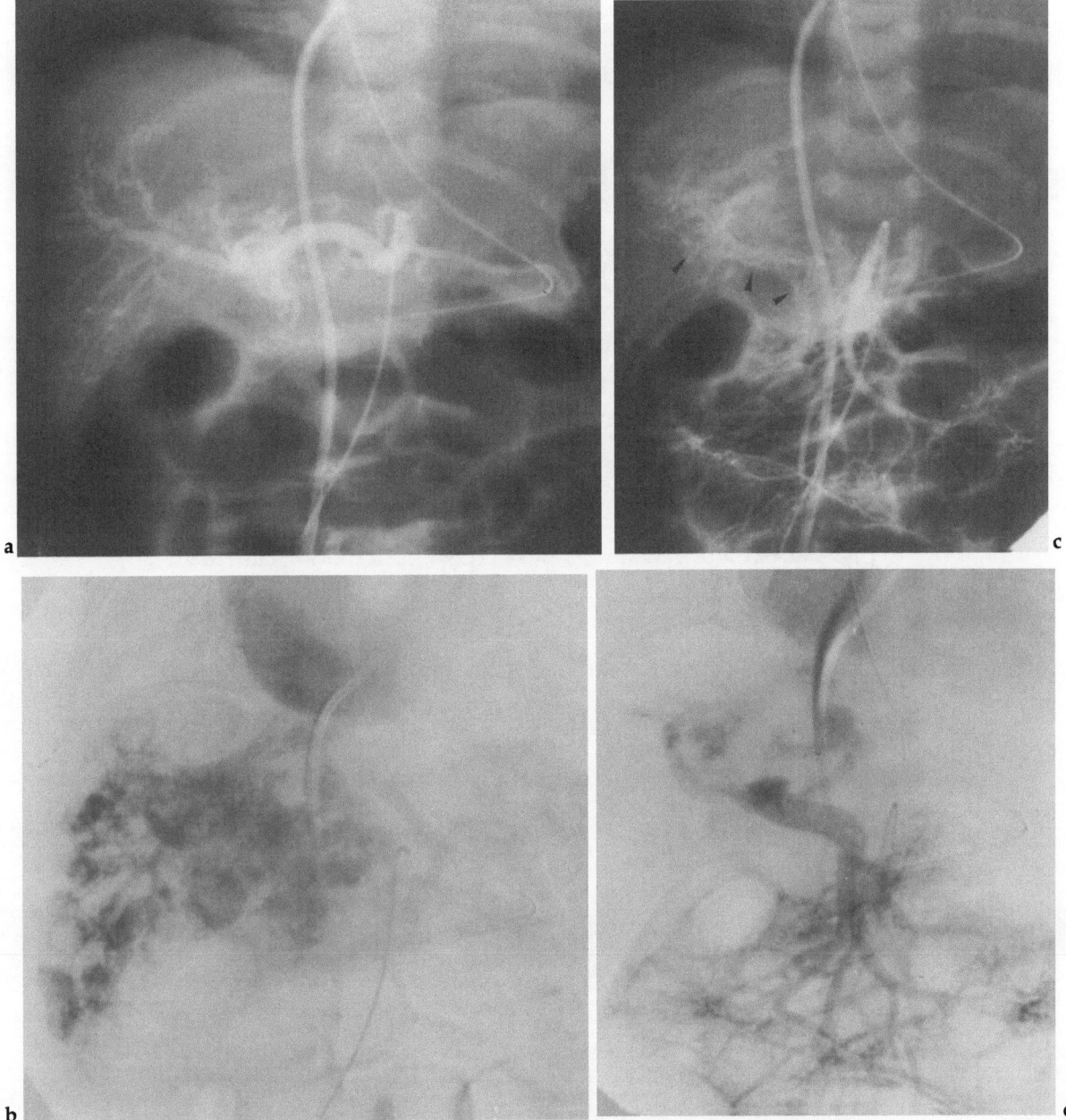

Fig. 4.4. Diffuse form: 2 years of age. **a** Coeliac trunk opacification. There is a diffuse hypervascularisation of the entire liver. **b** Late phase of the coeliac trunk injection. Multiple hypervascular nodules with peripheral enhancement are seen in the liver. **c** Selective injection of the superior mesenteric artery. Multiple collaterals from peribiliary arteries opacifying the liver (*arrowheads*). **d** On the late phase of the superior mesenteric artery injection, two porto sushepatic fistulas are seen without portal opacification of the liver.

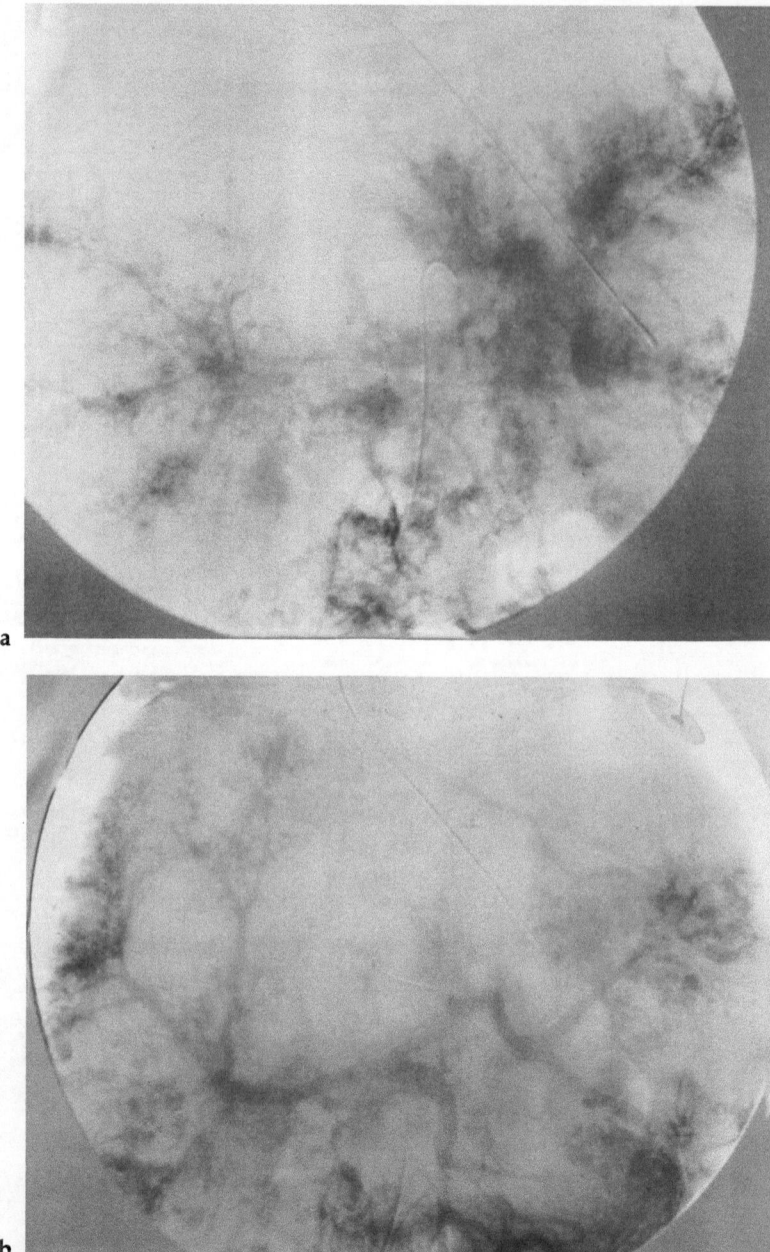

Fig. 4.5. Hepatic angioma: 1 month of age; diffuse form. **a** Late phase of hepatic artery injection. There is a diffuse hypervascularisation of the liver. The diaphragmatic arteries were also supplying the angiomatous liver. **b** Venous return of SMA injection. There is an unusual portal participation of the vascularisation of the angiomas.

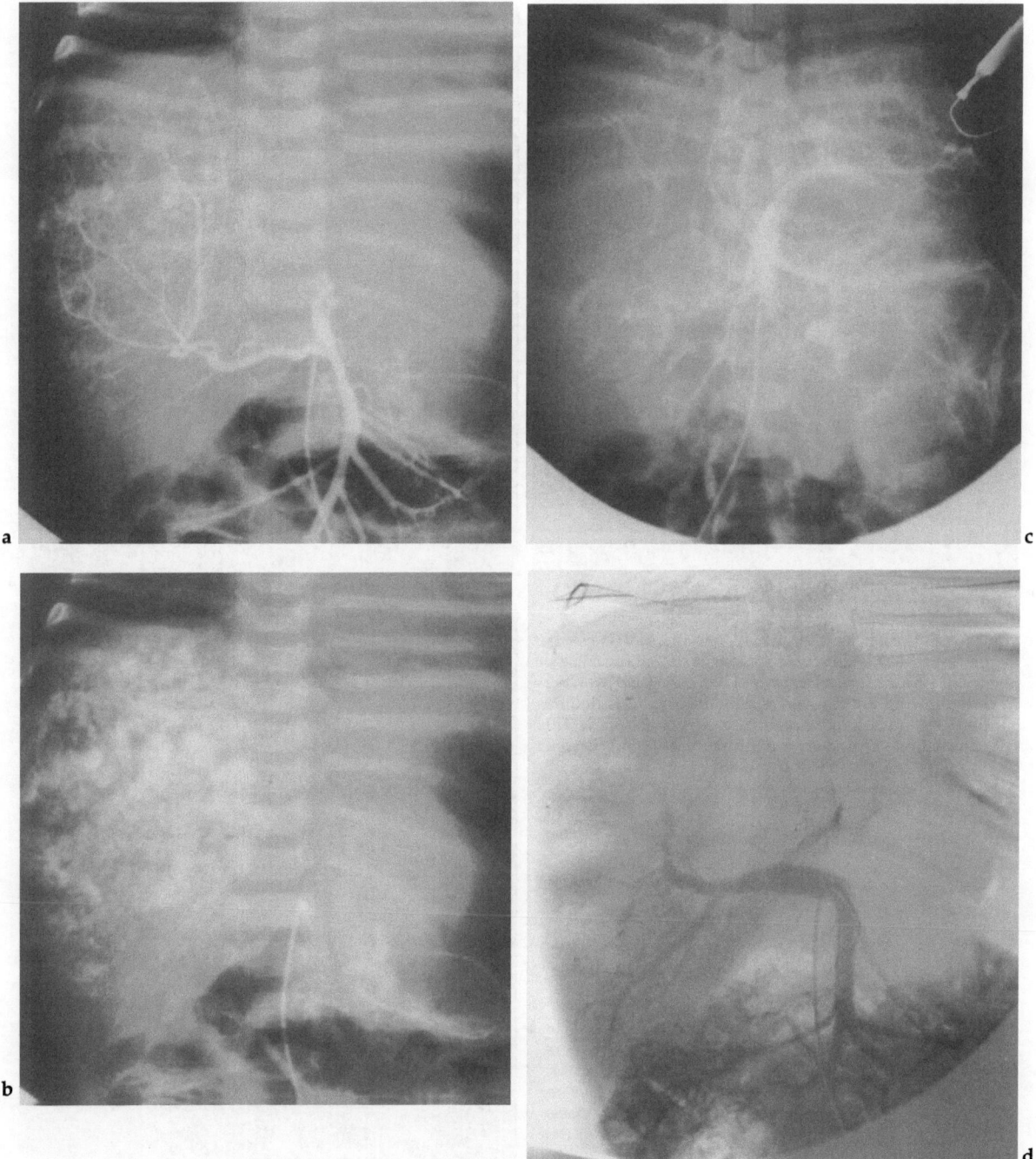

Fig. 4.6. Diffuse hepatic angioma: 2 months of age; cardiac insufficiency. **a** and **b** right hepatic artery injection. Multiple small hypervascular nodules are seen in both lobes of the liver. Radiotherapy. **c** Haemoperitoneum and respiratory failure; 2 months later. Coeliac trunk injection. The nodules have strikingly enlarged and present with a peripheral rim of enhancement. **d** Portal phase of superior mesenteric artery injection. Large defects of portography corresponding to the angiomatous nodules. Embolisation was performed. *Continued overleaf.*

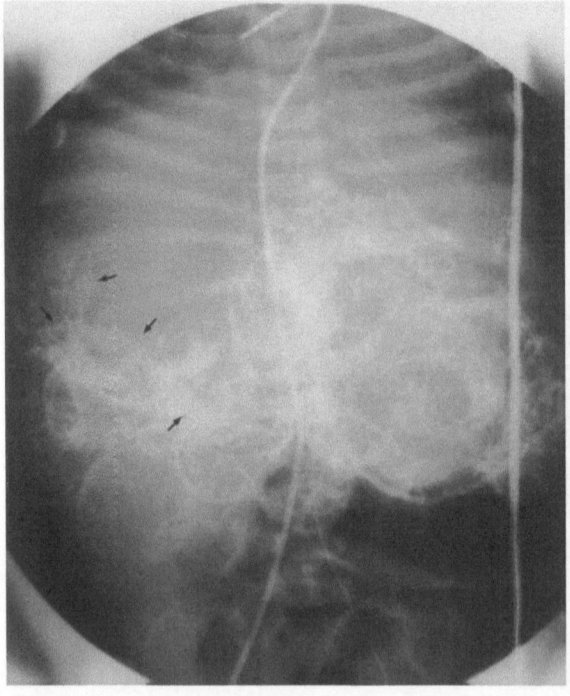

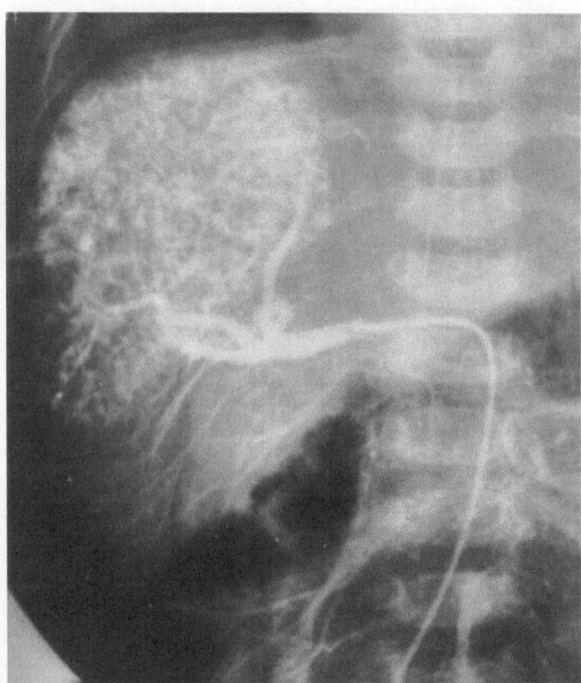

Fig. 4.6. Diffuse hepatic angioma: 2 months of age; cardiac insufficiency. (*continued*) **e** At 6 months of age, because of persistent cardiac insufficiency, a new angiogram was performed showing impressive residual angiomatous nodules supplied by an arterial collateral network (*arrows*). This patient died one year later of multiple diffuse angiomatous lesions in the brain, bones and ovaries.

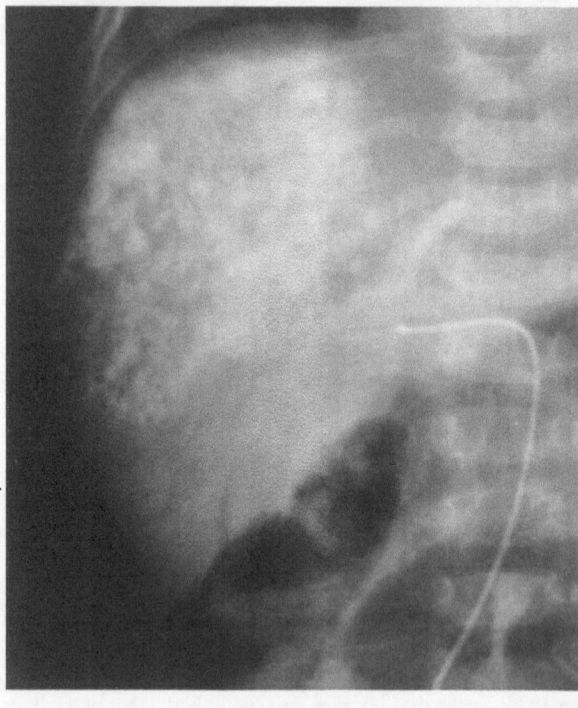

Fig. 4.7. Localised capillary form: 3 months of age. **a** The ▶ right hepatic artery injection shows a localised hypervascular mass in the right lobe of the liver. **b** Late phase. The mass is formed by multiple small nodules. At 2 years of age there was only slight regression of the mass. Embolisation was performed. Note that the pattern of the angiogram is similar to that observed in the first angiogram performed on the previous patient (Fig. 4.6). However, the evolution was quite different.

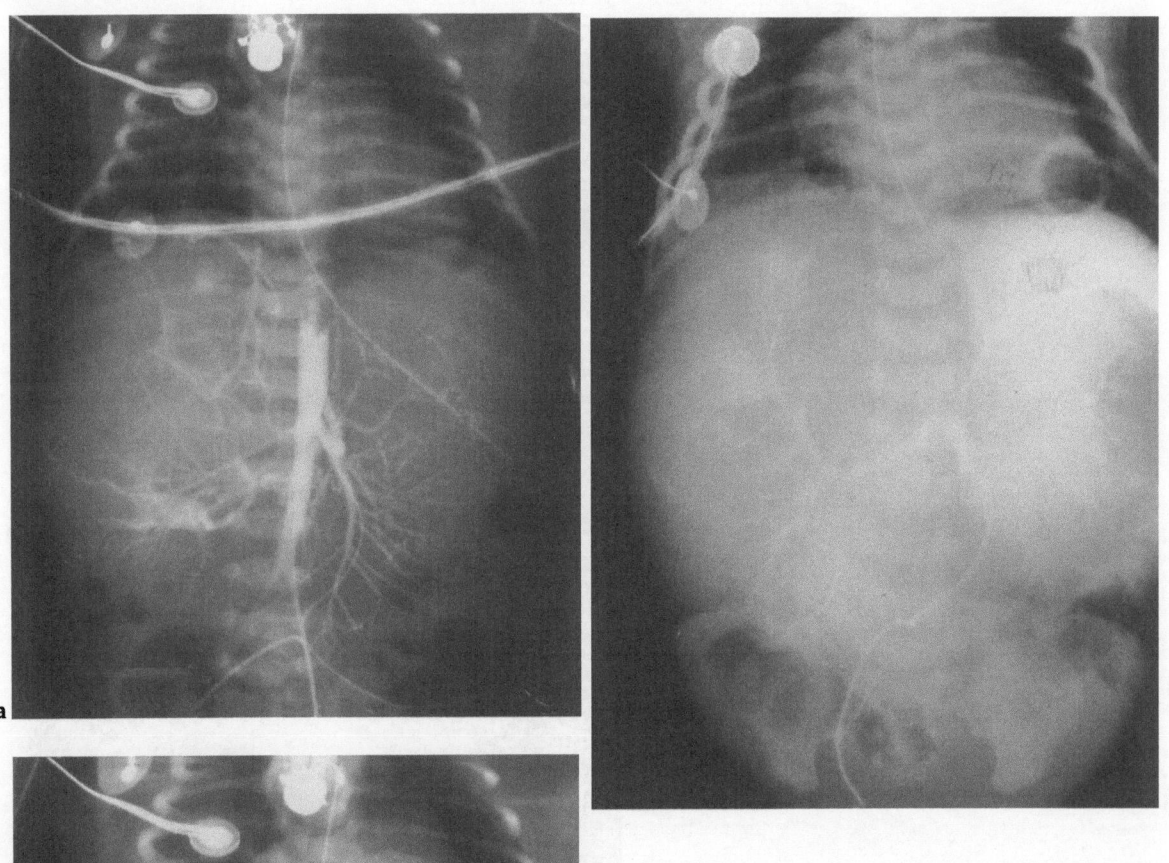

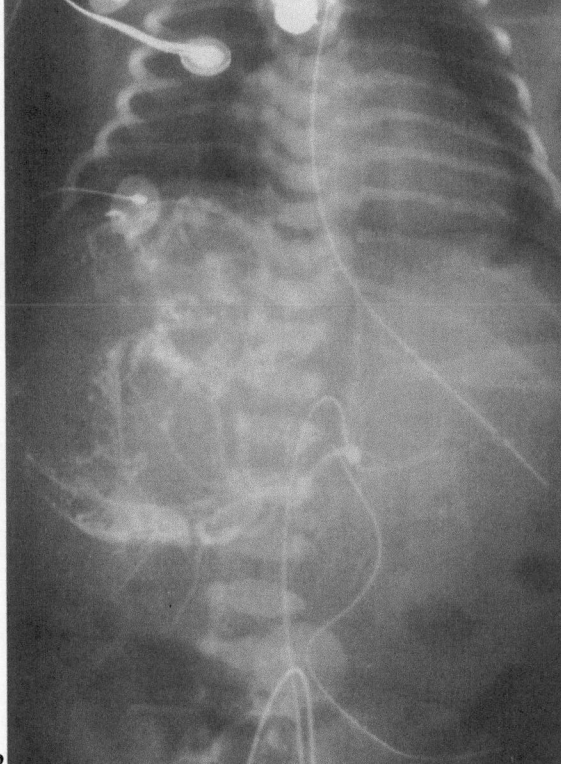

Fig. 4.8. Cardiac insufficiency and hepatomegaly; 1 day of age. Arteriography through catheterisation of the umbilical artery at bedside. **a** Aortography. **b** Selective hepatic artery injection. There is a hypervascular mass of the right lobe of the liver corresponding to the cavernous angioma type. The vascularisation is peripheral. There is opacification of venous lakes. **c** Portography via umbilical vein catheterisation. No portal vascularisation of the mass. In the following months, regression of the mass with calcifications.

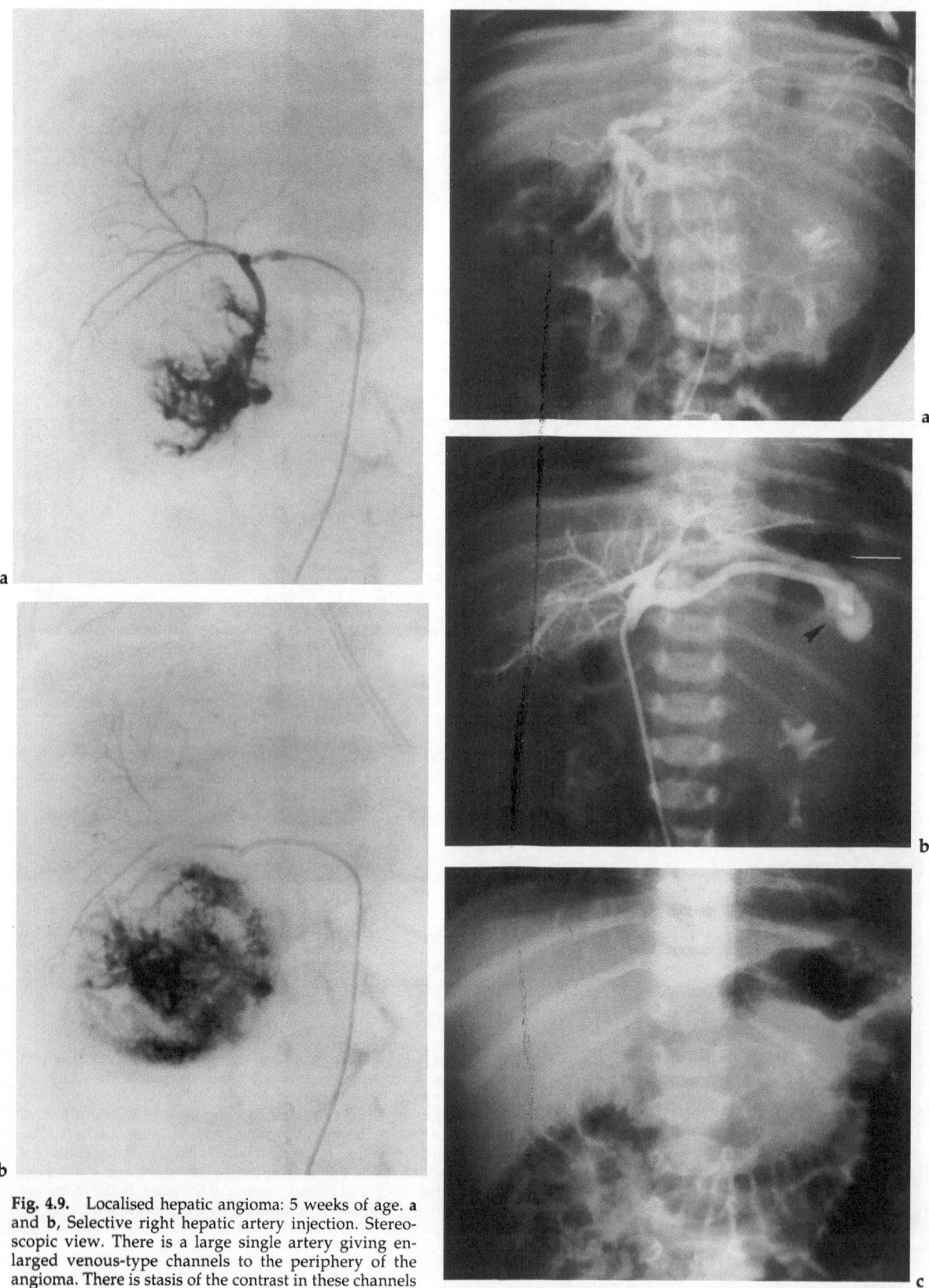

Fig. 4.9. Localised hepatic angioma: 5 weeks of age. **a** and **b**, Selective right hepatic artery injection. Stereoscopic view. There is a large single artery giving enlarged venous-type channels to the periphery of the angioma. There is stasis of the contrast in these channels without opacification of the hepatic veins. The rest of the liver is normal. Spontaneous regression of the angioma.

Fig. 4.10

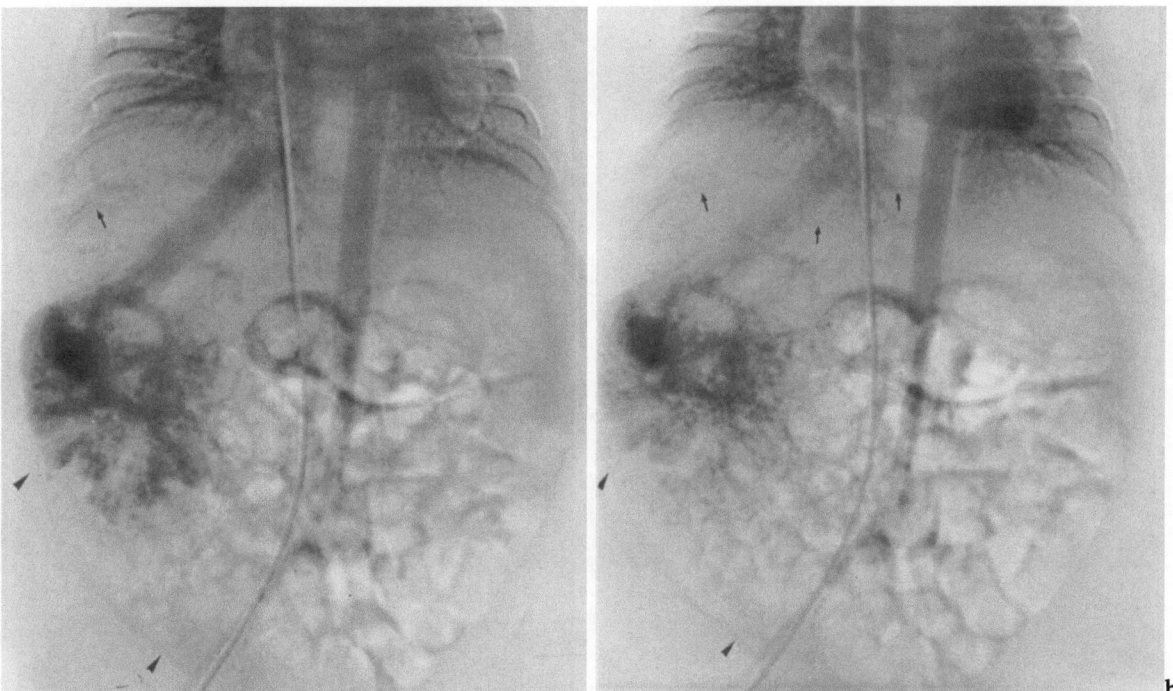

Fig. 4.11. Hepatomegaly with cardiac failure: 1 month of age. **a, b** Aortography obtained by injection in the right atrium just in front of a patent foramen ovale. There is a localised angioma vascularised by an enlarged hepatic artery had also by intercostal arteries (*arrows*) and a subcutaneous abdominal artery (*arrowheads*). The angiomatous mass is well-limited and there is early and massive opacification of an enlarged hepatic vein (2 s after the onset of the aortic injection). This mass regressed after radiotherapy. One year later the vascularisation of the liver was normal.

Fig. 4.10. Localised hepatic angioma: 5 days of age. **a** Hepatic artery injection through umbilical artery catheterisation. There is a localised hepatic angioma in the left lobe of the liver, with peripheral venous-type channels. **b** Portal opacification through umbilical vein catheterisation. There is a portohepatic shunt (*arrowhead*). **c** At 5 months later, there is a spontaneous regression of the mass with calcification of the left lobe of the liver.

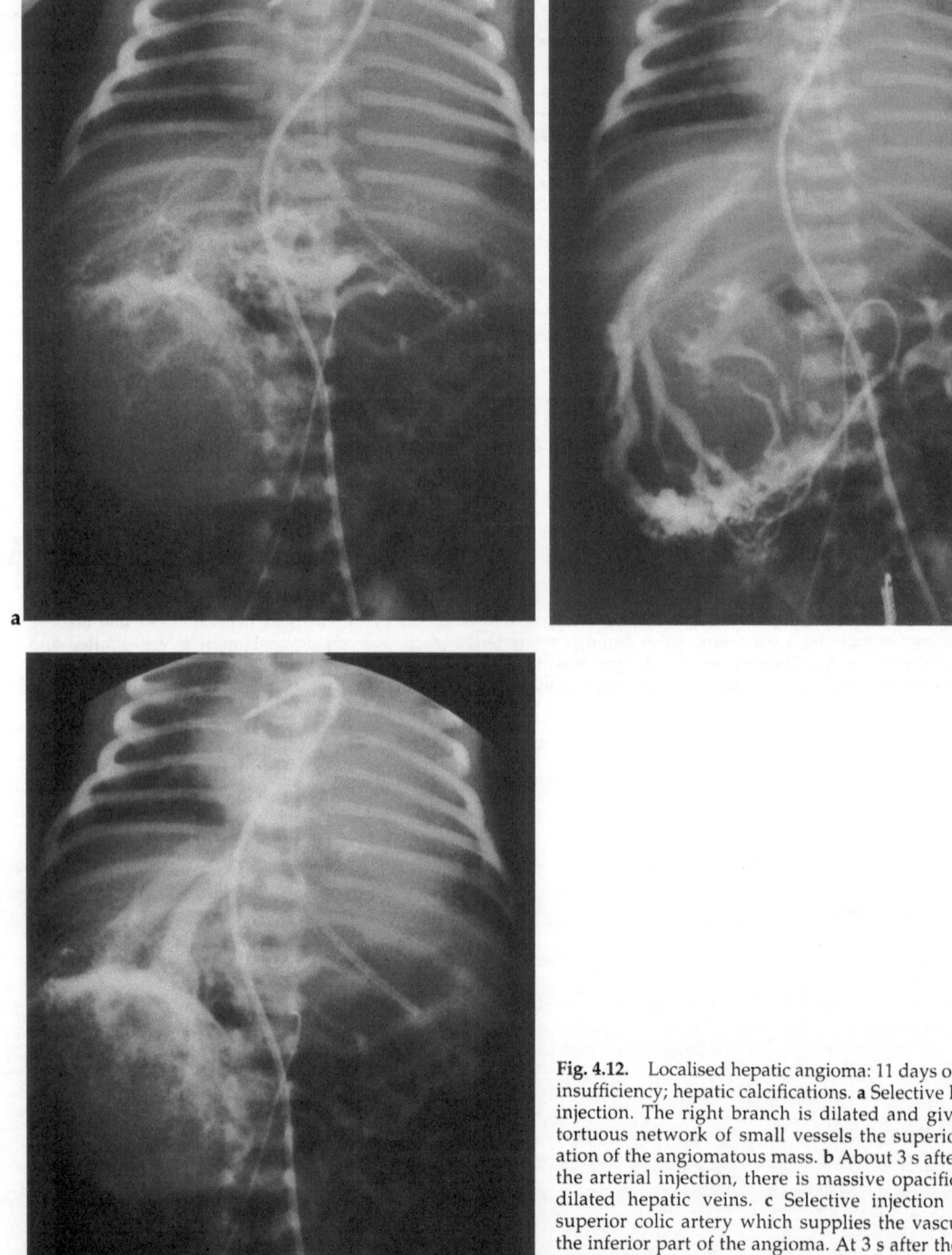

Fig. 4.12. Localised hepatic angioma: 11 days of age. Cardiac insufficiency; hepatic calcifications. **a** Selective hepatic artery injection. The right branch is dilated and gives through a tortuous network of small vessels the superior vascularisation of the angiomatous mass. **b** About 3 s after the onset of the arterial injection, there is massive opacification of two dilated hepatic veins. **c** Selective injection of the right superior colic artery which supplies the vascularisation of the inferior part of the angioma. At 3 s after the onset of the injection there is massive opacification of hepatic veins. A Swan–Ganz catheter was placed in the right pulmonary artery to control the cardiac output. Embolisation of the hepatic artery was performed. Regression of the mass.

Angiographic Findings (Figs. 4.13–37)

Angiography is now performed only as a pre-operative study after chemotherapy.

Technique

The complete angiographic work-up includes portal vein opacification via superior mesenteric arteriography, hepatic arteriography and also in cases of posterior and superior location of the tumour, opacification of the inferior vena cava and of the hepatic veins. Stereoangiography may be helpful to establish the relationship of the tumour and the main vessels.

Hepatoblastomas and Hepatocarcinomas

In our experience the arteriographic features of malignant hepatic tumours are not specific. Malignant tumours tend to be hypervascular but this is not always true, and after chemotherapy the hypervascularity of the tumour diminishes. The portal opacification on the other hand has a high diagnostic value. Portal invasion by the malignant tumour is a classic histological finding and is seen as a portal amputation on the portographic films. However, this finding is often less evident after chemotherapy. Thrombosis of the portal vein trunk or of the proximal branches leads to development of a cavernous hepatopetal network which may contraindicate or complicate surgery.

Invasion of the hepatic veins by the tumour can also be demonstrated.

Arterioportal shunt may be seen in malignant hepatic tumours and in our experience is suggestive of hepatocarcinomas.

Embolisation is not routinely performed. It was performed in two patients with rupture of the tumour and haemoperitoneum; but despite this procedure, the patients died shortly after.

Sarcomas

These are usually hypervascular (8/9 cases) but may be hypovascular (one case). There are no angiographic criteria to distinguish them from hepatoblastomas or hepatocarcinomas. It is very important to demonstrate the portal vein invasion in these cases as they are usually α-fetoprotein negative. Angiographic criteria are then very important to make the diagnosis of malignant tumour. In one case, an angiomyoliposarcoma was associated with jaundice.

Rhabdomyosarcoma is a rare form of sarcoma. It can invade the biliary ducts with intraluminal tumoral casts. The clinical presentation is jaundice and hepatic tumour. But it can present as a solitary hepatic mass. The α-fetoprotein level is normal. The arterial phase is that of a moderately hypervascular tumour. The superior mesenteric vein study demonstrates a portal vein amputation. In one case, bone metastases were present. If invasion of the bile ducts is suspected, cholangiography can be performed, to demonstrate the extension of the lesion.

Metastasis (11 cases)

The most frequent hepatic metastases in our series were from nephroblastoma (seven cases). Other primary tumours are: malignant teratoma, nasopharyngeal epithelioma, malignant ovarian teratoma and neuroblastoma.

The nephroblastoma metastases can be hypervascular or hypovascular. Portal amputation is usually seen in the same territory.

Angiographic investigation may exceptionally be necessary when metastases have close relationship to vessels and there may be a surgical problem.

Epithelioid Haemangioendothelioma

This rare type of malignant vascular tumour has been mainly reported in adults especially in females. We have had two cases in girls. There were diffuse masses with invasion of the hepatic veins in the presence of Budd–Chiari syndrome.

Hepatic Lymphomas

We have seen one case of lymphoma. Large lymph nodes may be present in the porta hepatis and can compress the bile ducts. Cholangiography with drainage may be indicated.

Benign Hepatic Tumours

Introduction

The clinical presentation is always as an isolated abdominal mass discovered by the family or the physician or on ultrasonography. Abdominal pain may be seen in girls with focal nodular hyperplasia.

The radiological diagnosis is based on US. Ultrasound usually easily localises the tumour within the liver. When cysts are present, the diagnosis of benign tumour can be confidently made in our experience. No truly cystic tumours are malignant. The differential diagnosis, however, is necrosis of highly malignant tumours such as sarcomas.

CT scan with bolus injection or MRI can be useful to further characterise the vascularity and structure of the lesion. Angiography is only performed as a preoperative work-up in the case of a large or central or hypervascularised lesion.

Anatomical variations of the hepatic arteries are frequent in this group of patients (19%).

The histopathology of the 32 patients in this group were:

Focal nodular hyperplasia	13
Adenoma	11
Cystic lymphangioma	8

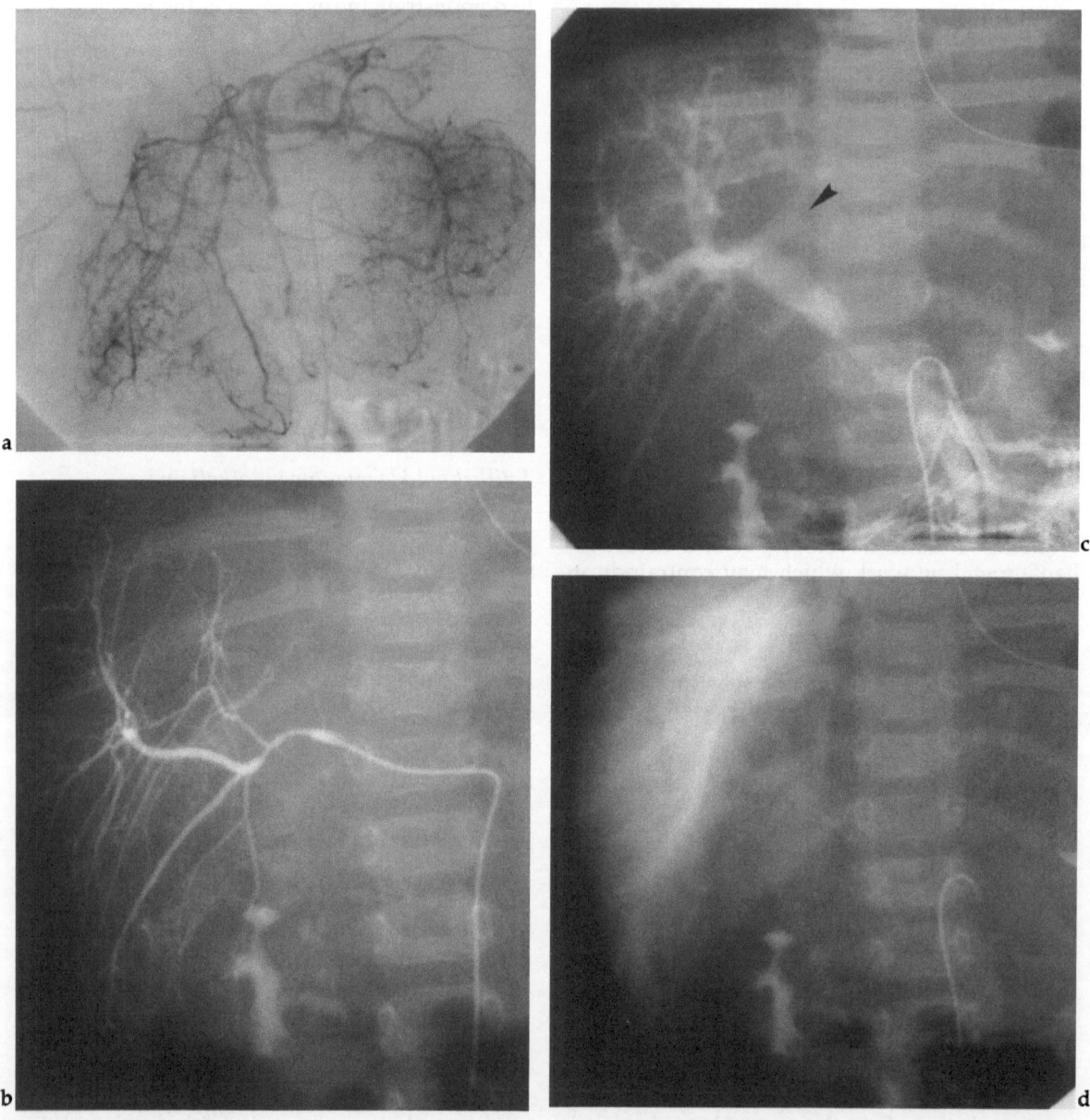

Fig. 4.13. Hepatoblastoma: 1 year of age. α-Fetoprotein positive; Chemotherapy; vascular work-up before surgery. **a** Selective injection of the left hepatic artery shows multiple hypervascular nodules in the left lobe of the liver. **b** The right hepatic artery is normal. **c** The venous return of a superior mesenteric artery injection shows that the left portal vein is obstructed (*arrowhead*). **d** Late phase. The left lobe of the liver is not perfused.

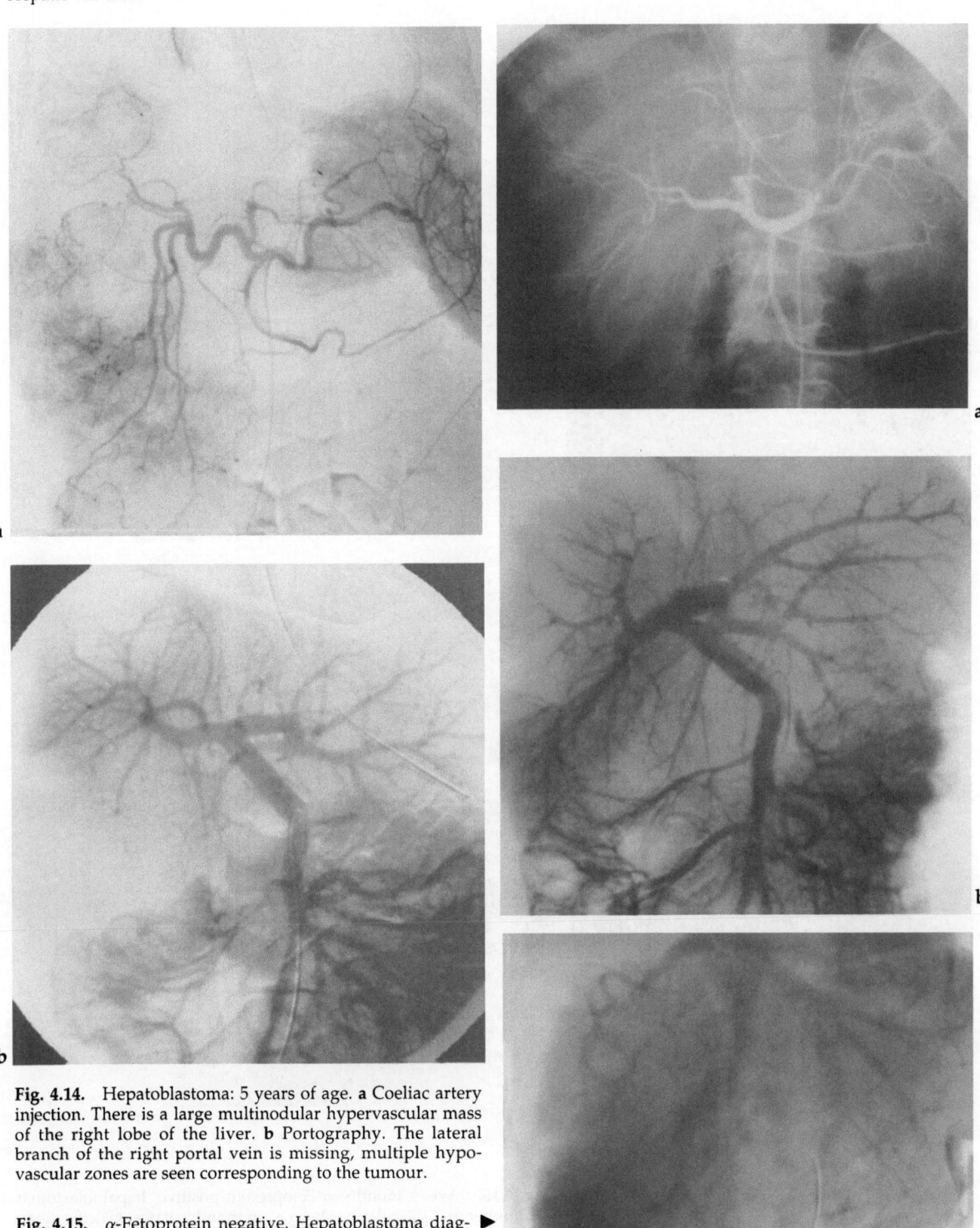

Fig. 4.14. Hepatoblastoma: 5 years of age. **a** Coeliac artery injection. There is a large multinodular hypervascular mass of the right lobe of the liver. **b** Portography. The lateral branch of the right portal vein is missing, multiple hypovascular zones are seen corresponding to the tumour.

Fig. 4.15. α-Fetoprotein negative. Hepatoblastoma diagnosed by biopsy. Vascular work-up after chemotherapy. **a** Coeliac trunk injection. After chemotherapy, the tumour is slightly hypervascular. **b** There are some hypovascular zones in the right lobe of the liver, but as usual after chemotherapy, the portal amputations are difficult to diagnose. There is hypertrophy of the left lobe. **c** Late phase of the superior mesenteric artery injection showing that the right hepatic vein is abnormal.

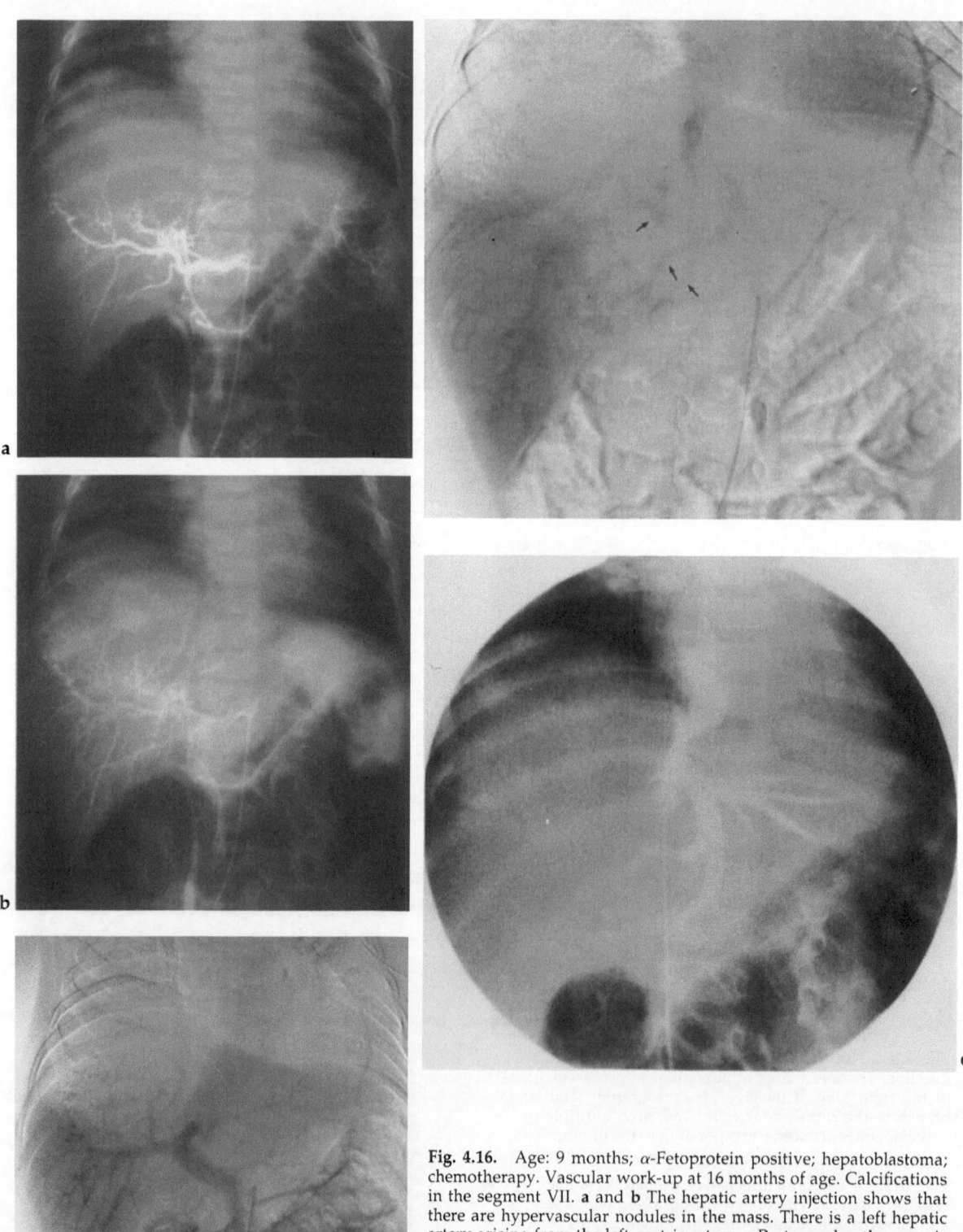

Fig. 4.16. Age: 9 months; α-Fetoprotein positive; hepatoblastoma; chemotherapy. Vascular work-up at 16 months of age. Calcifications in the segment VII. **a** and **b** The hepatic artery injection shows that there are hypervascular nodules in the mass. There is a left hepatic artery arising from the left gastric artery. **c** Portography: the mass is hypovascular on portography. **d** Late phase of portography. The right hepatic vein is not clearly seen, invaded by the tumour. There are interhepatic collateral veins (*arrows*). **e** Selective injection of the medial and left hepatic vein. The medial hepatic vein is displaced to the left, but patent. Surgery was performed, (bisegmentectomy segments VII and VIII).

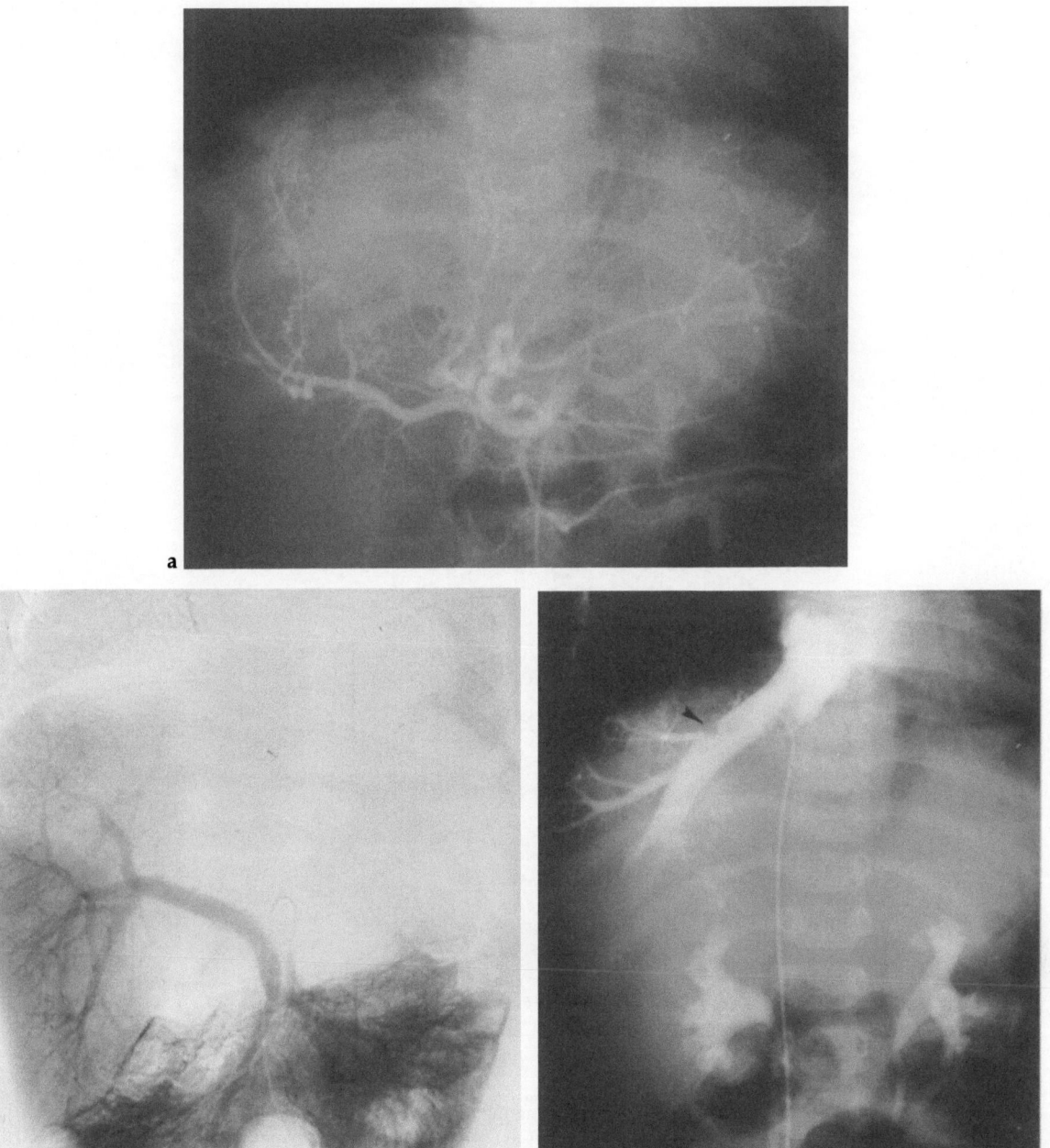

Fig. 4.17. Hepatoblastoma; vascular work-up after chemotherapy; 2 years of age. **a** Hepatic artery injection. This injection shows a large calcified hypervascular mass in the left lobe of the liver invading segments VII and VIII of the right of the liver. **b** Portography shows that there is complete amputation of the left portal system. There are some hypovascular regions in the dome of the right lobe. **c** Retrograde right hepatic vein injection showing a tumoral nodule in the right hepatic vein (*arrowhead*).

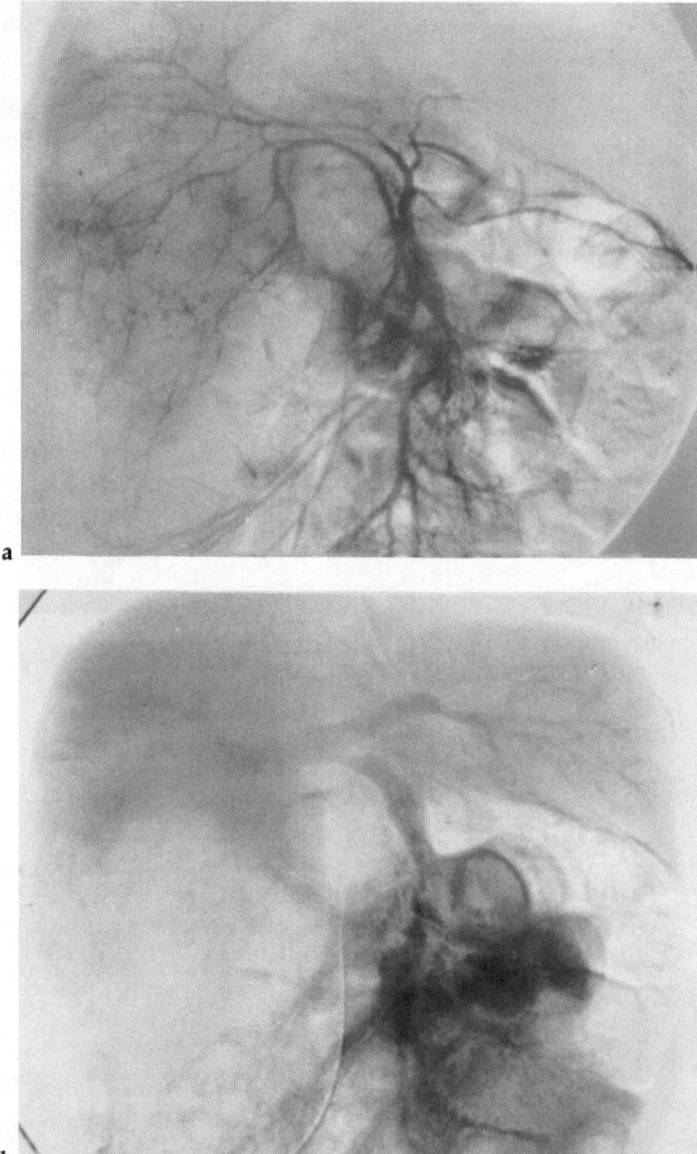

Fig. 4.18. α-Fetoprotein negative; hepatoblastoma with lung metastasis; 6 months of age. **a** Injection of a common coelio-mesenteric trunk. The right lobe of the liver is hypervascular. **b** Portography. There is an amputation of the inferior branches of the right portal vein (segment V and VI).

Fig. 4.19. Hepatoblastoma before chemotherapy: 11 years of age. **a** Coeliac trunk injection. There is a hypervascular mass of the right lobe of the liver. **b** Selective injection of the left branch of the hepatic artery showing that only segments II and III are normal. **c** Portography. There is a complete amputation of the right branch of the portal vein with a tumoral nodule in the lumen of the origin of the right portal vein (*arrow*).

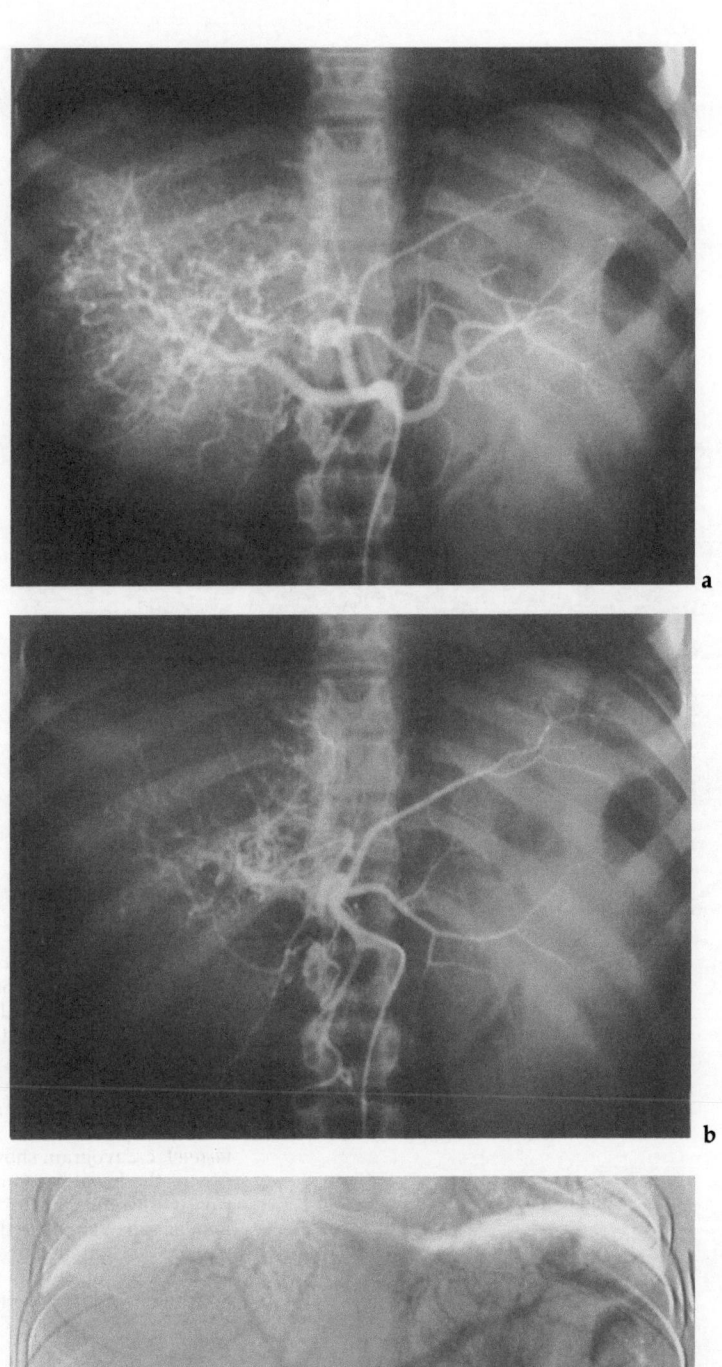

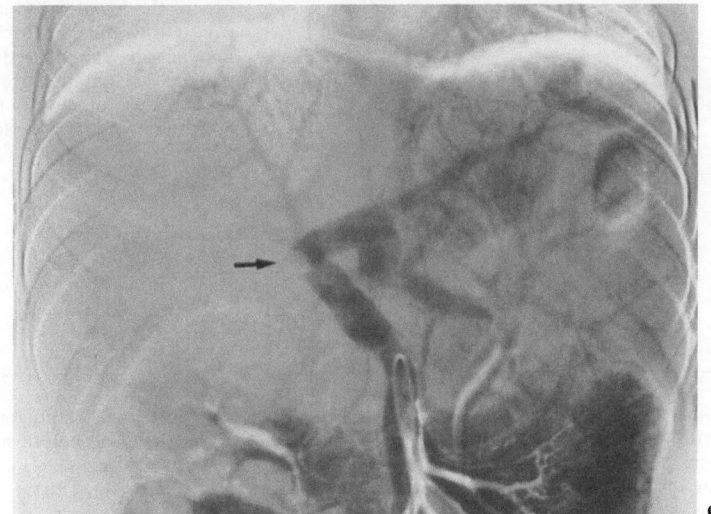

c   Fig. 4.19

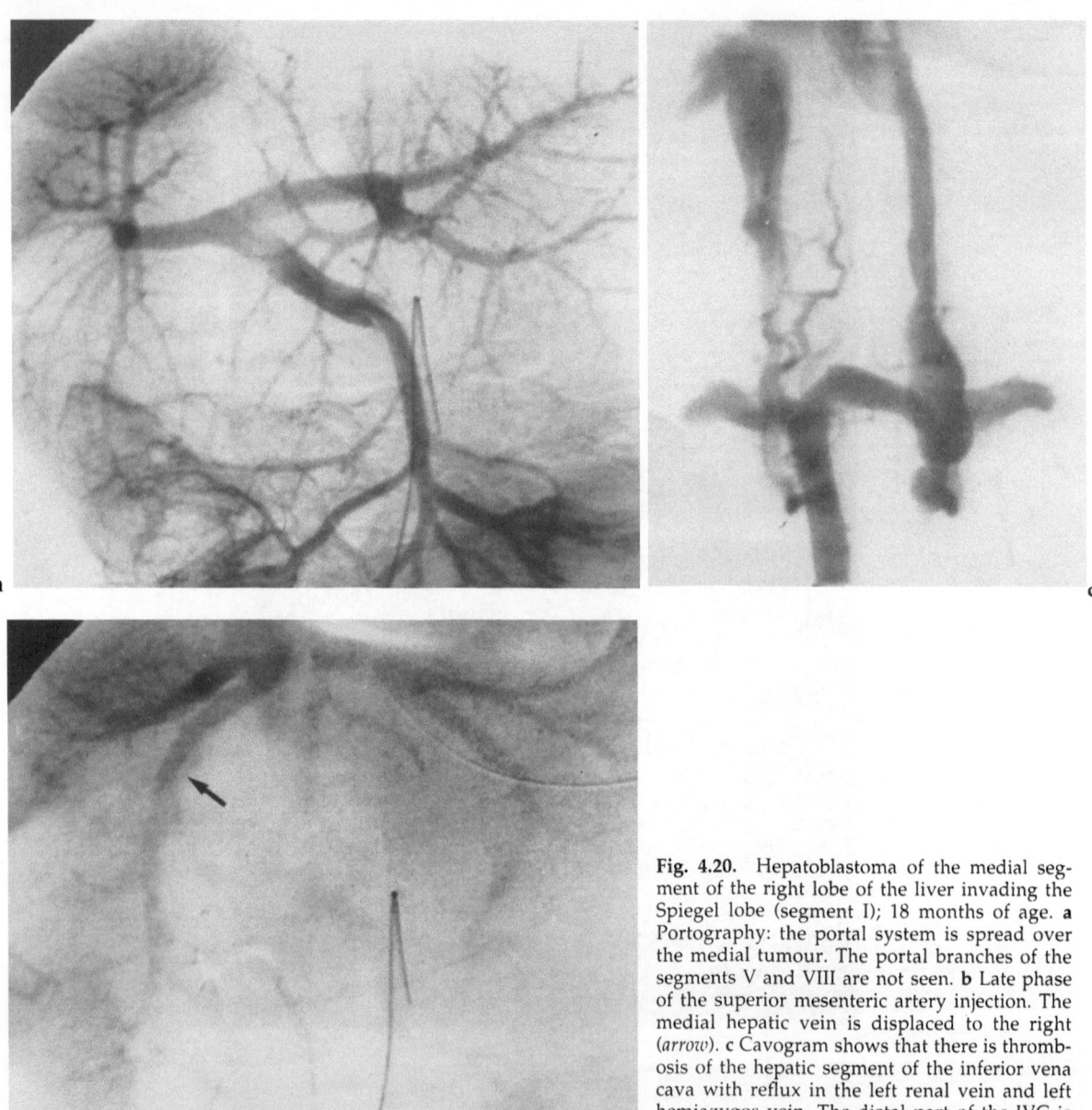

Fig. 4.20. Hepatoblastoma of the medial segment of the right lobe of the liver invading the Spiegel lobe (segment I); 18 months of age. **a** Portography: the portal system is spread over the medial tumour. The portal branches of the segments V and VIII are not seen. **b** Late phase of the superior mesenteric artery injection. The medial hepatic vein is displaced to the right (*arrow*). **c** Cavogram shows that there is thrombosis of the hepatic segment of the inferior vena cava with reflux in the left renal vein and left hemiazygos vein. The distal part of the IVC is patent. A right hepatectomy extended to the Spiegel lobe and to the thrombosed part of the IVC (segment I) was performed.

Fig. 4.21. Hepatoblastoma of the right lobe of the liver after chemotherapy. **a** The hepatic angiogram shows atrophy of the right lobe of the liver, with moderate hypervascularisation. **b** Portal phase of superior mesenteric artery injection. The left lobe of the liver is hypertrophied. The right lobe of the liver is atrophic and there are segmental amputations of the right branch of the portal vein (*arrow*). **c** Late phase of the superior mesenteric artery injection. The left and the medial (*arrow*) hepatic veins are displaced to the right. The right hepatic vein is not opacified.

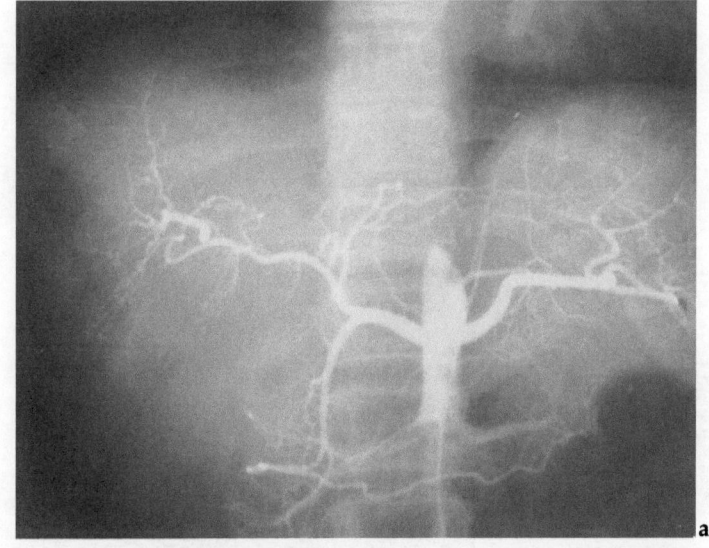

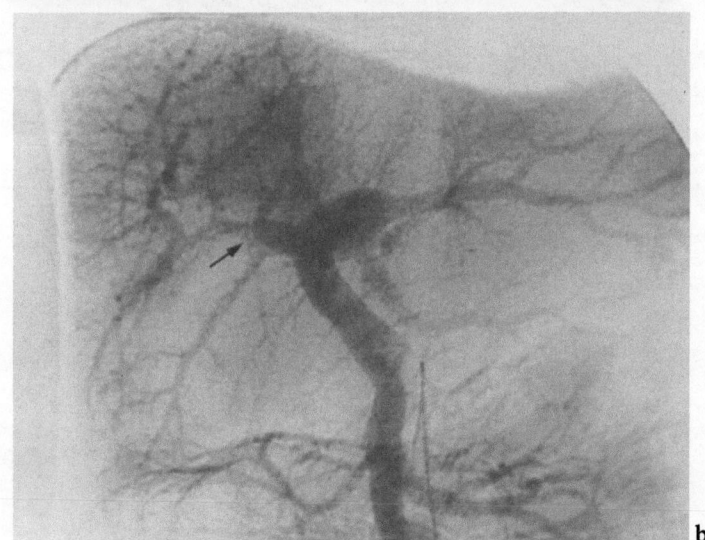

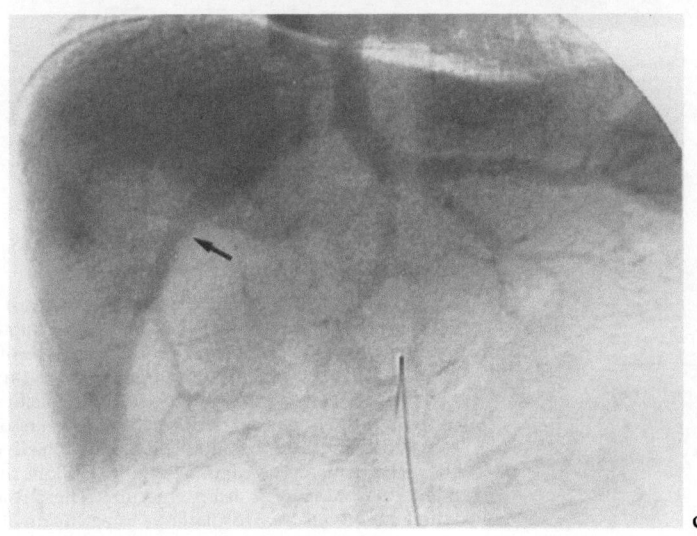

c   Fig. 4.21

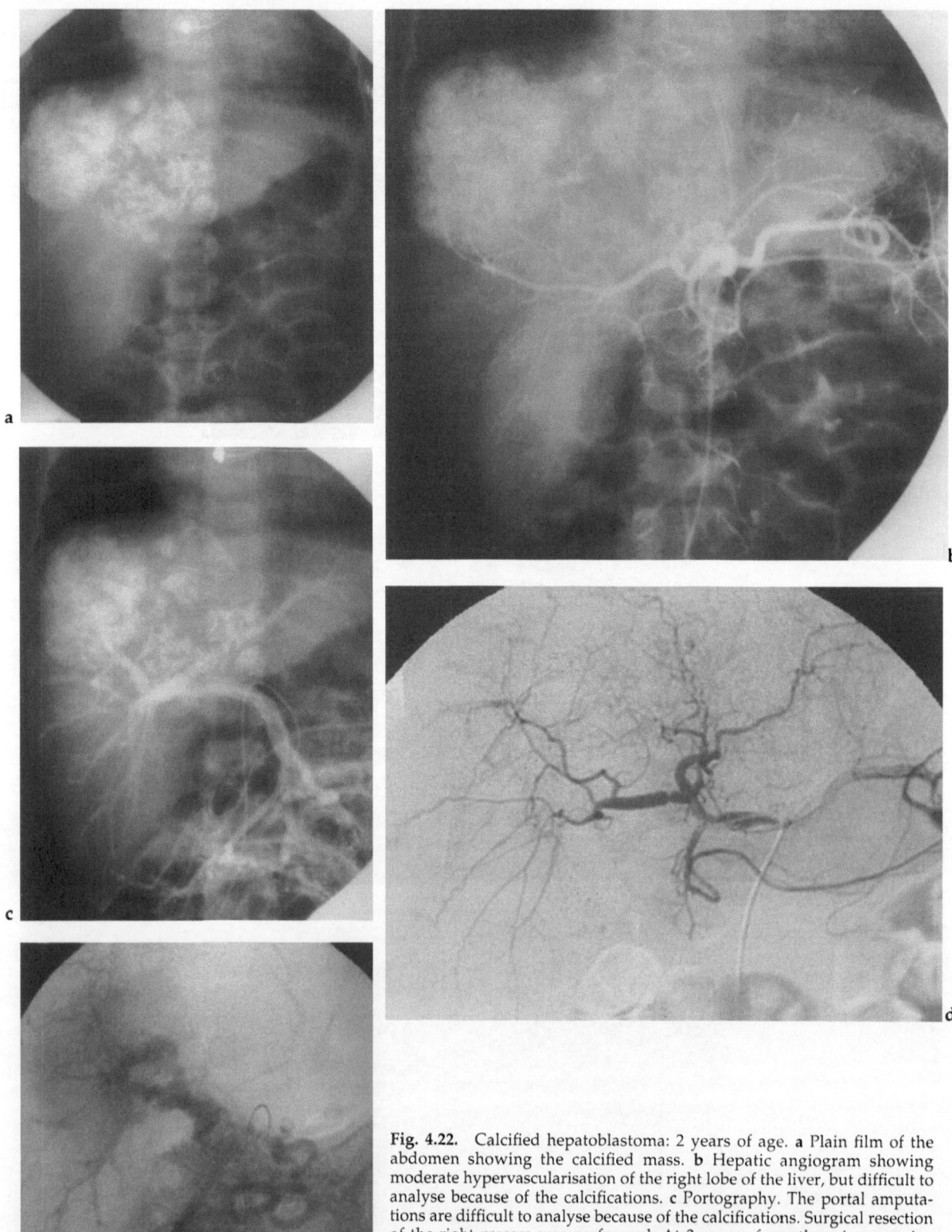

Fig. 4.22. Calcified hepatoblastoma: 2 years of age. **a** Plain film of the abdomen showing the calcified mass. **b** Hepatic angiogram showing moderate hypervascularisation of the right lobe of the liver, but difficult to analyse because of the calcifications. **c** Portography. The portal amputations are difficult to analyse because of the calcifications. Surgical resection of the right masses was performed. At 3 years of age there is a massive recurrence of the tumour in the left lobe of the liver. **d** Hepatic angiogram shows large hypervascular mass in the left lobe of the liver. **e** Portal phase of superior mesenteric artery injection. There is a portal vein thrombosis with a cavernous transformation. No perfusion of the left lobe of the liver.

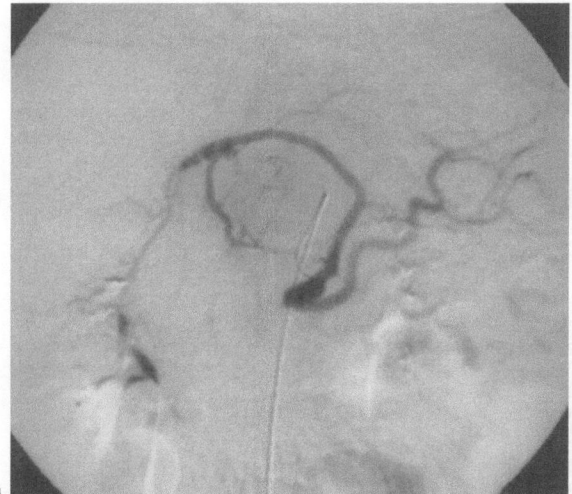

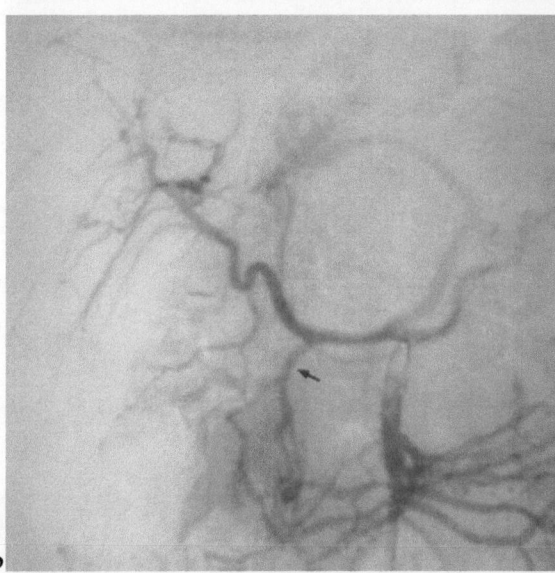

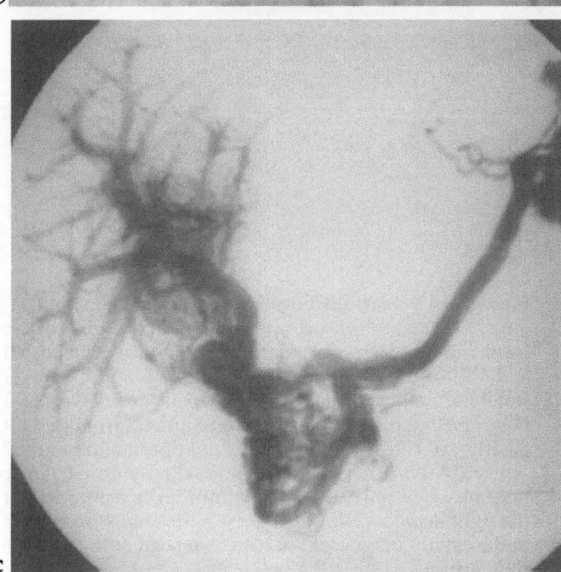

◄ Fig. 4.23. Hepatoblastoma plus portal vein thrombosis; 15-year-old boy. Vascular work-up after chemotherapy. **a** Selective injection of the left gastric artery giving the left hepatic artery. There is a hypervascular mass of the left lobe of the liver. **b** Selective injection of the superior mesenteric artery, opacifies the coeliac trunk through the gastroduodenal artery because of compression of the coeliac axis (*arrow*). **c** Splenoportography. Complete thrombosis of the left portal vein. Cavernous transformation of the portal vein. Hepatic transplantation was attempted but the child died.

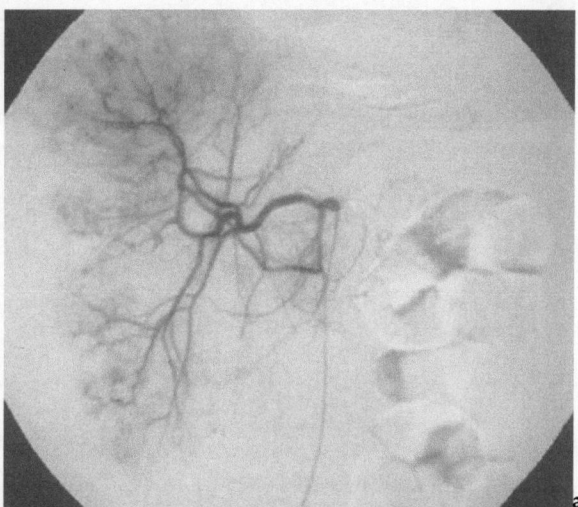

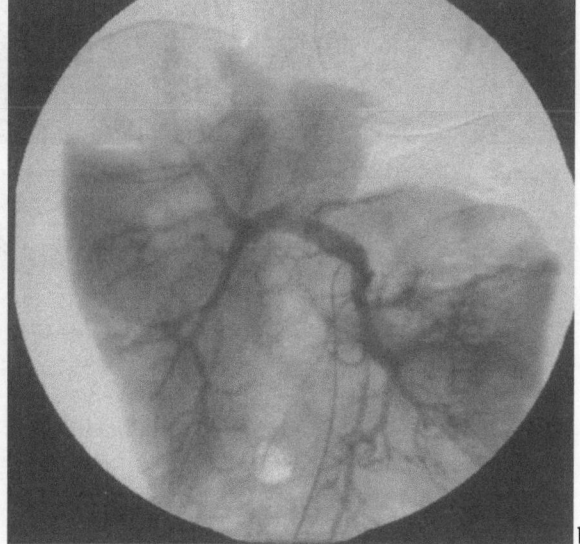

Fig. 4.24. Age 2 years. Recurrence of hepatoblastoma in the right lobe of the liver. This patient had been operated for a left-sided hepatoblastoma. **a** Right hepatic artery injection showing hypervascular masses of the right lobe of the liver. **b** Portography. The hypovascular masses are well seen. The patient died with lung metastasis, despite chemoembolisation.

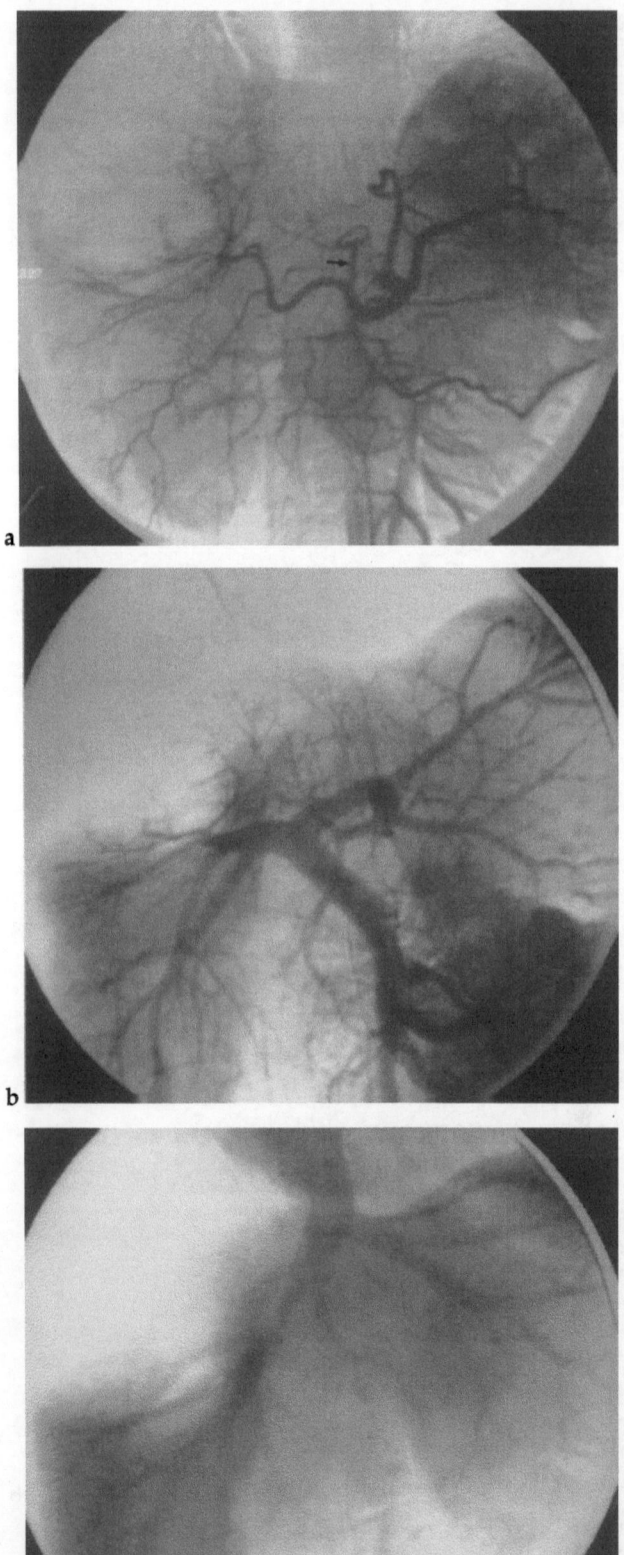

Fig. 4.25. 9-year-old boy. Non secreting hepatoblastoma; Vascular work-up after chemotherapy **a** Coeliac trunk injection: hypovascular tumour in the segments VII and VIII of the right lobe. The left lobe is supplied by a small left branch of the common hepatic artery (segment IV) (*arrow*) and a left hepatic artery arising from the left gastric artery. **b** Venous phase of superior mesenteric artery (SMA) injection. The tumour is hypovascular. **c** Late phase of SMA injection shows no opacification of the right hepatic vein. At surgery, a thrombus was found in the ostium of the right hepatic vein, extending into the right atrium.

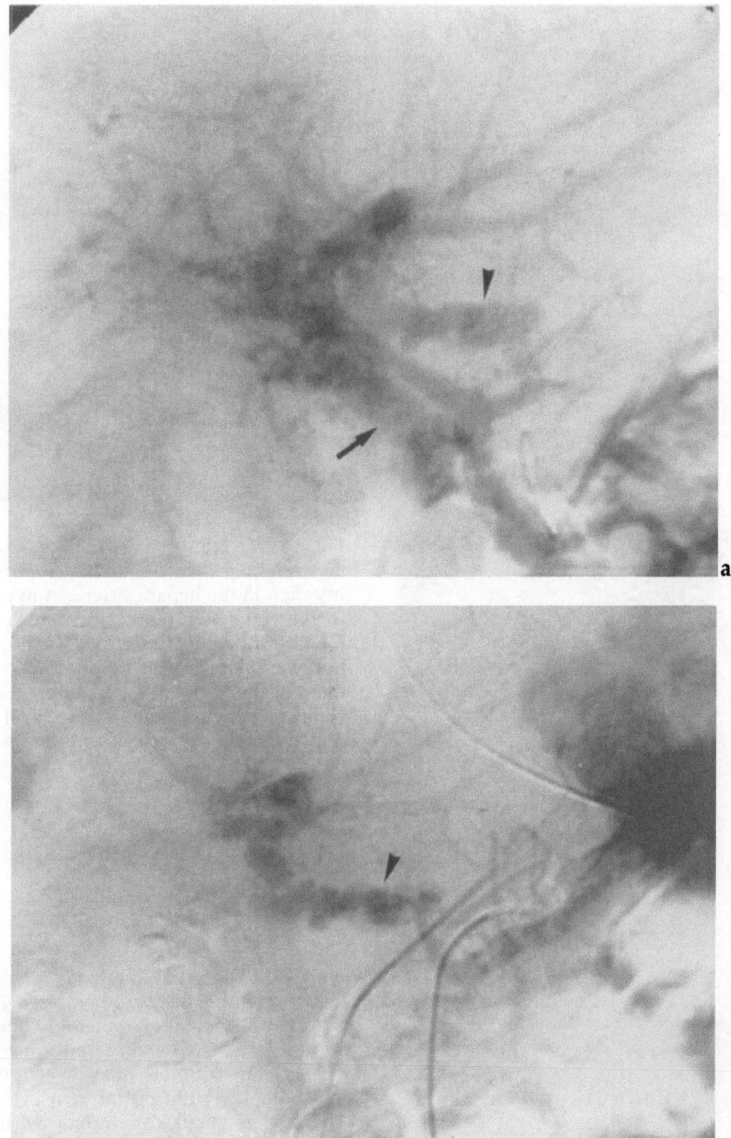

Fig. 4.26. A 1-year-old girl presenting with multinodular right hepatoblastoma. Vascular work-up after chemotherapy.
a, b Venous phase of the superior mesenteric artery injection. There is a right portal vein thrombosis and opacification of a double cavernomatous network. The superior mesenteric vein gives the inferior part of the cavernoma (*arrow*) and the splenic vein the superior part (*arrowhead*), as shown on the venous phase of the splenic artery injection (**b**). The tumour located in the right lobe was vascularised by a replaced right hepatic artery. Right hepatectomy was performed with ligation of the right hepatic artery, the small residual portal vein and the cavernomatous network arising from the superior mesenteric vein. The remaining left lobe is vascularised by the cavernoma arising from the splenic vein.

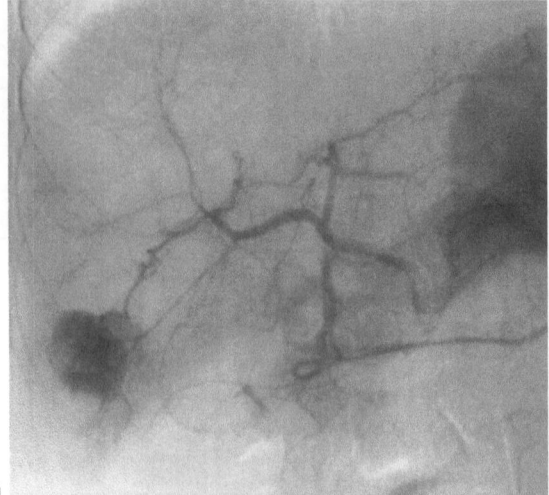

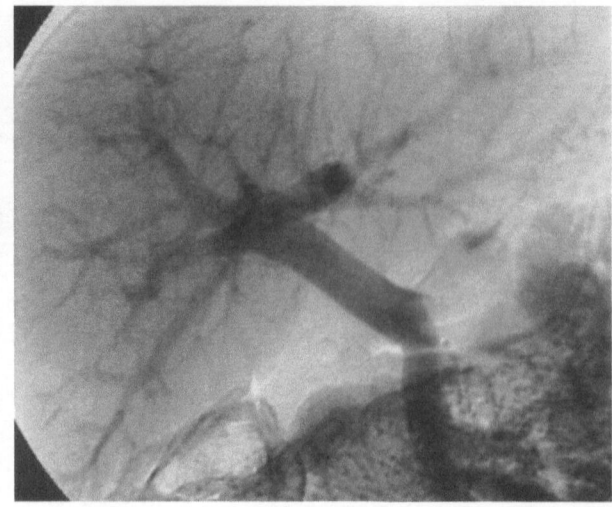

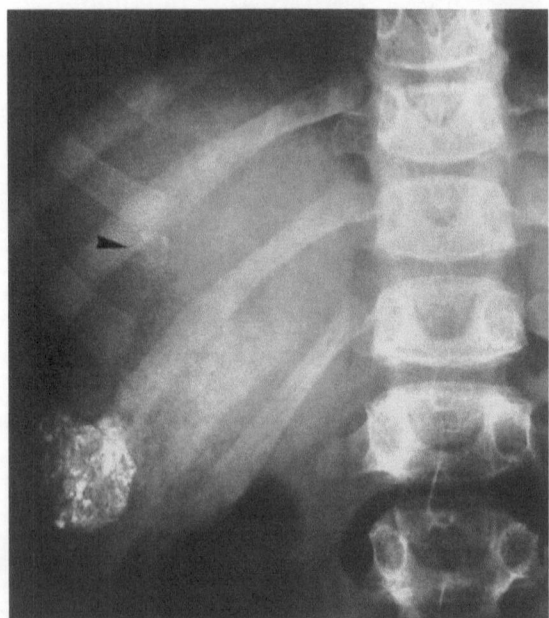

Fig. 4.27. Nine-year-old boy. Post-hepatitis (virus B) cirrhosis, hepatocarcinoma; α-fetoprotein positive. **a** Selective injection in the hepatic artery. A hypervascular mass is seen in the right lobe of the liver. **b** Portal phase of superior mesenteric artery injection. The tip of the liver appears hypovascular. **c** After lipiodol injection, not only the large mass of the segment VI is visible, but there is also another small lesion projection at the level of the tenth right rib which was not visible on the hepatic artery injection (*arrowhead*).

Fig. 4.28. Ten-year-old girl. Post-hepatitis (virus B) cirrhosis; hepatocarcinoma; chemotherapy. **a** Coeliac artery injection. The arterial anomalies of the right lobe of the liver are subtle. Some arteries have a corkscrew appearance. Normal left lobe of the liver. **b** Portal phase of superior mesenteric artery injection. The right portal vein is thrombosed (*arrowhead*). There is a small cavernoma with pancreaticoduodenal derivation parallel to the portal trunk.

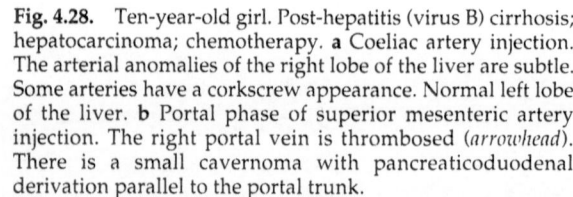

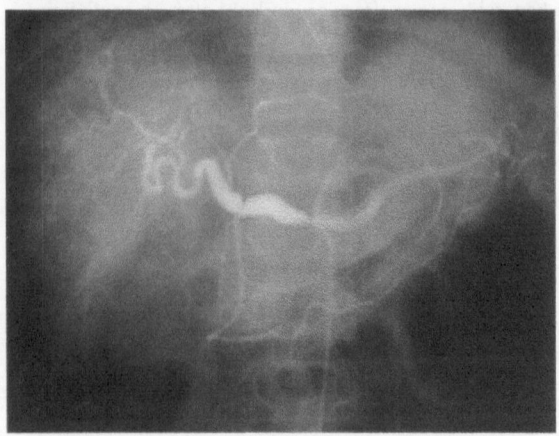

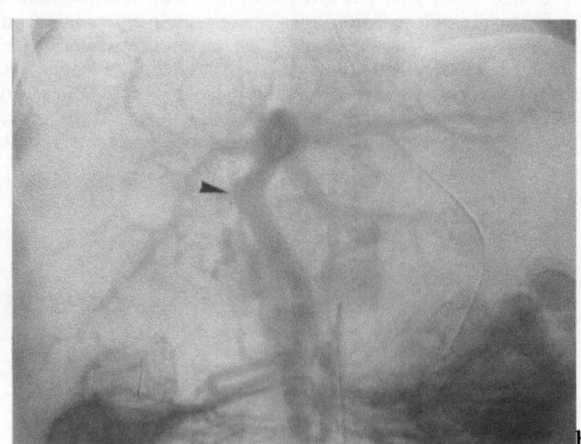

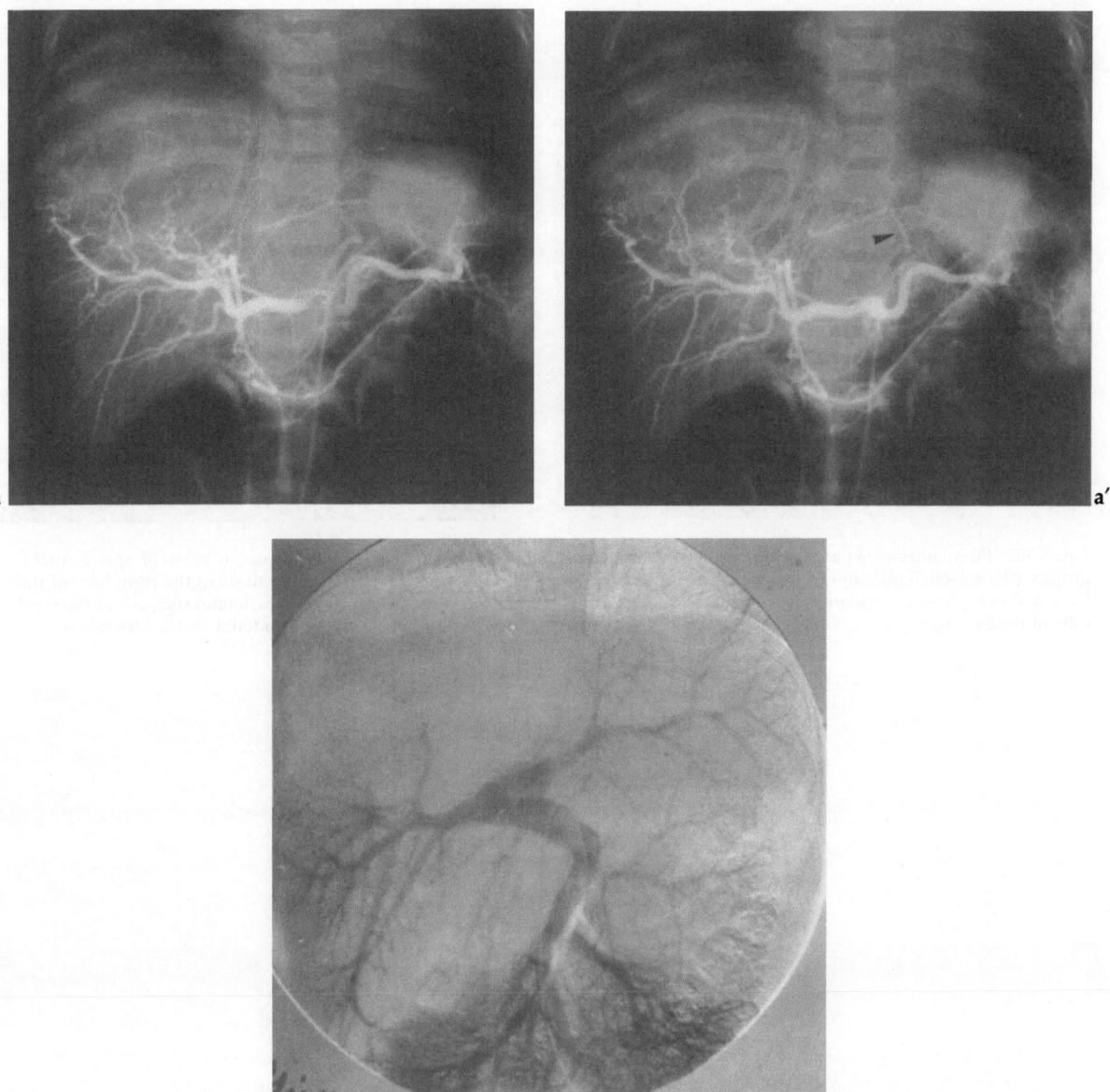

Fig. 4.29. Primitive hepatocarcinoma; 6 years of age. **a, a′** Coeliac artery injection showing a large hypervascular mass of the right lobe of the liver. Close to the left lobe there is a small left hepatic artery arising from the left gastric artery (*arrowhead*). Stereographic technique. **b** Portal phase of superior mesenteric artery injection. There is defect of the portography in the segments VII and VIII.

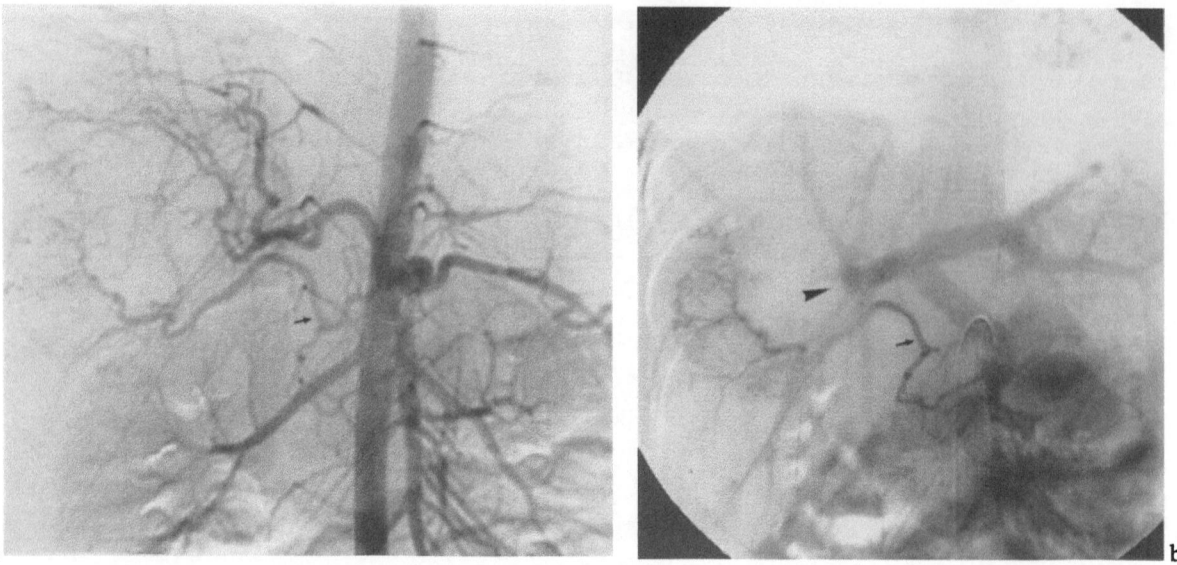

a   b

Fig. 4.30. Fibrolamellar hepatocarcinoma; hyperleucocytosis; clinical suspicion of a liver abcess; 6 years of age. **a** Aortography (the selective injection of the coeliac artery was not possible). There is a hypervascular mass of the right lobe of the liver. **b** Portal phase of superior mesenteric artery injection. There is a complete amputation of the lateral segment of the right lobe of the liver (*arrowhead*). Note a small replaced right hepatic artery coming off the gastroduodenal arcade (*arrow*).

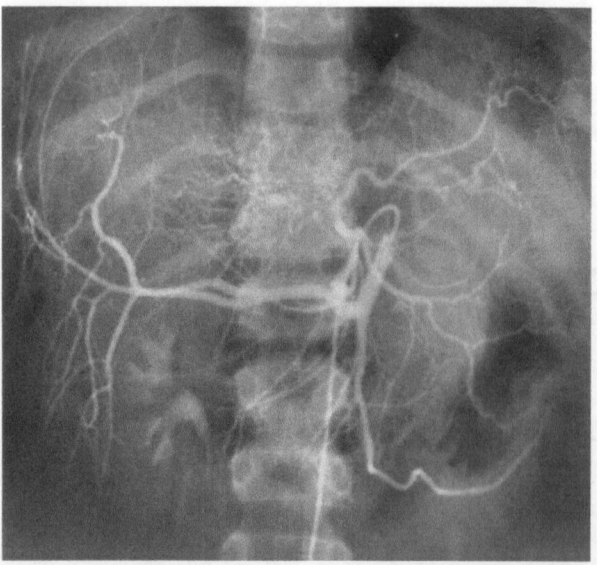

Fig. 4.31. Malignant mesenchymoma; 8 years of age. Hepatic artery injection. There is a spoke-wheel appearance of the medial segment of the liver. On the portal phase of splenic injection, there was a complete amputation of the left branch of the portal vein. After chemotherapy, the hypervascularisation regressed. The left portal vein thrombosis persisted. Surgery was performed.

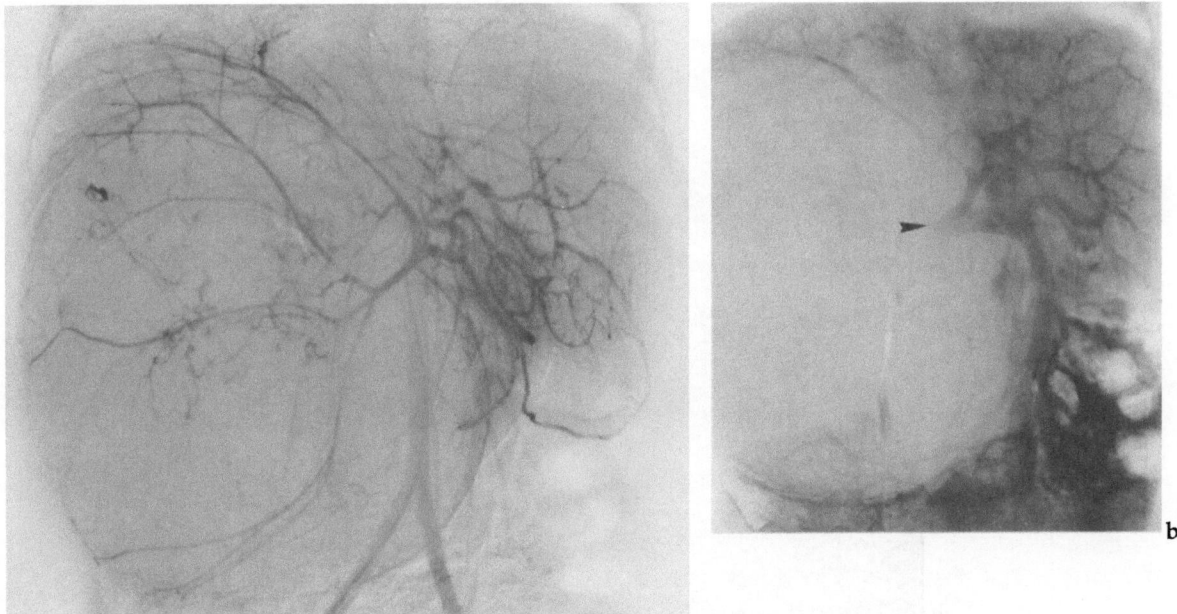

Fig. 4.32. Malignant mesenchymoma; 4 years of age. **a** Coeliac artery injection. There is a large hypovascular mass of the right lobe of the liver with many vascular lakes on the late phase. **b** The portal phase shows a complete amputation of the right branch of the portal vein (*arrowhead*).

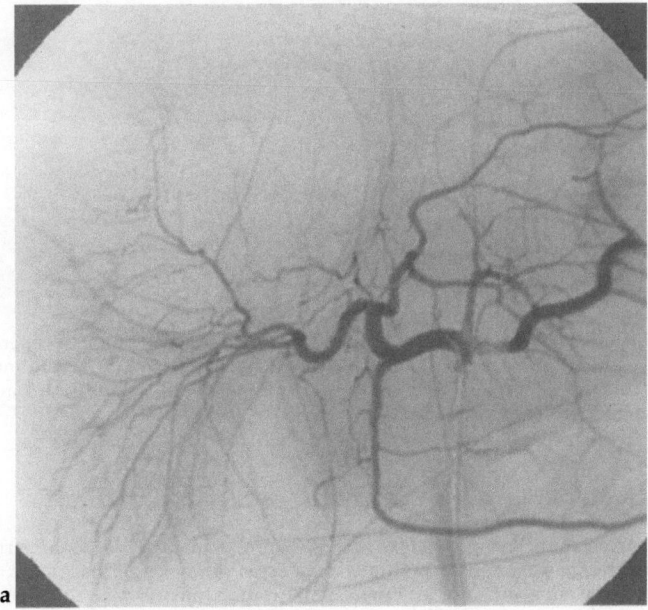

Fig. 4.33. Malignant sarcoma of the liver after chemotherapy. **a** Coeliac artery injection. There is a large hypovascular mass mainly located in segments VII and VIII, but also involving segments V and IV. *Continued overleaf.*

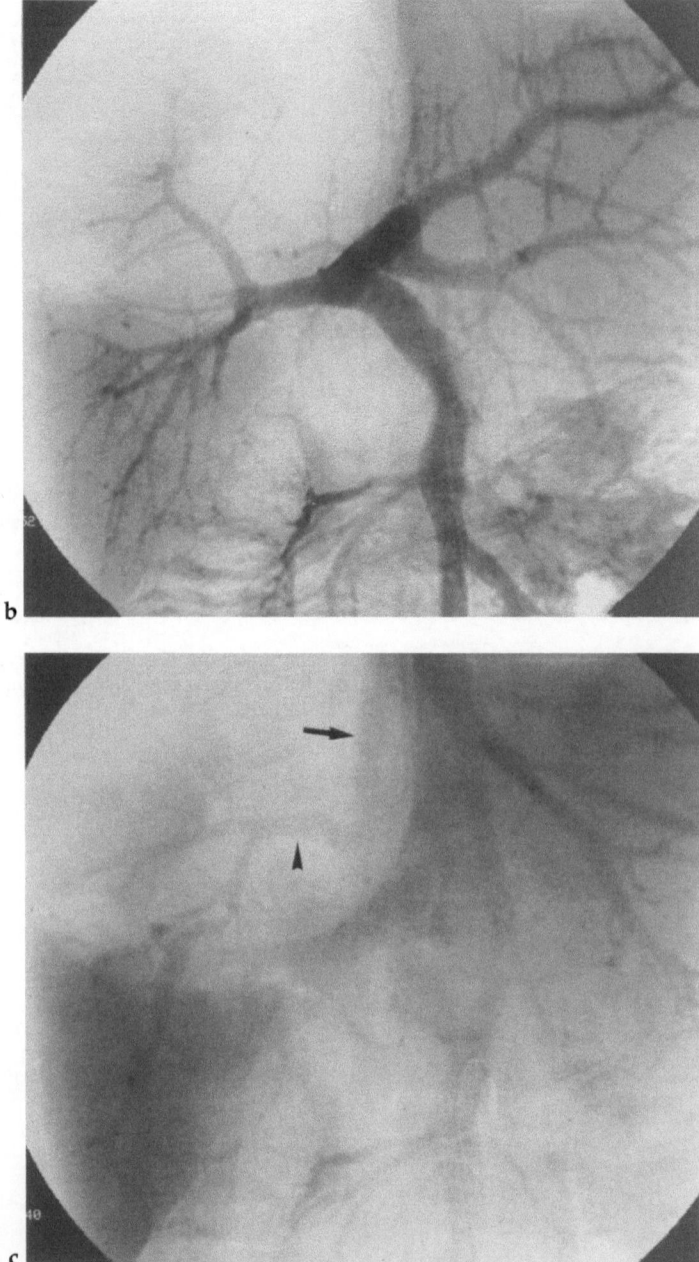

Fig. 4.33. Malignant sarcoma of the liver after chemotherapy. (*continued*) **b** Portal phase of superior mesenteric artery (SMA) injection. Only segments II and III are intact. **c** Late phase of the SMA injection. The left and medial hepatic veins are opacified but the right hepatic vein is amputated in its distal part. There is diversion toward an inferior right hepatic vein (*arrowhead*) opening into the inferior vena cava (*arrow*).

Fig. 4.34. Epithelioid hemangioendothelioma; 9 years of age; α-fetoprotein negative. **a** Coeliac artery opacification. There are diffuse abnormalities of the arterial system with multiple small areas of hypervascularisation. **b** Portal phase of superior mesenteric artery injection. There are some areas of hypovascularisation only in the medial portion of the liver. The main portal branches are normal. **c, c'** (stereographic films) (These two films can be viewed on stereoscopy.) Right hepatic vein injection through jugular vein approach. There is stenosis of the hepatic vein (*arrowhead*) and there are intrahepatic collateral veins joining a posterior spigelian vein (*arrow*) and diaphragmatic veins (*white arrow*) (Budd–Chiari syndrome).

Fig. 4.34

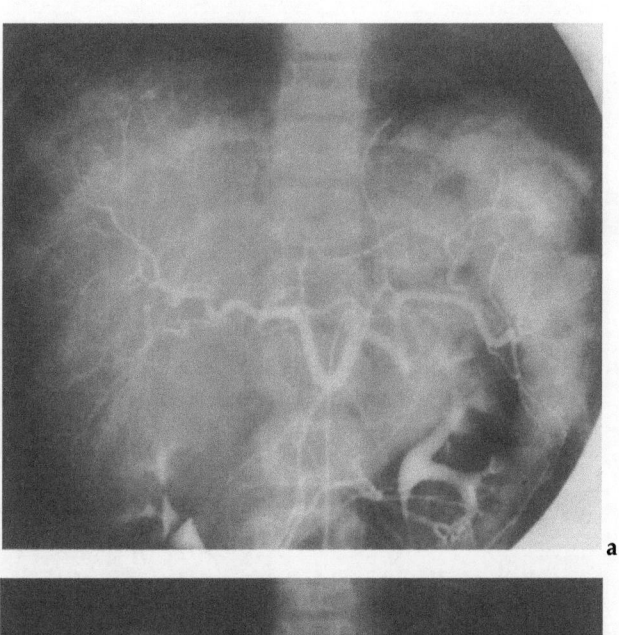

a

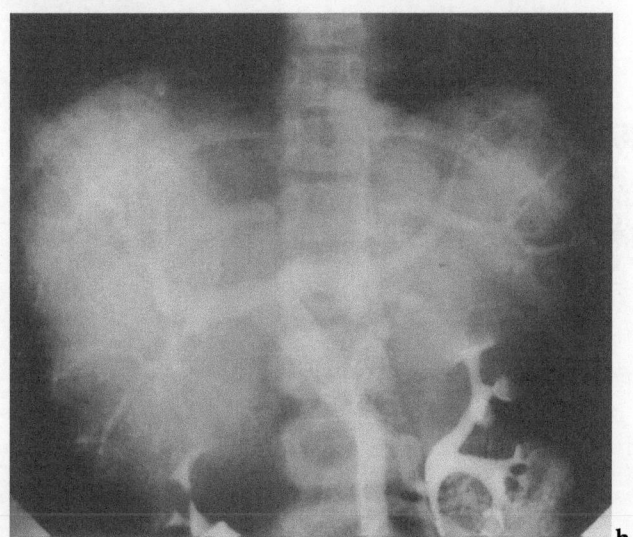

b

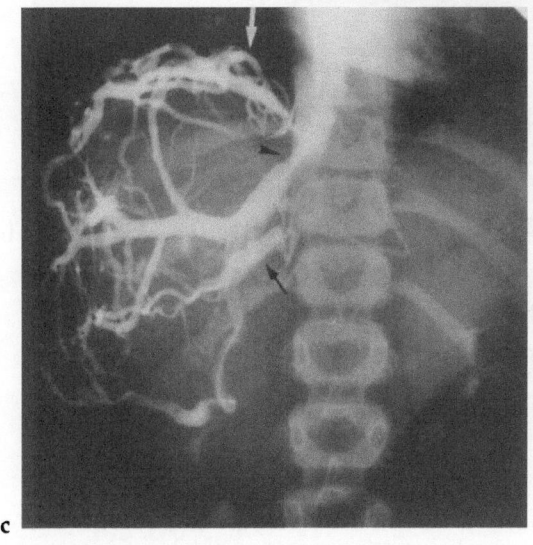

c

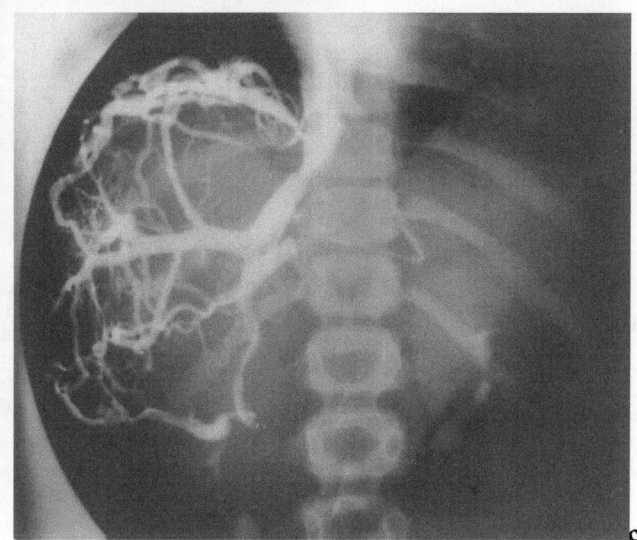

c'

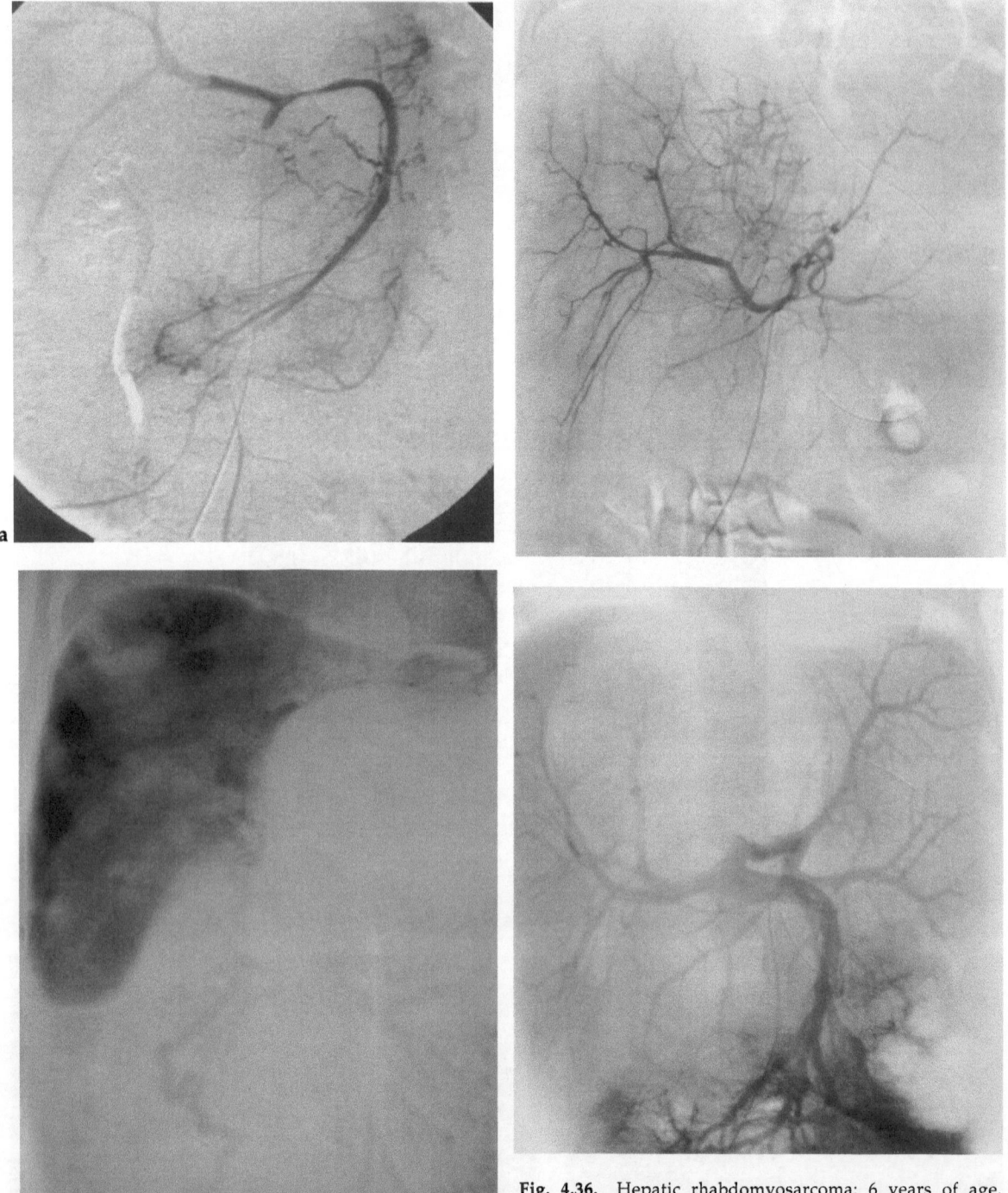

Fig. 4.35. Gastric leiyomyosarcoma with hepatic meta-stases. **a** Coeliac artery injection. The left gastric artery is dilated. There is diffuse hypervascularisation of the stomach. **b** Venous return of superior mesenteric artery injection. There is a complete occlusion of the portal vein. Some collaterals are seen in the hepatic hilum. There are multiple filing defects in the liver due to hepatic metastases.

Fig. 4.36. Hepatic rhabdomyosarcoma: 6 years of age. **a** Hepatic artery injection. There is a moderately hypervascular mass in the medial segment of the liver. **b** Portal phase of superior mesenteric artery injection. The medial tumour is hypovascular and spreads apart the left and right portal veins. *Continued opposite.*

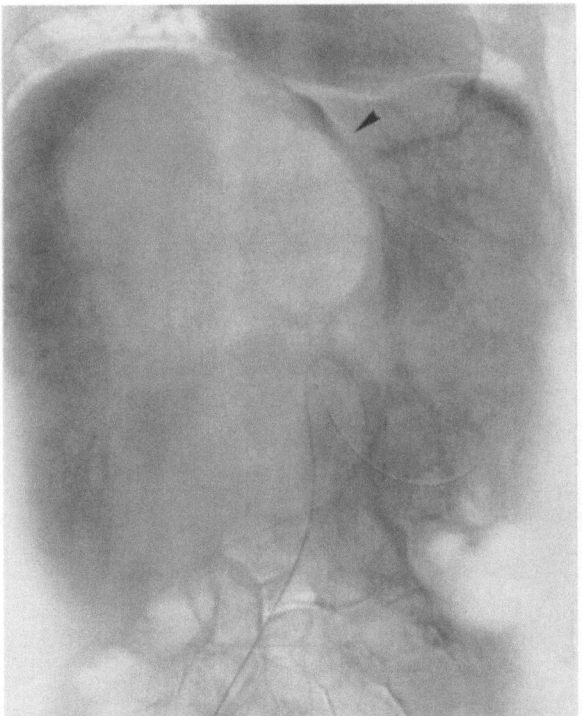

c

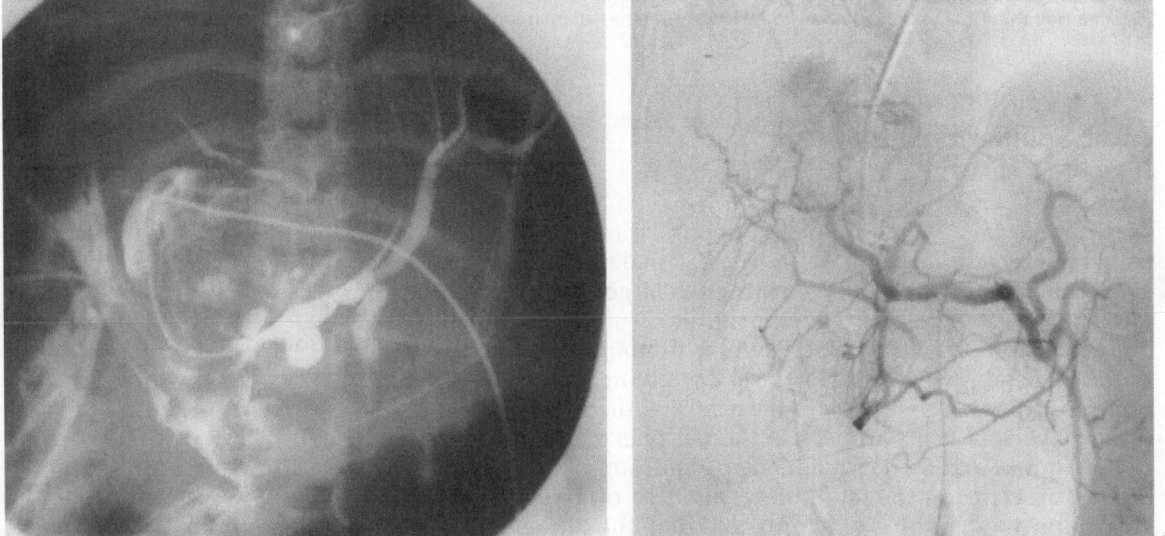

d   e

Fig. 4.36. Hepatic rhabdomyosarcoma: 6 years of age. (*continued*) **c** Late phase. The medial hepatic vein is displaced to the left (*arrowhead*). The right hepatic vein is not seen. **d** Surgical biopsy was performed. Biliary leak after surgery. Percutaneous drainage of the left and right biliary duct. The right biliary duct is opacified, there is a leak at the level of the common bile duct. The left biliary duct is drained with a separate catheter. **e** Same patient after chemotherapy. There is a dramatic diminution of the hepatic mass. There is still a hypervascular mass in the region of segment VIII.

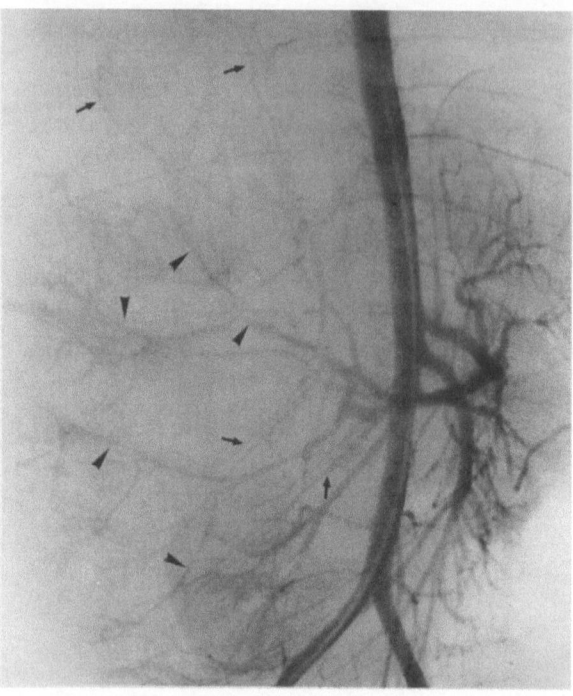

Fig. 4.37. Hepatic involvement of an adrenal neuroblastoma; 6-year-old boy. Aortography was performed to assess the operability of the tumour. The hepatic artery is enlarged and supplies posterior branches (*arrows*) to the adrenal tumour and also anterior abnormal branches (*arrowheads*) indicating the severe involvement of the liver (stereo angiography).

Focal Nodular Hyperplasia
(Figs. 4.38–4.40)

This tumour has been encountered in our series from between the ages of 1 and 13 years, females predominating (11 girls, 2 boys). It is often large, lobulated, superficial and may be painful.

Angiography shows a hypervascular tumour with one or two enlarged arteries giving branches from the periphery to the centre of the tumour. Dilated veins are seen at the periphery of the tumour and there is massive opacification of hepatic veins on the late films. This type of vascularisation gives the impression that the tumour is embedded in a vascular net.

The portal study shows that all branches of the portal vein are present and patent, merely displaced by the tumour that appears avascular during portography.

Embolisation was performed four times to reduce the vascularisation and volume of the tumour. Ivalon and alcohol were used most of the time. Prophylactic antibiotics must be given during the procedure and after the embolisation. One technical failure was encountered in a very tortuous hepatic artery.

A number of complications have been encountered. Liver abscesses were seen in two cases before antibiotics were systematically used. One complete cure was obtained after embolisation in a case in which the diagnosis was previously obtained by surgical biopsy. One case of gallbladder necrosis was seen. No malignant degeneration ever occurred with a follow-up of more than 15 years.

Adenomas (11 cases)

Three cases of adenoma were seen in boys treated by androgen therapy for Fanconi anaemia. They were seen because of complications: one rupture with haemoperitoneum, one intrahepatic haematoma and one hepatic abscess. The angiographic signs are similar to those seen in adenomas occurring in glycogen storage disease.

Embolisation was performed in one case on an emergency basis because of bleeding. Percutaneous drainage of the abscess was performed in another. Portal opacification shows portal vein compression by the rapidly growing intrahepatic haematoma in the patient with the intrahepatic bleed.

Adenomas may complicate glycogen storage disease (Chapter 8).

Adenoma may also occur without any underlying disease and was seen in a 5-year-old boy without any history.

Cystic Mesenchymatous Hamartomas
(eight cases)

Made of multiple cysts of variable size, in our series they are mainly seen in boys. The diagnosis is made on ultrasound, showing multiple cysts separated by thick septae.

When angiography is performed, the septae are hypervascular. The portal system is displaced, but patent. In one case, compression of an hepatic vein was responsible for segmental inversion of portal blood flow as in Budd–Chiari syndrome.

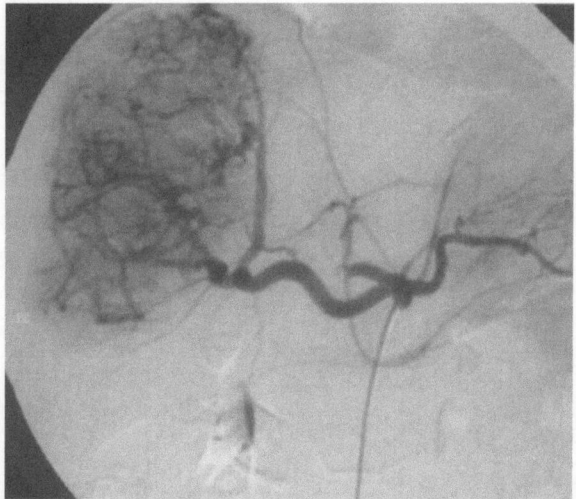

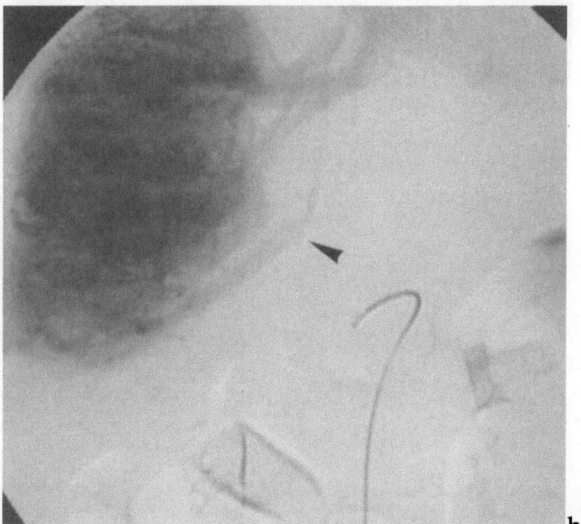

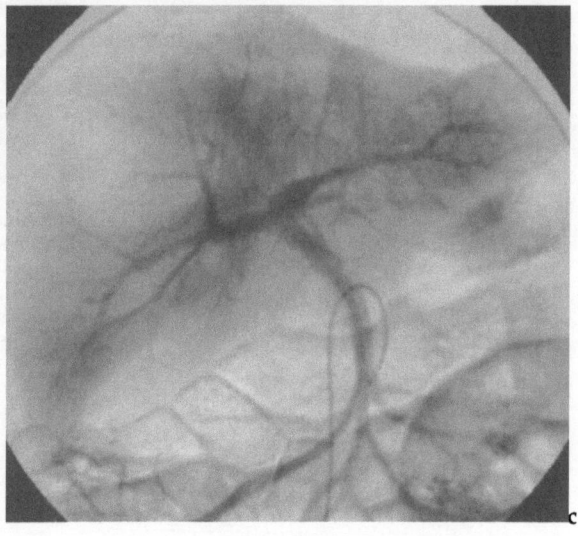

Fig. 4.38. Fortuitous discovery in a 2-year-old girl of a ▶ homogeneous solid hepatic mass. **a** Coeliac trunk injection: the tumour is supplied by an enlarged right branch of the hepatic artery. It is hypervascular with numerous dilated peripheral veins. The rest of the liver is hypoperfused. **b** The mass is well limited and there is rapid venous return in dilated right and right inferior hepatic veins (*arrowhead*). **c** The portography shows a defect corresponding to the mass. The portal branches are displaced. Liver biopsy confirmed the diagnosis. The mass was left in place and surgery is planned before puberty.

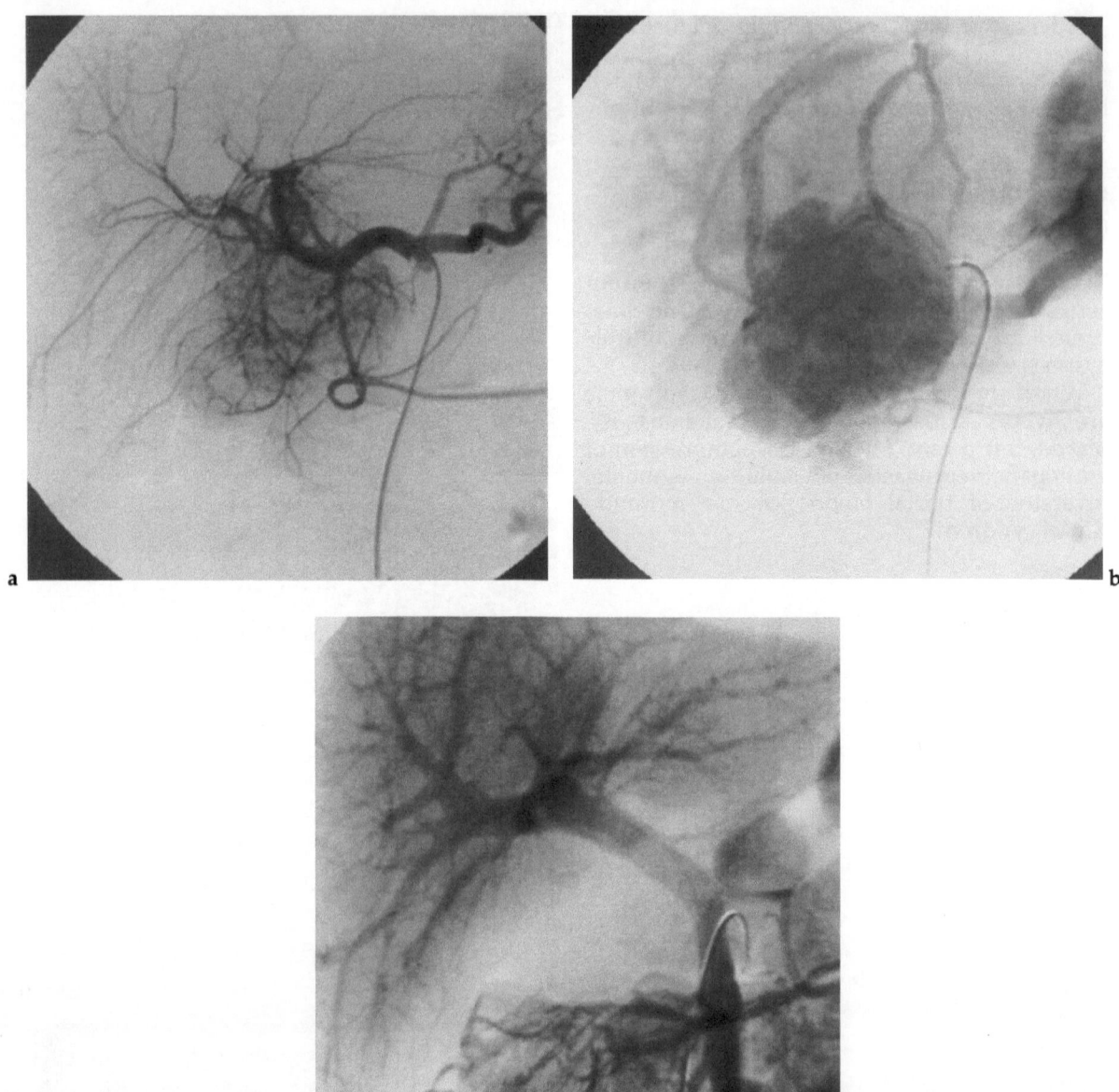

Fig. 4.39. A 7-year-old boy presenting with an asymptomatic abdominal mass. On ultrasound, CT and MRI, it was consistent with a focal nodular hyperplasia of segment IV, in spite of the sex of this patient. Preoperative work-up. **a** Coeliac trunk injection: early phase. The mass is hypervascular, supplied by a dilated arterial branch coming from the left branch of the hepatic artery. **b** Later phase. The mass is well limited, bilobulated. Enlarged peripheral veins are visible, rapidly draining (8 s) into dilated hepatic veins. **c** Portography: the portal branches are displaced by the tumour.

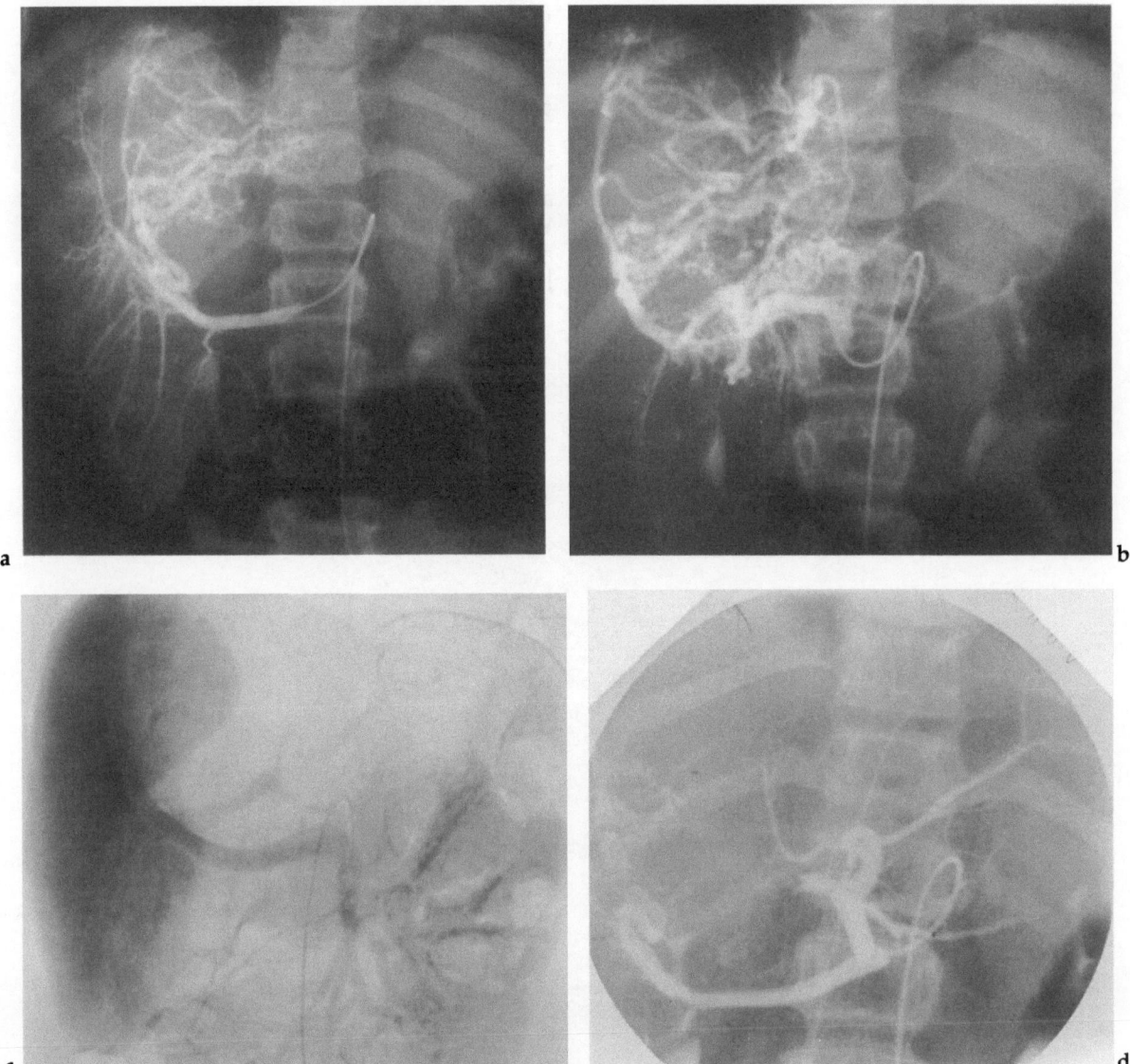

a   b   c   d

Fig. 4.40. A 3-year-old girl with abdominal pain. Liver tumour localised in segment 1 (Spiegel lobe). **a, b** The tumour is hypervascular, supplied by a right hepatic artery (**a**) and a left hepatic artery (**b**). The arterial branches have a radiating pattern, from the periphery to the centre of the mass. **c** Venous phase of the superior mesenteric arteriogram. There is compression and displacement of the left portal branch, but no amputation. **d** Because of the hypervascularity and the location of the lesion, surgery was not undertaken. Embolisation was successfully performed and massive calcification appeared later on. The patient was finally operated at 20 years of age.

Others

Hydatid Cysts

Invasive radiology is rarely necessary preoperatively. If angiography is performed the masses are seen to be hypovascular. Alveolar ecchinococcosis (Fig. 4.41), on the other hand, may invade the lumen of the bile ducts and vascular structures despite the medical treatment. Portal

vein thrombosis, intra-arterial nodules and vascular incasement can be seen (one case).

Hepatic Abscesses

Seven cases of hepatic abscess were seen on angiography before the advent of ultrasound. When angiography is performed, the wall of the abscess is hypervascular. In one case, the abscess had a pseudotumoral aspect. On the other hand

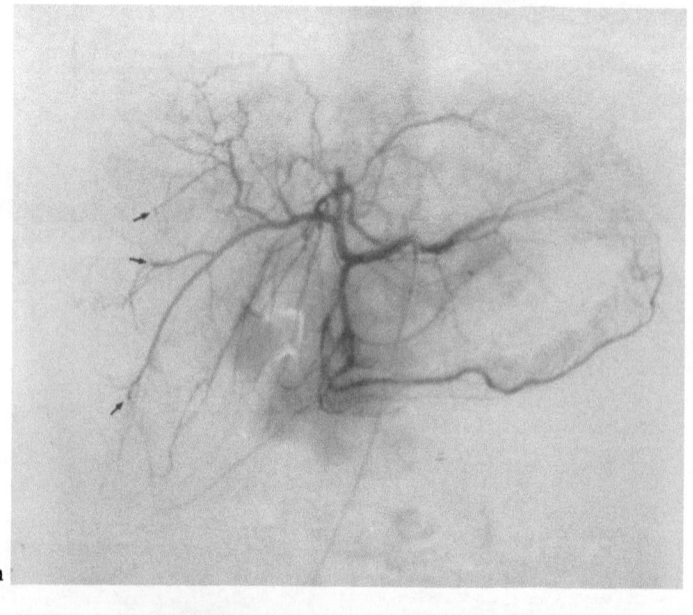

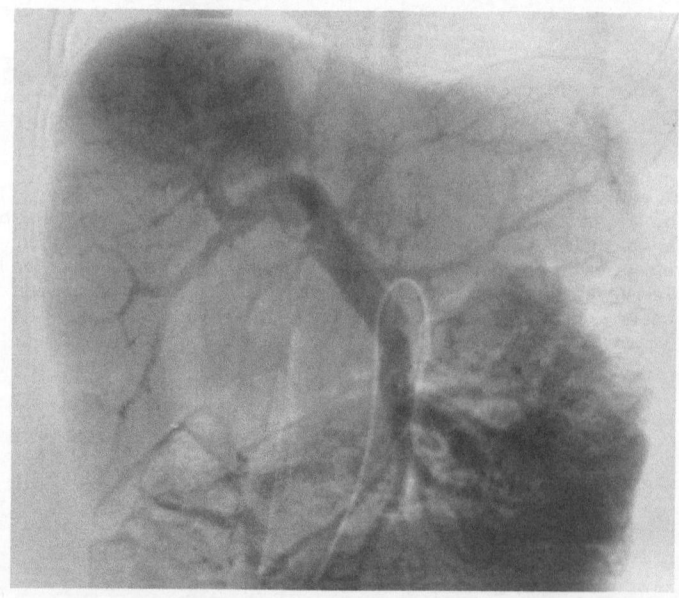

Fig. 4.41.   Alveolar ecchinococcosis. **a** Hepatic artery injection. Multiple distal arterial obstruction and stenosis (*arrows*). **b** Portal phase of superior mesenteric artery injection. The portal branch of segment V is missing. Multiple hypovascularised foci.

one malignant necrotic hepatic tumour presented clinically and on ultrasound as an hepatic abscess.

Bibliography

General

Boechat I, Kangarloo H, Gilsanz V (1988) Hepatic masses in children. Semin Roentgenol 23: 185–193

Boechat I, Kangarloo H, Ortega J et al. (1988) Primary liver tumors in children: comparison of CT and MRI. Radiology 169: 727–732

Jabra AA, Fishman EK, Taylor GA (1992) Hepatic masses in infants and children: CT evaluation. AJR 158: 143–149

Taylor GA, Perlman EJ, Scherer LR et al. (1991) Vascularity of tumors in children: evaluation with color doppler imaging. AJR 157: 1267–1271

Tonkin ILD, Wrenn EL, Hollabaugh RS (1988) The continued value of angiography in planning surgical resection of benign and malignant hepatic tumors in children. Pediatr Radiol 18: 35–44

Angiomas

Burrows PE (1991) Variations in the vascular supply to infantile hepatic hemangioendotheliomas. Radiology 181: 631–632

Burrows PE, Mulliken JB, Fellows KE, Strand RD (1983) Childhood hemangiomas and vascular malformations: angiographic differentiation. AJR 141: 483–488

Dachman AH, Lichtenstein JE, Friedman AC, Hartman DS (1983) Infantile hemangioendothelioma of the liver: a radiologic – pathologic – clinical correlation. AJR 140: 1091–1096

Fellows KE, Hoffer FA, Markowitz RI, O'Neill JA (1991) Multiple collaterals to hepatic infantile hemangioendotheliomas and arteriovenous malformations: effect on embolization. Radiology 181: 813–818

Kirchner SG, Heller RM, Kasselberg AG, Greene HL (1981) Infantile hepatic hemangioendothelioma with subsequent malignant degeneration. Pediatr Radiol 11: 42–45

Mazoit JX, Brunelle F, Danel P, De Victor D (1985) Therapeutic embolization of hemangiomas and hemangio-endotheliomas of the liver in infants: a hemodynamic study. Ann Radiol 28: 283–288

Stanley P, Geer GD, Miller JH et al. (1989) Infantile hepatic hemangiomas. Cancer 64: 936–949

Malignant Tumours

Brunelle F, Garel L, Harry G, Chaumont P (1979) L'angiographie portale des tumeurs hépatiques de l'enfant. Ann Radiol 22: 142–149

Dachamn A, Pakter RL, Ros PR et al. (1987) Hepatoblastoma: radiologic–pathologic correlation in 50 cases. Radiology 164: 15–19

Furin S, Itai Y, Ohtomo K et al. (1989) Hepatic epitheloïd hemangioendothelioma: report of five cases. Radiology 171: 63–68

Ros PR, Olmsted WW, Dachman AH et al. (1986) Undifferentiated (embryonal) sarcoma of the liver: radiologic and pathologic correlations. Radiology 161: 141–145

Ruyman FB, Raney RB, Crist WM et al. (1985) Rhabdomyosarcoma of the biliary tree in childhood: a report from the intergroup rhabdomyosarcoma study. Cancer 56: 575–580

Verstanding A, Bar-ziv J, Abu-Dalu KI, Granot E, Schiller M, (1991) Sarcoma botryoides of the common bile duct: preoperative diagnosis by coronal CT and PTC. Pediatr Radiol 21: 152–153

Benign Tumours

Bourliere-Najean B, Panuel M, Guys JM et al. (1989) Spontaneous liver adenoma in a child. Pediatr Radiol 20: 95

Brunelle F, Tammam S, Odièvre M, Chaumont P (1984) Liver adenomas in glycogen storage disease in children. Pediatr Radiol 14: 94–101

Didier D, Weiler S, Rohmer P et al. (1985) Hepatic alveolar echinococcosis: correlative US and CT study. Radiology 154: 179–186

Garel L, Kalifa G, Buriot D, Sauvegrain J (1981) Multiple adenomas of the liver and Franconi's anaemia. Ann Radiol 24: 53–54

Ros PR, Goodman ZD, Ishak KG et al. (1986) Mesenchymal hamartoma of the liver: radiologic–pathologic correlation. Radiology 158: 619–624

Sawhney S, Jain R, Safaya R, Berry M (1992) Pedunculated focal nodular hyperplasia. Pediatr Radiol 22: 231–232

Stocker JT, Shak DG (1981) Focal nodular hyperplasia of the liver: a study of 21 pediatric cases. Cancer 48: 336–345

5 Bile Ducts

Biliary Atresia

Definition

This is a congenital anomaly consisting of interruption of the extrahepatic bile ducts. It is the single most common cause of neonatal cholestasis and accounts for approximately half the cases in our series. The atresia may be complete (60% of cases) or partial with preservation of the gallbladder and, in some cases, of the common bile duct. The intrahepatic bile ducts have been shown to be always abnormal with a plexiform and moniliform appearance on cholangiography. The aetiology is still unknown.

Diagnosis

In most of the cases the diagnosis is evident, because the faeces are always white and the liver feels hard.

Ultrasonography shows no dilatation of the bile ducts. It may also fail to show a gallbladder, but this is not a completely reliable finding, as it may be found in other types of intrahepatic cholestasis. Moreover a large gallbladder may be present in some cases. In 5%–10% of cases, ultrasonography demonstrates the presence of a biliary cyst at the porta hepatis, at the remnant of the common bile duct. The size of the cyst varies from 0.5 to 3–4 cm. In 10% of cases, ultrasonography is diagnostic of biliary atresia by showing one or several anomalies of the so-called non-cardiac polysplenia syndrome (cf. Chapter 3).

Isotope studies may be used and many radionuclides have been employed. However, false results are frequent. Percutaneous liver biopsy may help the diagnosis.

Surgery has to be performed as soon as possible, preferably before 40 days of age, to provide the best chance of clearing the jaundice, and achieving survival with a good quality of life as well as delaying the definitive treatment which is liver transplantation. The surgical procedure (Kasai procedure) consists of a hepatoportoenterostomy or a hepatoportocholecystostomy when the gallbladder and the choledochus are patent.

Cholangiography

Preoperative Cholangiography (four cases)
(Figs. 5.1–5.3)

This is only rarely performed. In the cystic forms, when ultrasound and the clinical presentation are not conclusive, it may help to diagnose or to exclude a choledochal cyst. The intrahepatic ducts may be opacified above the cyst showing a typical moniliform pattern. The cyst may communicate with the gallbladder but the extrahepatic bile duct is never opacified on its entire length by definition.

When the gallbladder is large enough and the diagnosis uncertain, bile duct percutaneous cholecystography can be performed. In biliary atresia the bile is uncoloured and there may be opacification of the choledochus and the duodenum, but there is absence of opacification of the common hepatic duct and the intrahepatic ducts.

Differential diagnoses such as sclerosing cholangitis or ductular hypoplasia can also be made by this technique.

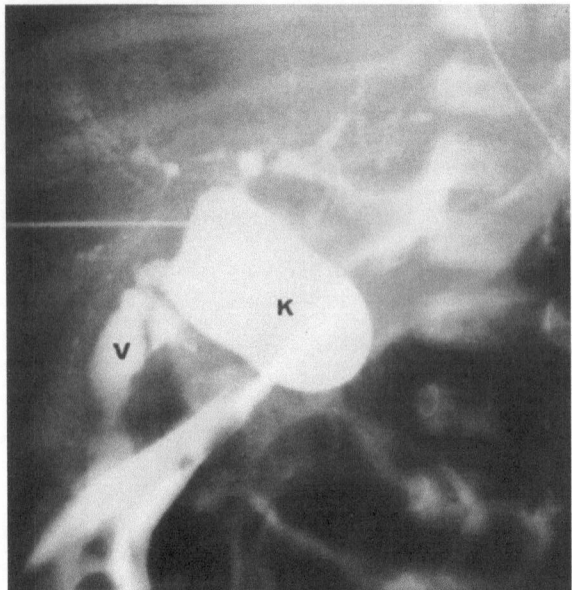

Fig. 5.1. Biliary atresia with hilar cyst. Preoperative biliary opacification (3 weeks of age). The cyst (K) is punctured and communicates with a small gall-bladder (V) and intrahepatic neocanalicules. No communication with the distal common bile duct seen.

Fig. 5.3. Biliary atresia. Preoperative biliary opacification. The gallbladder (V) communicates with a cyst (K) and with small biliary canalicules.

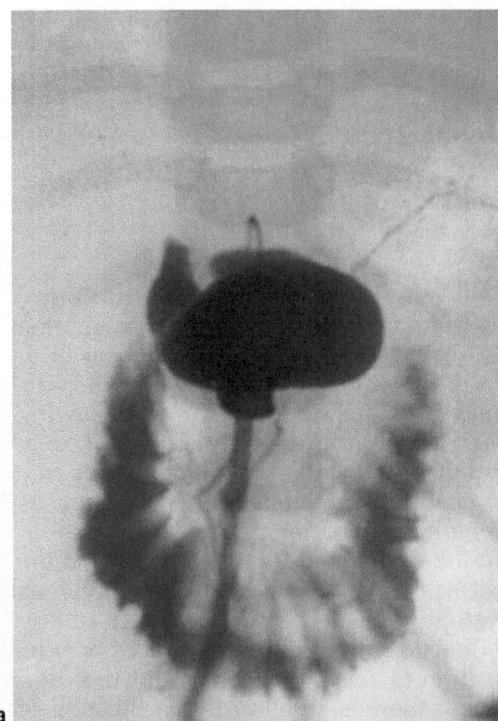

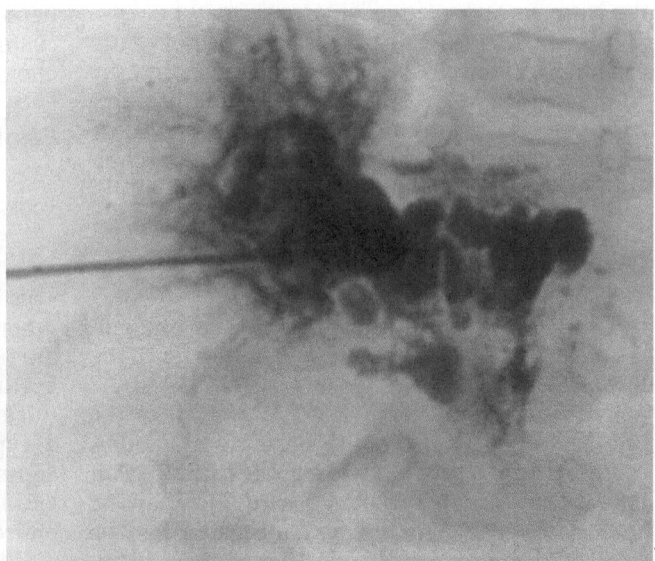

Fig. 5.2. Biliary atresia; 4.5 months of age. **a** Percutaneous opacification of the gallbladder. The gallbladder and the common bile duct are patent, there is a reflux in the Wirsung duct. There is opacification of the intrahepatic bile ducts. **b** PTC. Multiple cysts are seen with neocanalicules and no opacification of the extrahepatic bile duct.

Postoperative Cholangiography (97 cases)
(Figs. 5.4–5.14)

Performed systematically early in our experience, cholangiography is nowadays only indicated when there is suspicion of bilio-digestive anastomosis obstruction or stenosis or to drain large necrotic cavities in cases of persistent cholangitis.

Technique (Table 5.1). As the bile ducts are usually not dilated in biliary atresia, the technique for bile-duct opacification is special.

Under general anaesthesia, the liver is punctured at the mid-axillary line with a Chiba needle. A connecting tube is fixed to the hub of the needle and small amounts of contrast medium injected while the needle is slowly withdrawn. Films are taken when the bile ducts are opacified: they slowly drain towards the hepatic hilum with a roughly segmental distribution. They may present segmental stenoses and dilatations. The lymphatics are often opacified: they have a moniliform appearance and drain rapidly towards the hepatic hilum. Lymph nodes and thoracic duct may also be opacified. Another drainage pathway is along the surface

Table 5.1. Cholangiographic appearance of lymphatics versus bile ducts

Lymphatics	Bile ducts
Regular	Irregular
Valvulae	Stenosis
Rapidly clear	Segmental dilatations
Lymph nodes	Collaterals
Thoracic duct	Slowly clear
	Digestive anastomosis opacified

of the liver toward the mediastinum. The hepatic artery, as well as the portal or hepatic vein branches, can be punctured: they are easily recognised when opacified.

Findings. The typical appearance is similar to sclerosing cholangitis with an association of stenoses, collaterals and segmental dilatations (Fig 5.15). Opacification of the bile ducts was successful in a third of the postoperative cases. In six cases, they were frankly dilated. In two cases, there was associated intrahepatic lithiasis.

Percutaneous drainage was performed in some cases because of persistent cholangitis. It brought about significant clinical improvement.

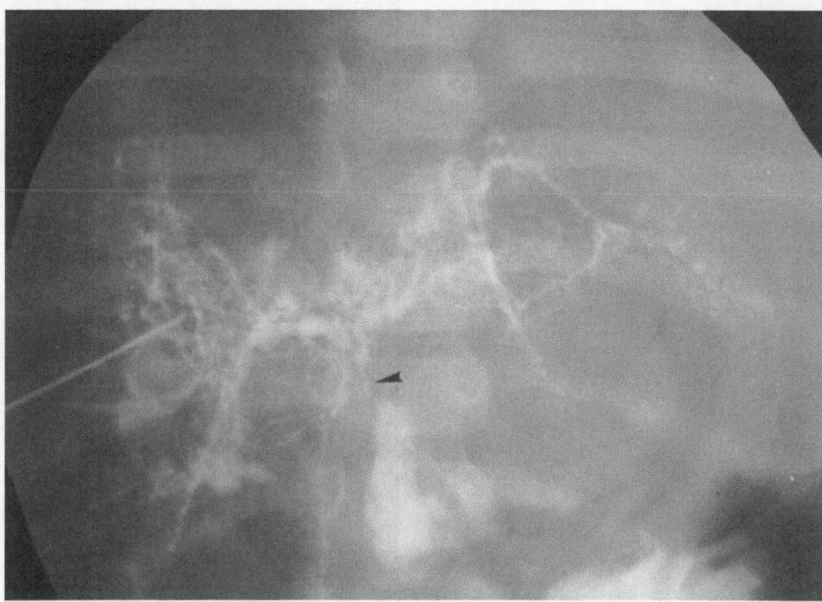

Fig. 5.4. Biliary atresia, hepato-porto-enterostomy, postoperative PTC; 22 months of age. The Chiba needle opacifies multiple neocanalicules in the liver. They communicate with the jejunal loop through a narrow canal (*arrowhead*).

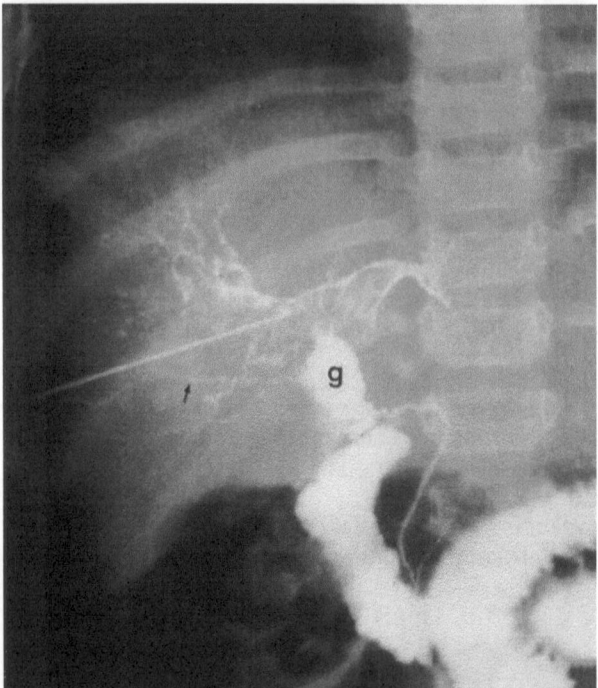

Fig. 5.5. Biliary atresia, postoperative PTC at 14 months of age. A first puncture (*arrow*) opacified the gallbladder (g). A second puncture opacifies the intrahepatic biliary neocanalicules. They drain into the gallbladder. The common bile duct is opacified. There is a small reflux in the pancreatic duct. Stereoangiographic films show that the neocanalicules are situated in the portal spaces.

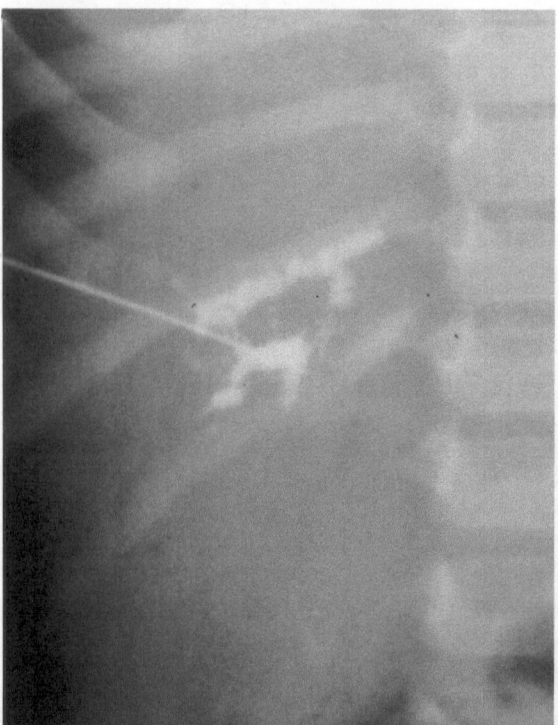

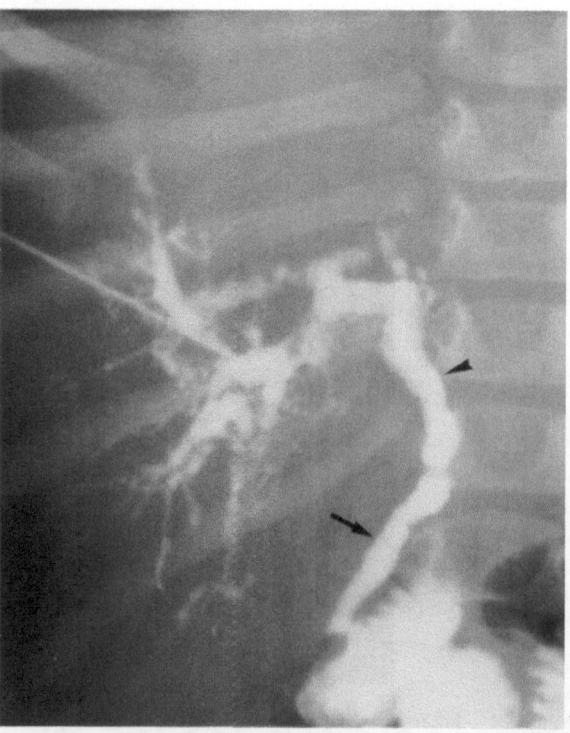

a   b

Fig. 5.6. Biliary atresia. The gallbladder was patent. The common bile duct was atretic with patency of the hepatic duct. Surgery consisted of anastomosis between the common hepatic duct (*arrowhead*) and a jejunal loop through the gallbladder (*arrow*). PTC at 17 months of age, (**a, b**). Multiple irregular dilated intrahepatic bile ducts are seen draining through the gallbladder into the jejunal loop. Stereography shows that it persists dilated segments of bile ducts connected to each other by multiple neoductules in the portal space. *Continued opposite.*

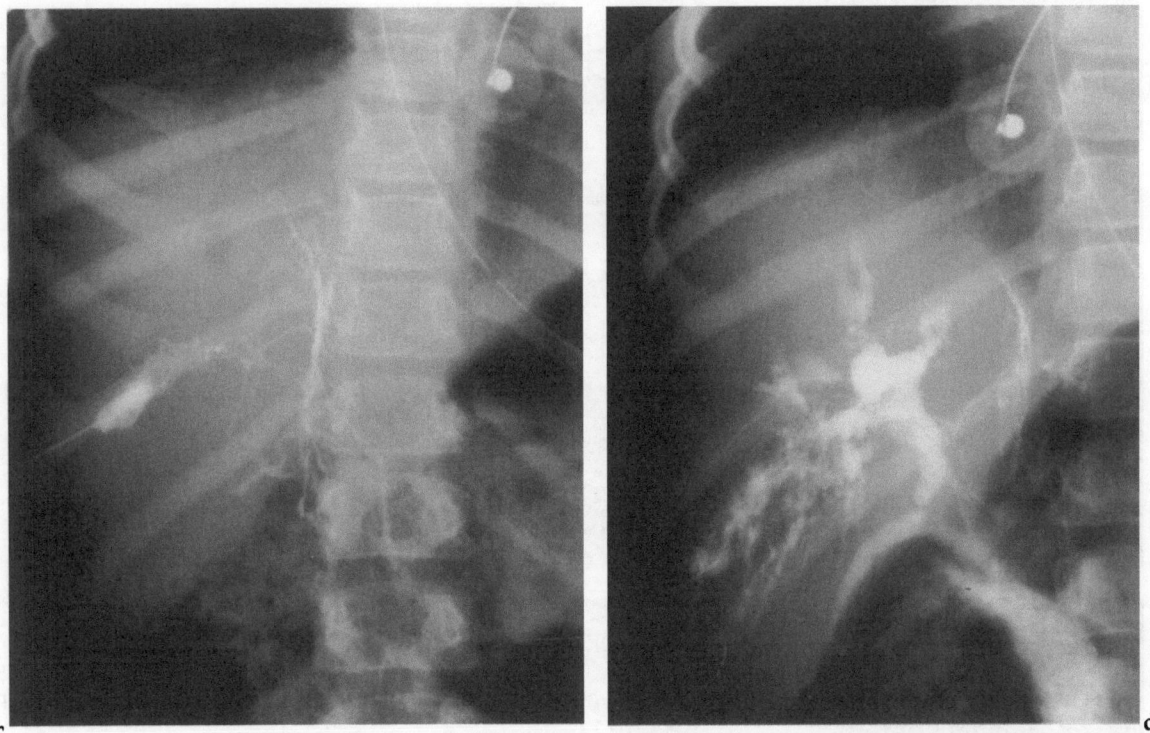

c   d

Fig. 5.6. Biliary atresia. The gallbladder was patent. The common bile duct was atretic with patency of the hepatic duct.
Surgery consisted of anastomosis between the common hepatic duct (*arrowhead*) and a jejunal loop through the gallbladder
(*arrow*). PTC at 17 months of age (*continued*) **c** Same patient at 5 years of age. The PTC opacifies multiple lymphatics that
drain into the hilum of the liver, parallel to the common hepatic duct. They differ from bile ducts which are more irregular. **d**
Opacification of the intrahepatic bile duct is similar to **b** at 17 months of age.

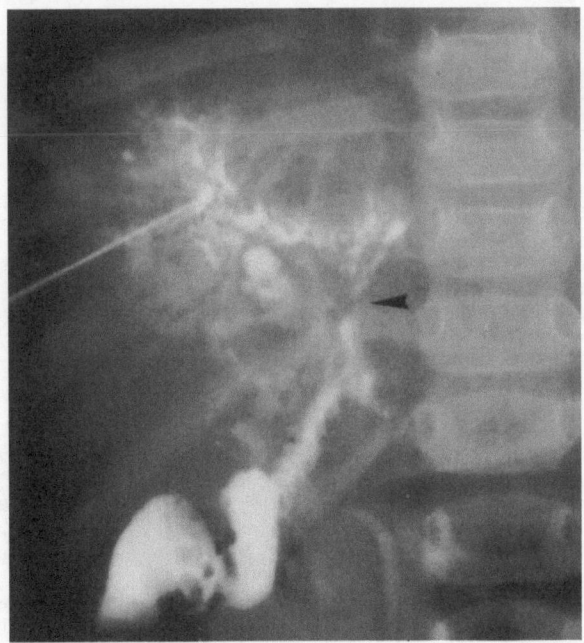

Fig. 5.7. Biliary atresia. Hepato-porto-enterostomy. PTC at 22 months. Multiple intrahepatic canalicules are seen opacifying
the enterostomy (*arrowhead*).

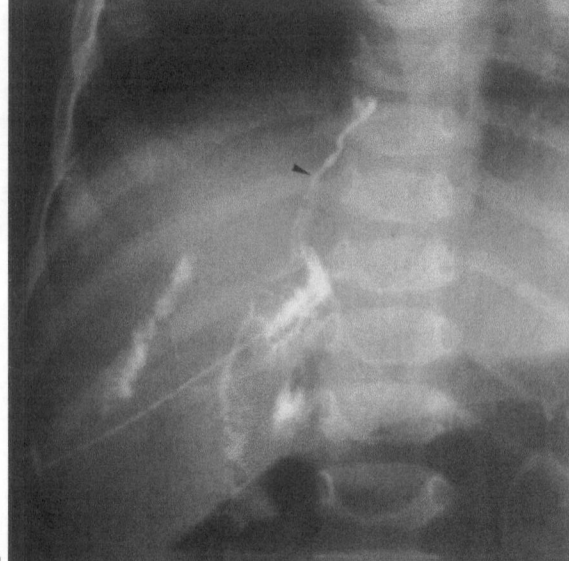

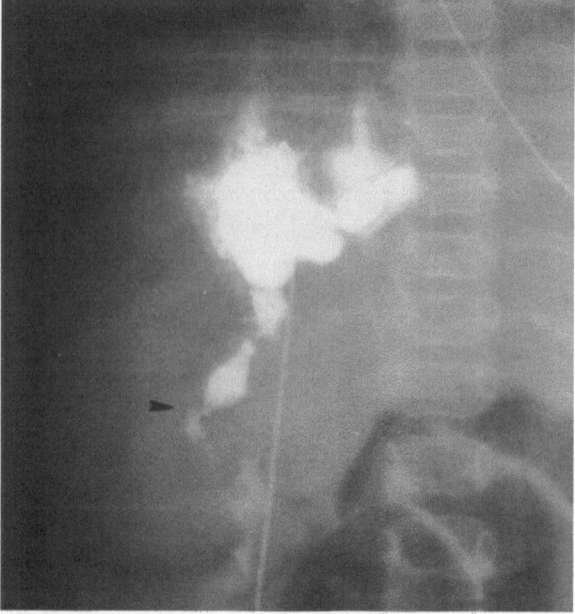

Fig. 5.9. Biliary atresia. Hepato-enterostomy. PTC at 9 months of age. A large cyst draining into the jejunal loop (*arrowhead*). Another segmental dilatation is seen in the left lobe of the liver.

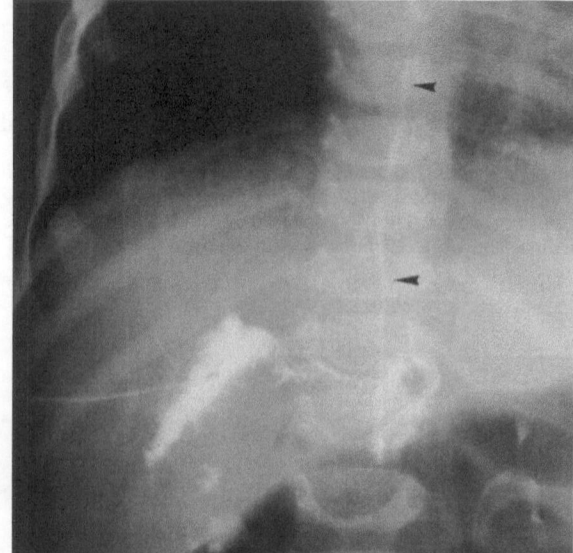

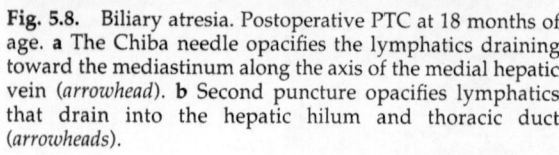

Fig. 5.8. Biliary atresia. Postoperative PTC at 18 months of age. **a** The Chiba needle opacifies the lymphatics draining toward the mediastinum along the axis of the medial hepatic vein (*arrowhead*). **b** Second puncture opacifies lymphatics that drain into the hepatic hilum and thoracic duct (*arrowheads*).

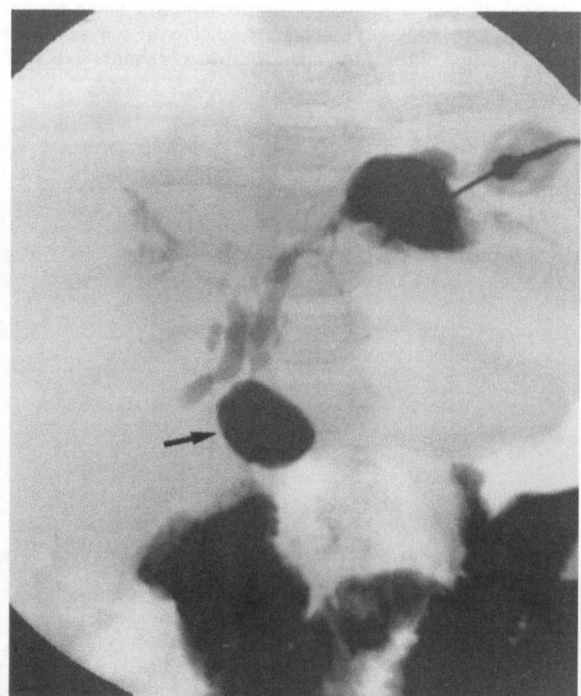

Fig. 5.10. Biliary atresia with hilar cyst diagnosed as choledochal cyst. A cystojejunostomy has been performed. Portal hypertension and biliary cirrhosis. Ultrasound shows biliary cyst. At 1 year of age PTC. The left intrahepatic cyst communicates with abnormal bile ducts and the hilar cyst (*arrow*) and the jejunostomy. Typical aspect of biliary atresia.

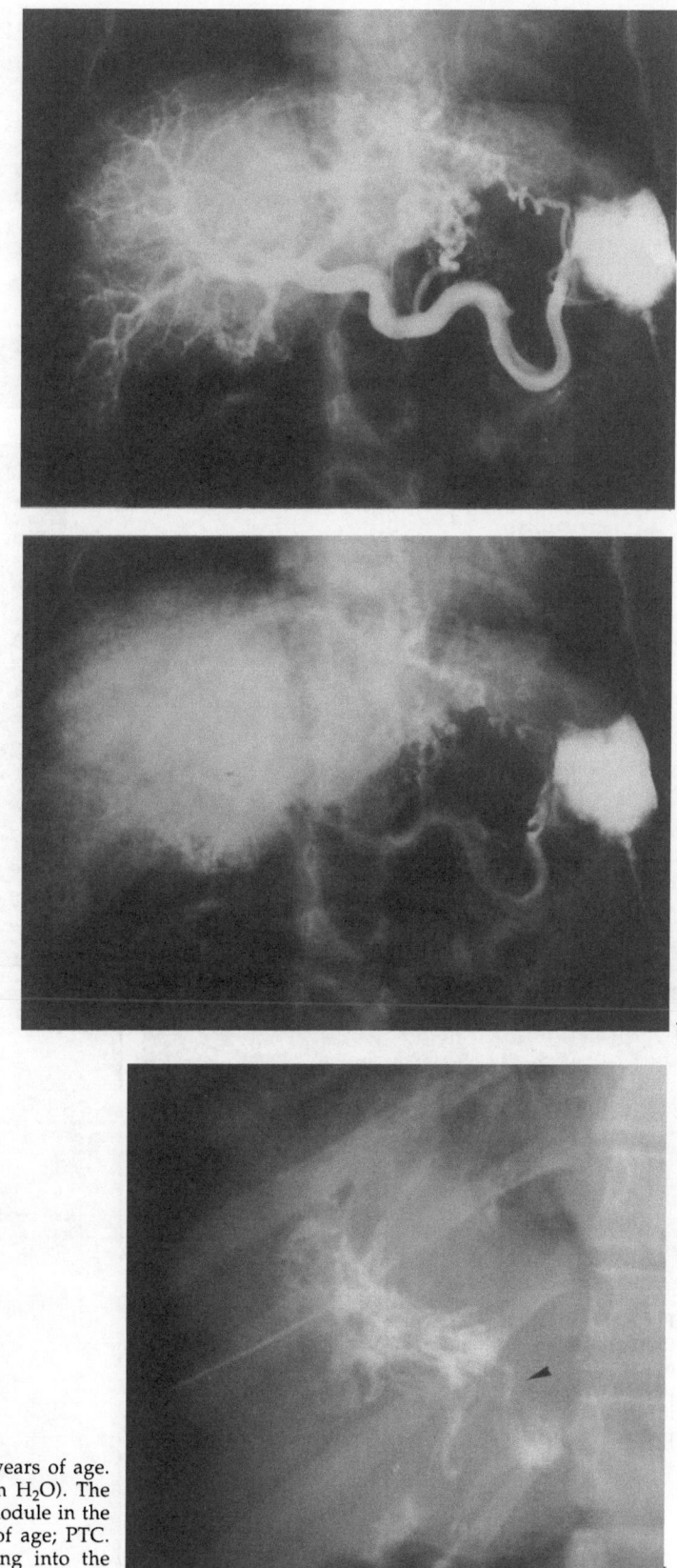

Fig. 5.11. Biliary atresia, biliary cirrhosis; 4 years of age.
a, b Splenoportogram (splenic pressure 39 cm H$_2$O). The
liver is nodular. There is large hypervascular nodule in the
middle of the liver. **c** Same patient; 5 years of age; PTC.
Multiple abnormal biliary canalicules draining into the
jejunostomy (*arrowhead*).

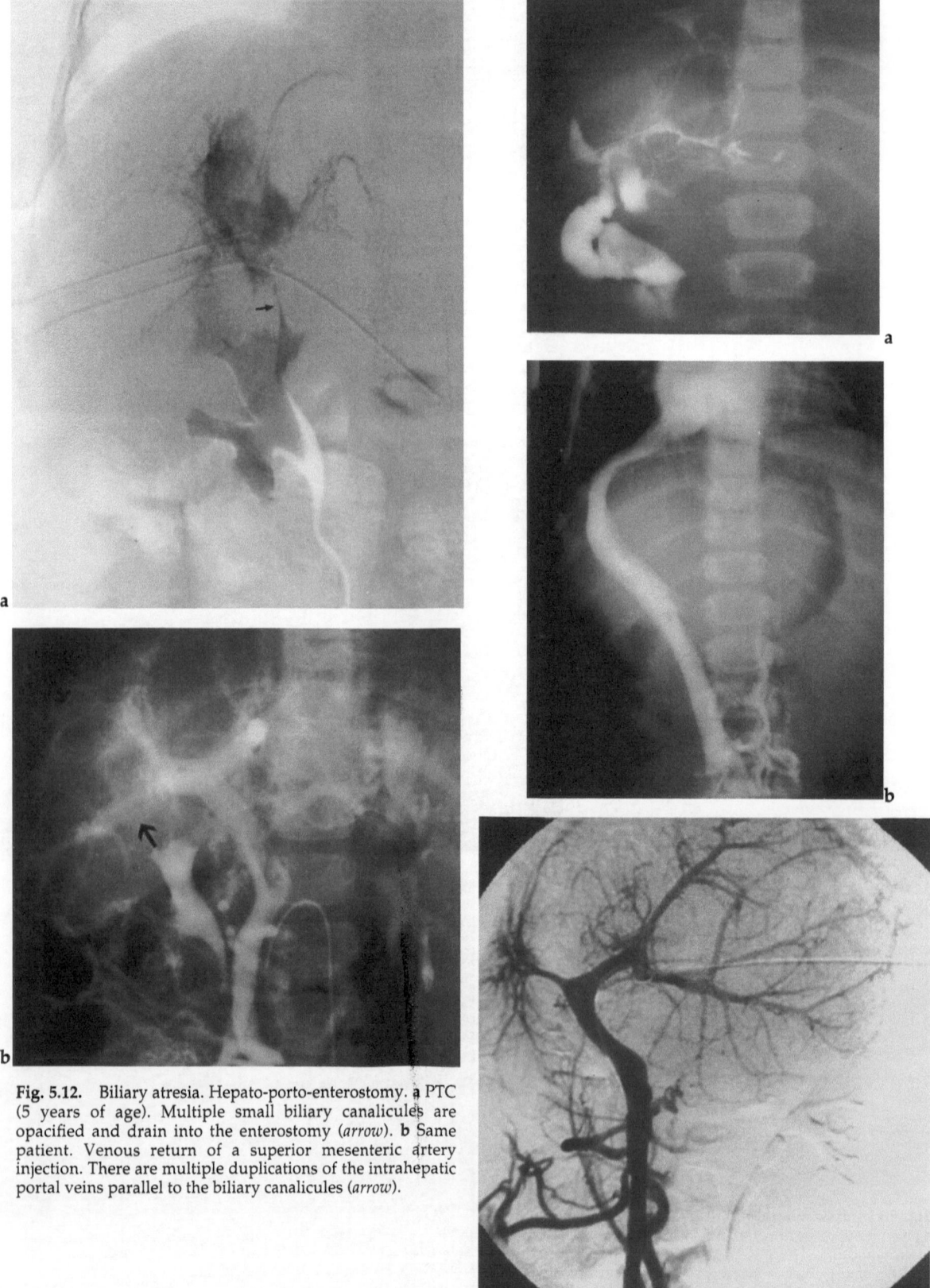

Fig. 5.12. Biliary atresia. Hepato-porto-enterostomy. **a** PTC (5 years of age). Multiple small biliary canalicules are opacified and drain into the enterostomy (*arrow*). **b** Same patient. Venous return of a superior mesenteric artery injection. There are multiple duplications of the intrahepatic portal veins parallel to the biliary canalicules (*arrow*).

Fig. 5.13

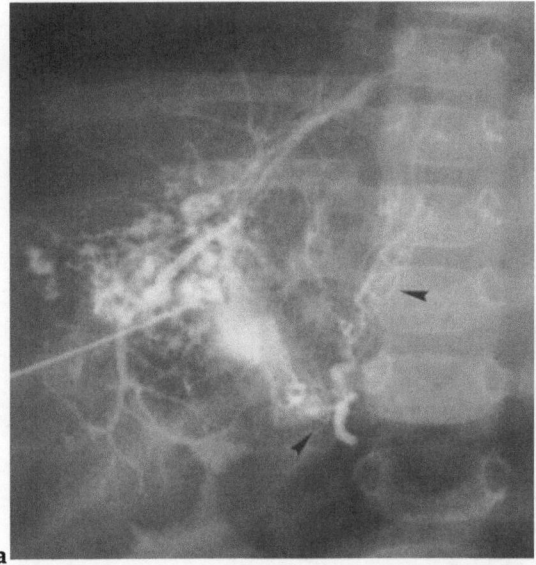
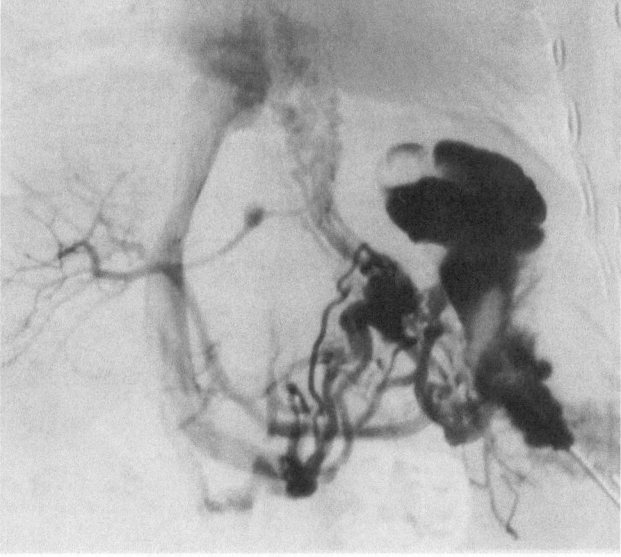

a
b

Fig. 5.14. Biliary atresia. Postoperative PTC; 4 years of age. **a** Simultaneous opacification of portal vein branches, hepatic vein and lymphatics. The hepatic vein drains towards the right atrium, the lymphatics are draining towards the hepatic hilum (*arrowhead*). **b** Same patient. Splenoportography (splenic pressure 31 cm H_2O). The splenic vein, the portal trunk and the intrahepatic portal vein branches are small. There is opacification of the renal vein through posterior gastric and adrenal vein. The inferior vena cava is opacified.

Sclerosing Cholangitis (47 cases)

Definition

This is a rare disease in children characterised by an inflammatory obliterative fibrosis affecting the intra- and extrahepatic biliary tree.

The pathogenesis remains unknown but the disease has been encountered in association mainly with chronic inflammatory bowel disease, histiocytosis X and immunodeficiency disorders.

The clinical findings, liver function tests and histological changes are often non-specific, and, as in adults, the diagnosis is based on cholangiographic features.

The prognosis is poor with progressive evolution to biliary cirrhosis. Liver transplantation has been performed in six out of our patients without recurrence with a maximal follow-up of 5 years.

Cholangiography (Figs. 5.15–5.21)

We have used percutaneous cholecystography (32) or cholangiography (6), endoscopic retrograde cholangiography (2) and preoperative cholangiography (7). In all cases the cholangiographic features included several strictures with intervening dilatations of bile ducts.

The intrahepatic bile ducts were always abnormal, whereas the extrahepatic bile ducts were abnormal in 65% of cases. Different patterns were found depending on the associated disease.

Histiocytosis X (13 cases)

Sclerosing cholangitis was the presenting sign of the disease in three cases. Findings include stenosis of the hepatic ducts junction, frequent lithiasis and rare involvement of the extrahepatic bile duct. The prognosis is poor; 60% of our patients died.

Fig. 5.13. Biliary atresia. Kasaïa procedure at 3 months of age. **a** PTC. Multiple abnormal biliary canalicules are seen draining into the enterostomy. **b** Inferior vena cava opacification. There is a massive distortion of the inferior vena cava due to right lobe atrophy. **c** Percutaneous transhepatic portography. The right lobe of the liver is atrophic. Note the hypertrophy of the left lobe. Portal pressure 41 cm H_2O.

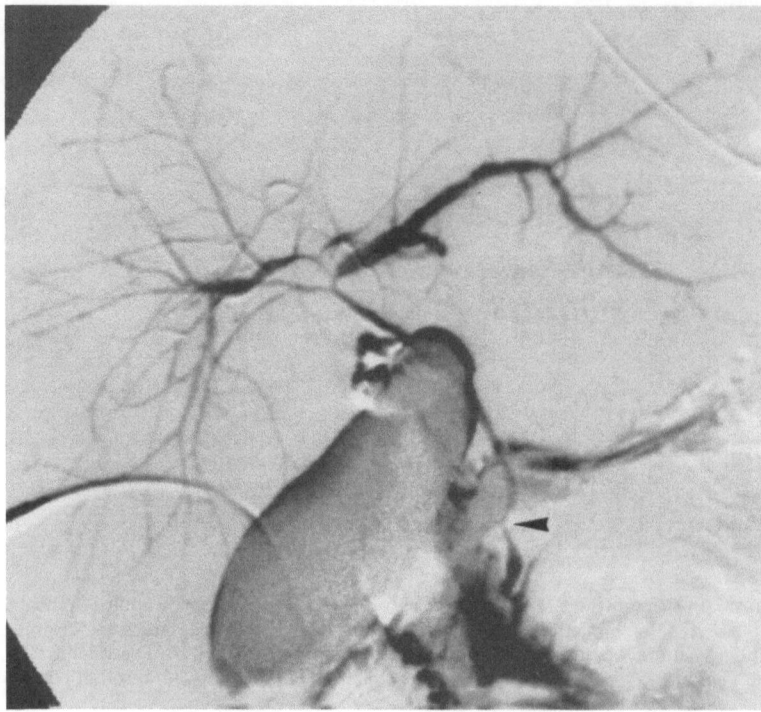

Fig. 5.15. Onset of jaundice at 4 months of age. Percutaneous cholecystography at 14 months of age. There are multiple stenoses in the region of the hepatic hilum and there is also stenosis of the choledochus (*arrowhead*).

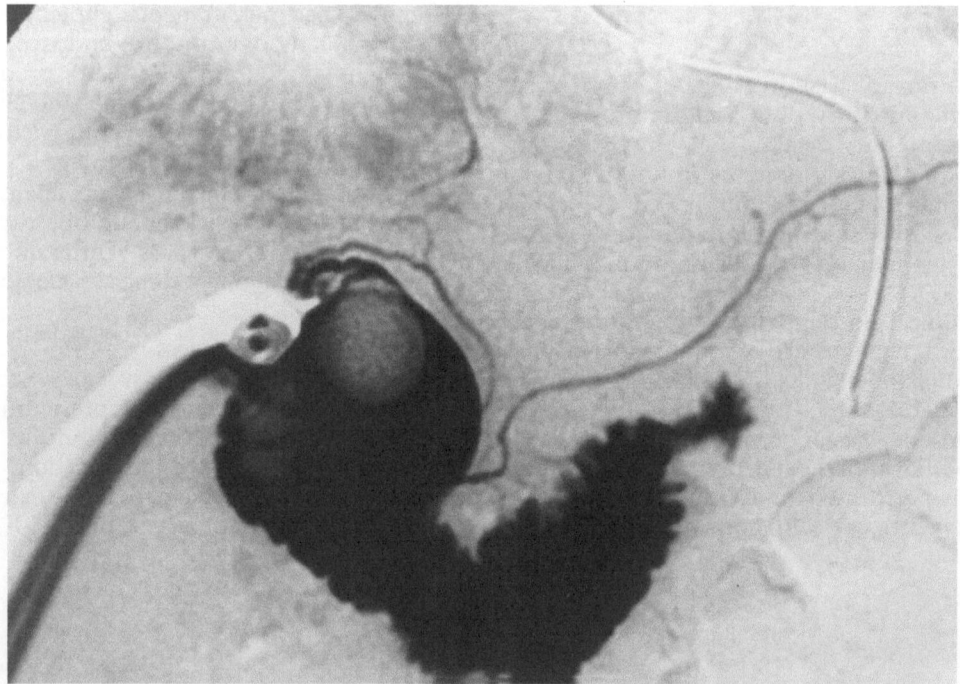

Fig. 5.16. Neonatal sclerosing cholangitis. Percutaneous cholecystography at 2 years of age. The cystic duct and the common bile duct are normal. There is a reflux in the Wirsung duct. There is opacification of very abnormal intrahepatic bile ducts, with irregularities of calibre and network of neoductules. This intrahepatic pattern is very close to that found in biliary atresia.

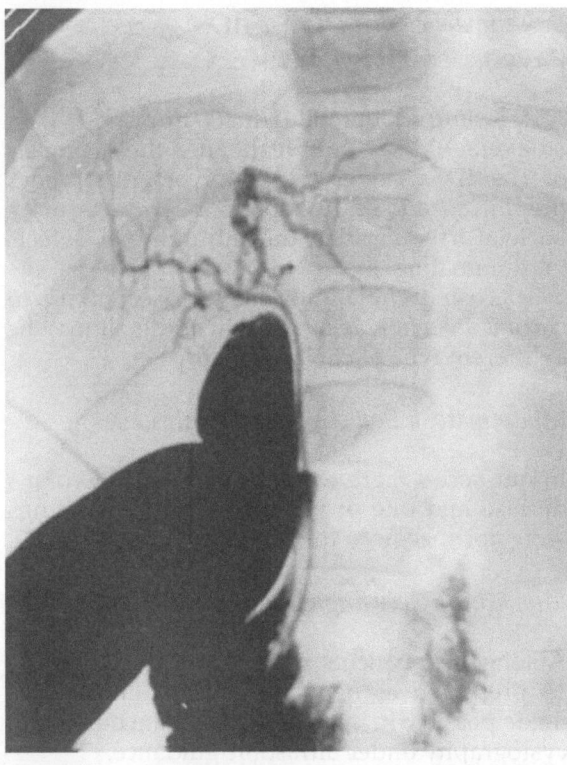

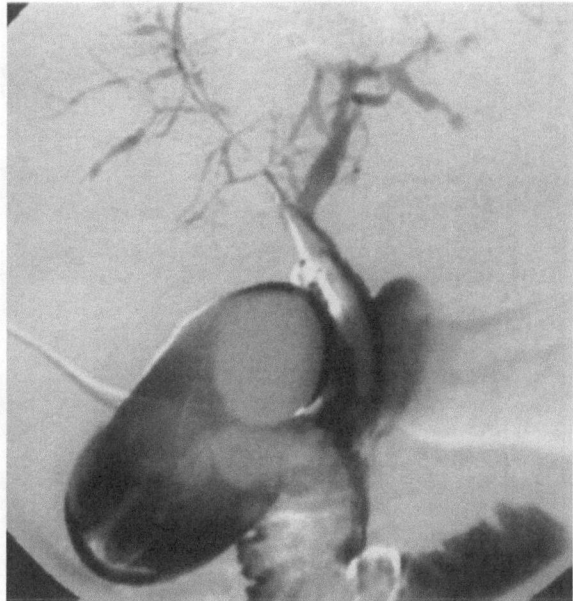

Fig. 5.19. Idiopathic sclerosing cholangitis, 19 years of age. Percutaneous cholecystography. Multiple stenosis and segmental dilatations of the intrahepatic biliary ducts are seen.

Fig. 5.17. Idiopathic sclerosing cholangitis; 10 years of age. Percutaneous cholecystography. Multiple stenosis and irregularities of the intrahepatic bile ducts are seen. The common bile duct is very thin.

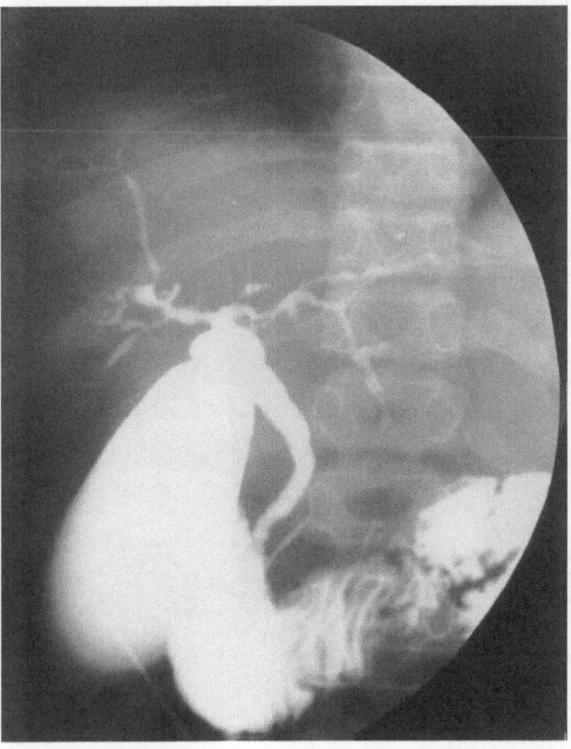

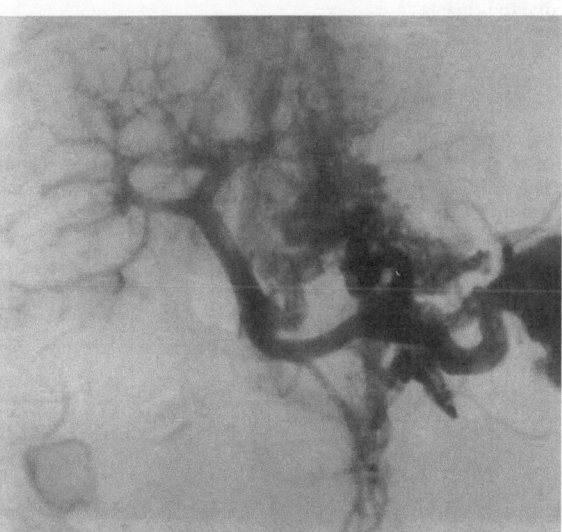

Fig. 5.20. Sclerosing cholangitis, portal hypertension. Splenoportography (splenic pressure 31 cm H$_2$O). There are multiple oeosophageal derivations. The intrahepatic portal branches are rare and some are duplicated.

◀ **Fig. 5.18.** Sclerosing cholangitis associated with Crohn's disease; 12 years of age. Percutaneous cholecystography. Multiple irregularities and stenosis of the intrahepatic bile ducts are seen. The common bile duct is dilated above a zone of irregularities.

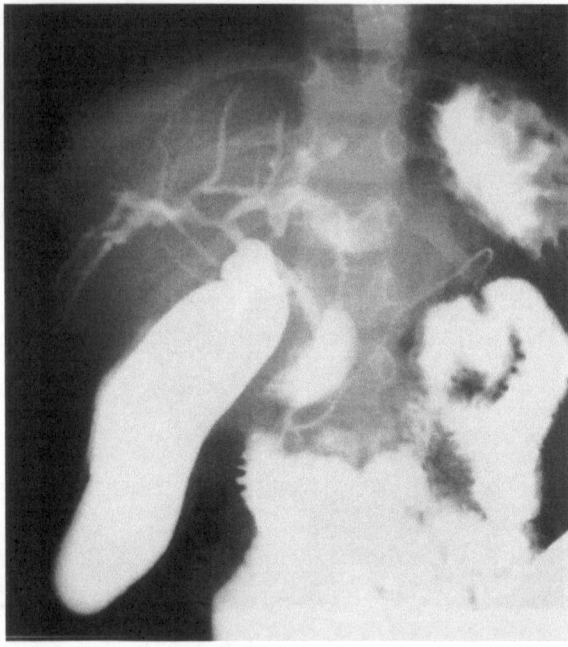

Fig. 5.21. Sclerosing cholangitis associated with histio-cytosis X; 3 years of age. Percutaneous cholecystography. Segmental stenosis and marked dilatations are seen in the intrahepatic bile ducts. There are also intraluminal defects due to lithiasis.

Fig. 5.22. Immunodeficiency syndrome (lack of expression of HLA); 20 months of age. Percutaneous cholecystography. The intrahepatic bile ducts are moderately dilated and irregular. The common bile duct is normal.

▼

Immunodeficiency Disease (IDS) (seven cases) (Figs. 5.22–5.24)

The lesion in the bile ducts appeared with an average delay of 5 years after the diagnosis of the IDS. There was involvement of both the intra- and extrahepatic bile ducts with parietal irregularities and intraluminal defects predominating.

Sclerosing cholangitis may be secondary to chronic infection as in AIDS in adults. It may be a different type of cholangiopathy.

Inflammatory Bowel Disease (four cases)

In our series there were three cases of Crohn's disease and one of ulcerative colitis. Findings were not specific in this small group.

Idiopathic Sclerosing Cholangitis (23 cases)

Among these patients, with no associated disease, 14 presented as neonates. The diagnosis was made possible in infancy by percutaneous chole-cystography under ultrasonic guidance.

These neonatal forms were characterised by the tiny and beaded appearance of the bile ducts, focal lack of opacification of peripheral bile ducts and frequent presence of an irregular network of neoductules. The appearance of the biliary tree was very similar to that observed in biliary atresia, except that the extrahepatic bile duct was always patent.

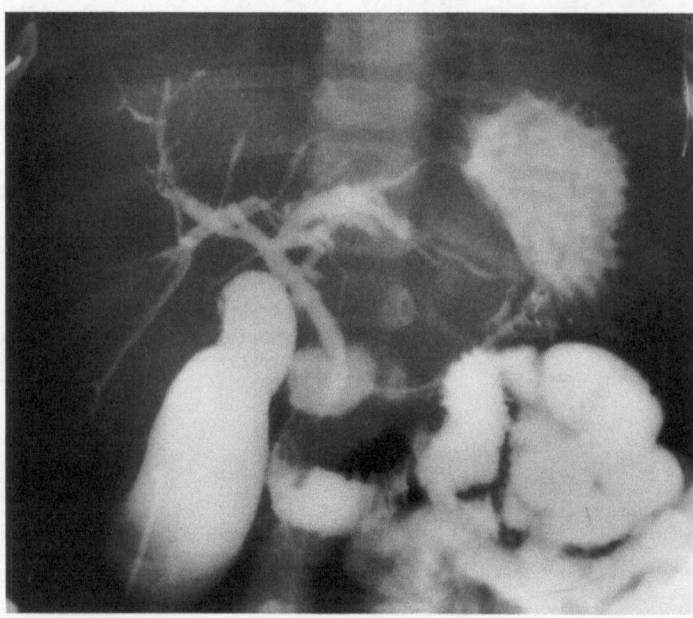

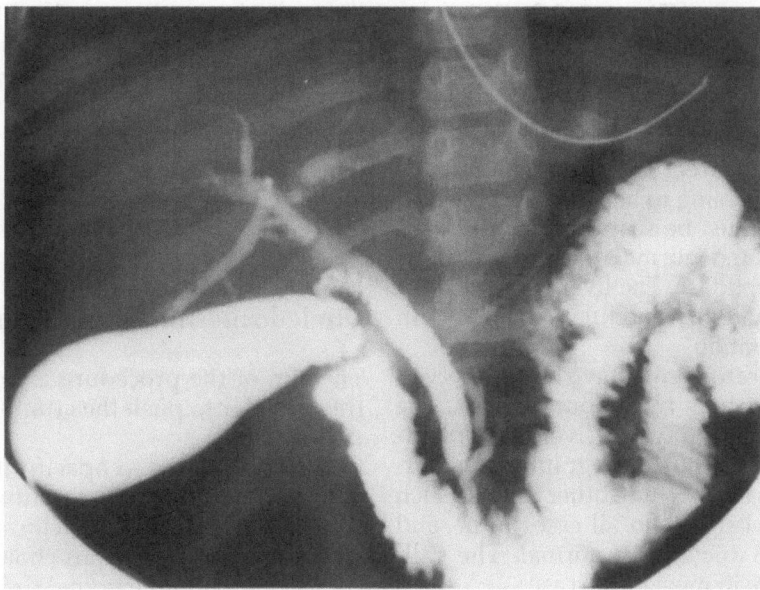

Fig. 5.23. Immunodeficiency syndrome (lack of expression of HLA); 6 years of age; hepatomegaly. Percutaneous cholecystography. The common bile duct is dilated with parietal irregularities. The intrahepatic bile ducts are irregular and slightly dilated.

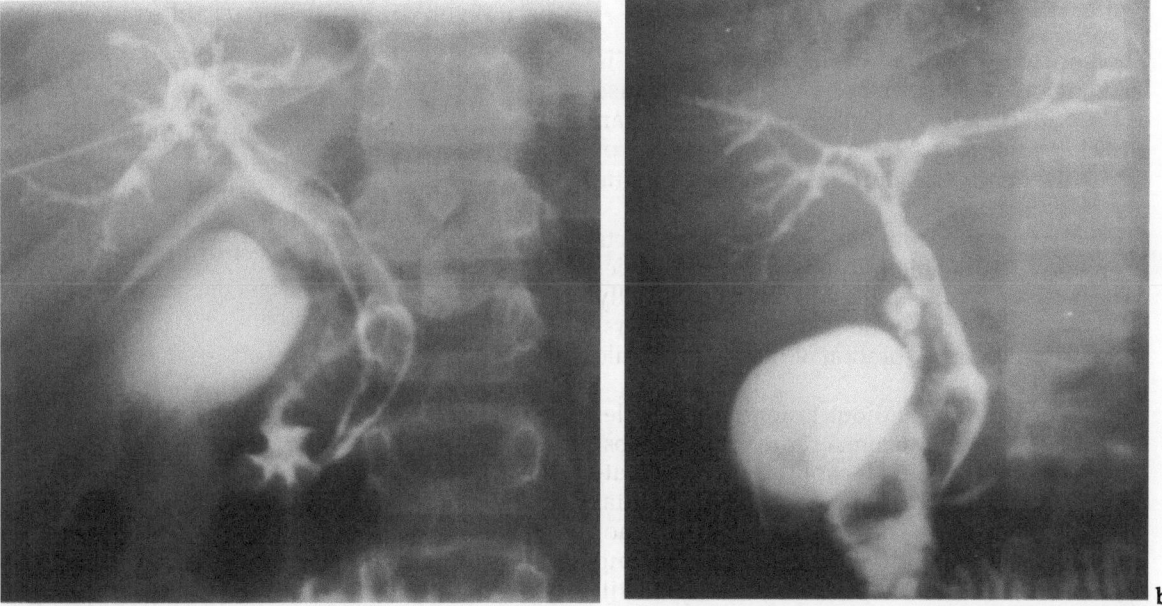

a   b

Fig. 5.24. Immunodeficiency syndrome. **a** 10 years of age, percutaneous transhepatic cholecystography. The intra- and extrahepatic bile ducts are dilated. The filling defect corresponds to a non-mixing thick bile. **b** 13 years of age; percutaneous transhepatic cholecystography. The intrahepatic bile ducts are narrowed and irregular. The common bile duct is moderately dilated. Thick bile is again seen.

Byler's Disease (Figs. 5.25–5.26)

Byler's disease, also known as familial progressive intrahepatic cholestasis, is an autosomal recessive disease, often presenting in infancy and rapidly progressing to hepatic insufficiency.

The diagnosis must be suspected in an infant with cholestasis and normal serum level of γ-glutamyl transpeptidase. The liver biopsy shows marked fibrosis and micronodular cirrhosis with nearly no regeneration.

Diffuse hepatocarcinomas have been observed before 2 years of age in two of our patients. The only treatment nowadays is liver transplantation. Percutaneous cholecystography was performed in 16 cases to exclude other disease such as sclerosing cholangitis. In all cases intra- and extrahepatic bile ducts were normal. The gallbladder was large in most of the cases.

Choledocholithiasis

Introduction

Choledocholithiasis is rare in children but it is being reported with increasing frequency because of the widespead use of ultrasonography. It can be either secondary to an anatomical anomaly of the choledochus (stricture or dilatation) or due to a bile disturbance.

In our series anomalies of the bile ducts associated with choledolithiasis include choledochal cysts, sclerosing cholangitis (especially histiocytosis X and immunodeficiency disorders) and spontaneous perforation of the common bile duct (three cases).

In older children without lesion of the choledochus, haemolytic anaemia represents the most common cause of choledocholithiasis. The treatment is surgical and may include partial or total splenectomy. In infants primary choledocholithiasis was first described as the "bile plug syndrome". The aetiology of this entity is still unclear but some causative factors have been described: prematurity, infection, dehydration, parenteral nutrition, furosemide treatment, gastrointestinal dysfunction. The disease is thought to be due to immaturity of the glucurono-conjugation.

In our institution 20 cases have been seen with an age range from 10 days to 11 months. Spontaneous elimination of the lithiasis has been documented on ultrasonography in three cases. However, cholangitis was present in four and hepatic abscess in one. Fifteen cases were successfully treated by radiological percutaneous treatment. This is the treatment of choice and surgery is only indicated in case of hepatic failure.

Radiological-interventional Treatment of Choledocholithiasis in Infants

The aim of the procedure is to flush the biliary tree in order to push the crumbly stones into the duodenum.

The first step is to opacify the biliary tree to confirm that there is no anatomical obstacle on the choledochus. This opacification can be easily obtained by percutaneous cholecystography.

Placement of an external drainage in the gallbladder and/or the common bile duct is recommended to allow washing of the biliary tree with contrast and saline and to check, the following day, that complete clearing of the lithiasis has been obtained (Figs. 5.27–5.31).

The use of intravenous glucagon or other spasmolytic drugs may be useful to reduce the spasm of the sphincter of Oddi.

Two of our cases have been cured by placement of a catheter in the gallbladder. In the other cases a drainage of the common bile duct was also used. In two cases the common bile duct was entered via the cystic duct.

Sampling of the bile for bacteriological analysis and antibiotic cover during the procedure are recommended.

Choledochal Cysts and Pancreatico Biliary Ducts Anomalies

Initially published in 1969 by Babbitt, the pathogenesis of the choledochal cysts is now well recognised. The abnormal junction of the choledochal duct and Wirsung's duct before the sphincter of Oddi allows mixing of the two secretions and activation of pancreatic enzymes in the bile duct. The dilatation of the common bile duct is a result of this chronic chemical injury and is associated with dysplastic changes of the bile duct wall.

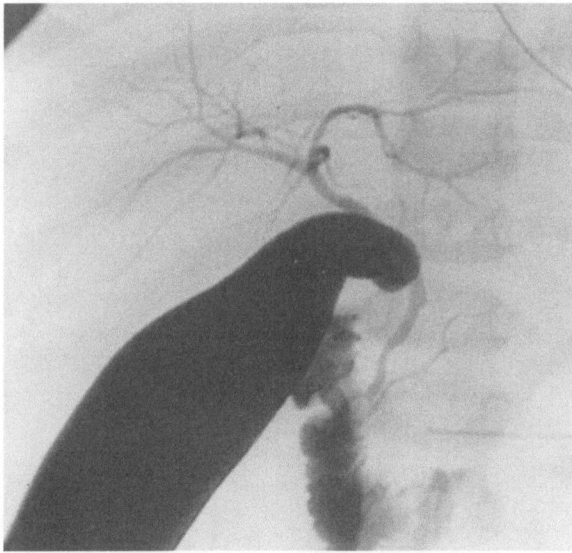

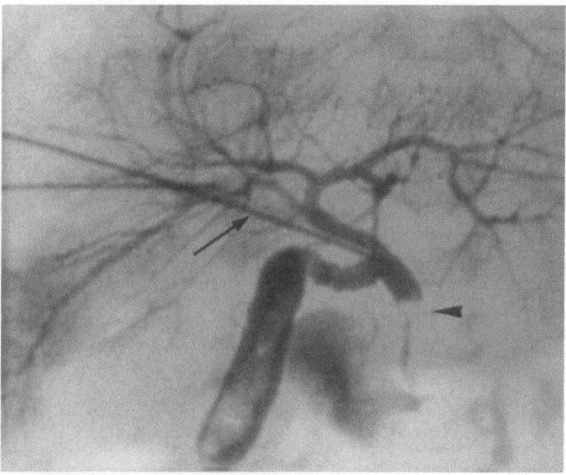

Fig. 5.25. Byler's disease. Biliary cirrhosis. Percutaneous cholecystography opacifies normal intrahepatic ducts. This opacification eliminates the diagnosis of sclerosing cholangitis.

Fig 5.27. A 2-month-old baby boy with cholestasis. The diagnosis of choledocholithiasis is made by ultrasonography. Percutaneous cholangiography shows mild dilatation of the common bile duct above the lithiasis (*arrowhead*). There is also a large intraluminal defect into the gallbladder. An external drainage was placed into the common bile duct via a second puncture of the common hepatic duct (*arrow*). After two sessions of lavage the calculus was eliminated into the duodenum and the dilatation resolved.

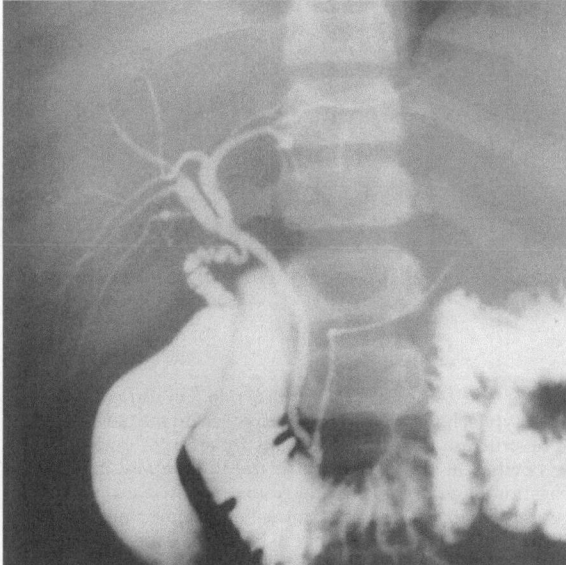

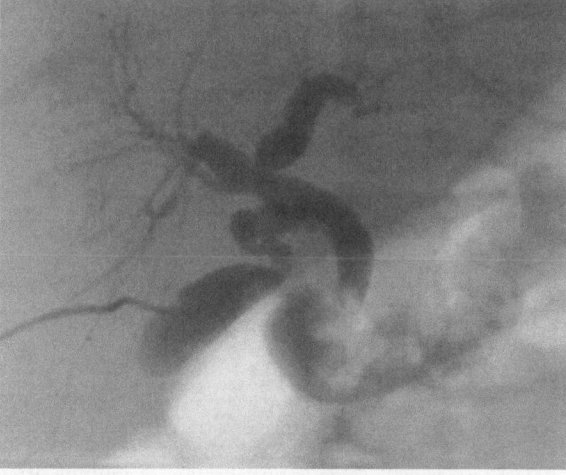

Fig. 5.26. 9 years old, biliary cirrhosis, suspicion of sclerosing cholangitis. Percutaneous cholecystography. Normal anatomy of the intrahepatic bile ducts.

Fig. 5.28. A 3-month-old boy with cholestasis and bile ducts dilatation. Percutaneous cholecystography shows moderate dilatation of the biliary tree due to a calculus of the distal choledochus. There is also sludge in the gallbladder. Transhepatic puncture of the right hepatic duct and placement of an external drainage. Lavage of the biliary tree with saline and contrast medium. Expulsion of the lithiasis at the end of the examination.

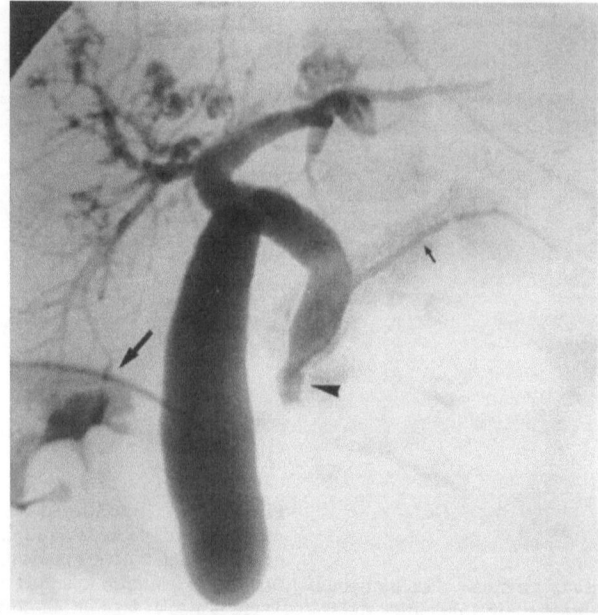

a

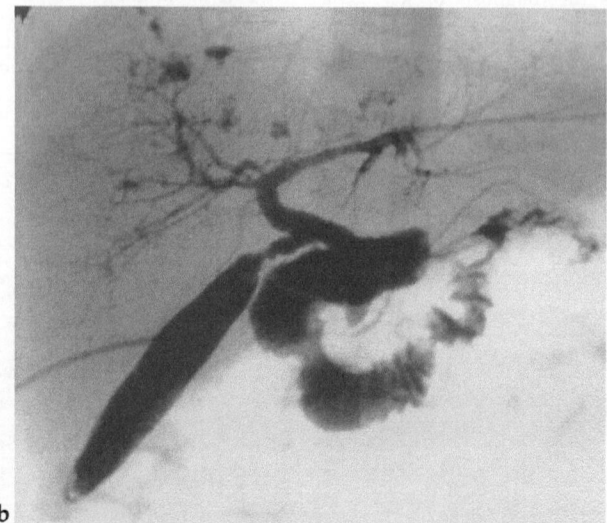

b

Fig. 5.29. A 1-month-old baby girl presenting with cholestasis, fever and *Escherichia coli* septicaemia. On ultrasound there were bile ducts dilatation, lithiasis in the choledochus and multiple hypoechoic areas in the liver parenchyma, suggestive of abscesses. **a** Percutaneous cholecystography. There is complete obstruction of the choledochus by an intraluminal filling defect (*arrowhead*). There is opacification of multiple irregular cavities at the periphery of the intrahepatic bile ducts, corresponding to abscesses and there is also subcapsular extravasation (*large arrow*) coming from one of these cavities. The pancreatic canal is dilated (*small arrow*). After very gentle lavage of the biliary tree with contrast and saline, the calculus is pushed into the duodenum. **b** Control opacification 2 days later shows complete clearing of the biliary tree, resolution of the dilatation and evident decrease in size of the parenchymal cavities. The drainage was taken off. One week later the liver was homogeneous on ultrasound.

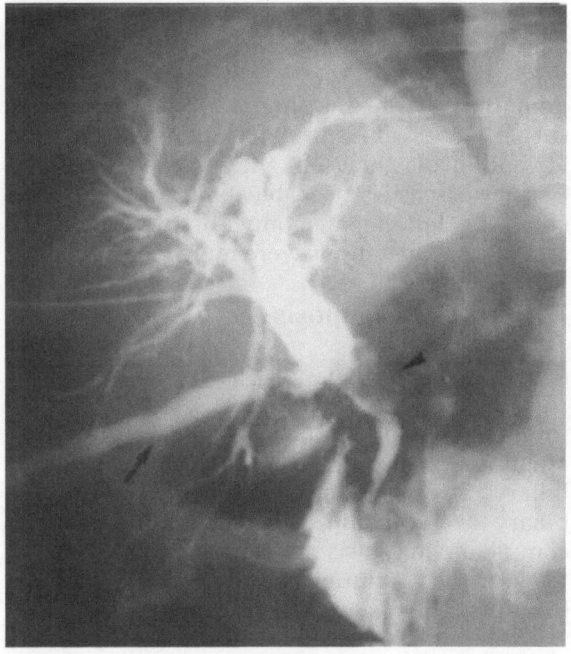

Fig. 5.30. Spontaneous perforation of the common bile duct: a 6-month-old baby boy presenting with cholestasis. Percutaneous transhepatic cholangiography shows dilatation of the intrahepatic bile ducts and of the common bile duct. There is lithiasis in the choledochus above a mild stenosis (*arrowhead*). The gallbladder is very narrow (*arrow*). These lesions were thought to be secondary to spontaneous perforation of the common bile duct.

Clinical Presentation

Although rare, this entity represents the most frequent cause of extrahepatic cholestasis in childhood. It is mainly encountered in the first decade of life, with a strong female predominance. Adult and antenatal cases have been reported, as early as in the 15th week of gestation. For some authors, there must be another pathophysiology in these cases, as secretion of pancreatic enzymes is not yet established.

Clinical presentation is recurrent episodes of abdominal pain and jaundice. The right upper quadrant mass is not frequently palpated. Single or recurrent episodes of pancreatitis are also presenting findings. Complications include cholangitis, complete obstruction of the distal choledochus by lithiasis, biliary cirrhosis, rupture of the cyst with biliary peritonitis and degeneration in late childhood.

Diagnosis is made by ultrasonography. Percutaneous or preoperative cholangiography is performed to identify the precise anatomy of the lesion. Treatment is surgical and consists of complete resection of the cyst and hepaticojejunostomy.

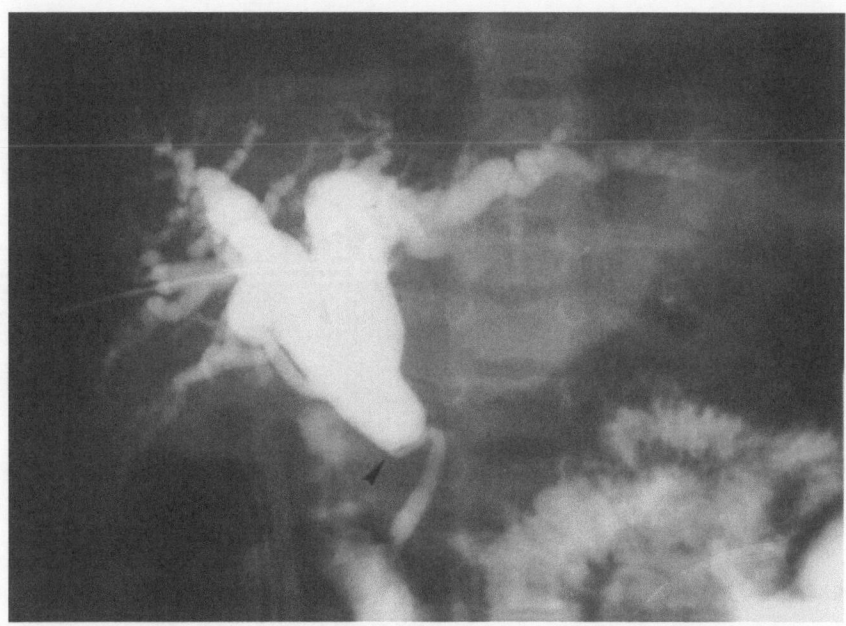

Fig. 5.31. Spontaneous perforation of the common bile duct: 6-month-old baby boy. Percutaneous cholangiography. Massive dilatation of the bile ducts above a stenosis of the choledochus (*arrowhead*). No opacification of the gallbladder. At surgery the stenosis was consistent with sequelae of spontaneous perforation of the common bile duct.

Cholangiography (44 cases)
(Figs. 5.32–5.44)

Opacification can be performed by percutaneous cholecysto- or cholangiography.

The size and the morphology of the dilatation are variable – cystic or fusiform or only mild dilatation – and the degree of dilatation is not related to the age of the child. In all except two cases there was associated dilatation of intrahepatic bile ducts. The left hepatic duct is usually larger than the right probably due to its extrahepatic situation in the proximal portion.

The gallbladder and the cystic duct are often dilated.

The abnormal junction of the choledochus and the pancreatic duct with a long common channel was observed in every case where it was opacified. Rather than measurements, the criterion used was the union of the two ducts above the sphincter. This sphincter can be localised in two ways, either by the irregularity of the wall of the common bile duct due to the muscular fibres or by its contraction during fluoroscopy. However, in a few cases with very large cystic dilatation and obstruction of the bottom of the cyst by lithiasis, opacification of this common channel was not obtained. Reflux pancreatic secretion in the CBD was demon-strated by measuring the enzyme level in the bile, after i.v. injection of cholecystokinin.

In three cases there was persistent cystic dilatation of the intrahepatic bile ducts after surgery with episodes of cholangitis and the formation of stones. In these cases associated Caroli's disease is probable. One child has been cured by left hepatectomy. In the two other cases cystic dilatations were more diffuse.

Differential Diagnosis

Cystic Form of Biliary Atresia

In the neonatal period the main differential diagnosis of choledochal cyst is a cystic form of biliary atresia. The clinical presentation of biliary atresia is quite different because there is complete cholestasis and ultrasonography fails to show the communication of the cyst with the bile ducts.

Choledochocele

Choledochocele is extremely rare. It is the consequence of an intraluminal duodenal duplication in which the common bile duct ends. The relationship of the common bile duct and Wirsung's duct is normal.

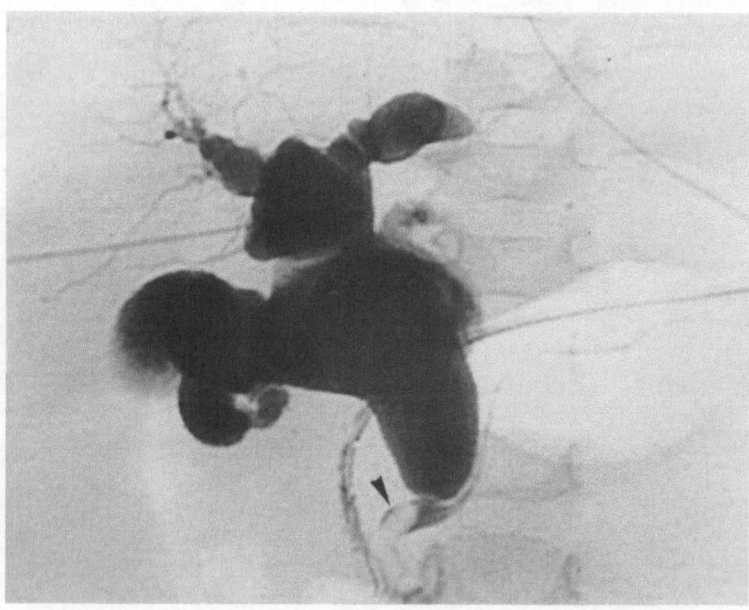

Fig. 5.32. Choledochal cyst; 8 months of age. Percutaneous transhepatic cholecystography. Important dilatation of the intrahepatic and extrahepatic bile ducts. Stenosis is seen at the junction between the common bile duct and the common channel. Filling defect is seen in the common channel (lithiasis) (*arrowhead*). Reflux in the Wirsung duct.

Caroli's Syndrome

Caroli's disease is characterised by cystic, non-obstructive dilatation of the intrahepatic bile ducts. It is a complicated spectrum of disease.

In most cases it is diffuse and associated with congenital hepatic fibrosis and recessive polycystic kidney disease.

In a few cases it is associated with a choledochal cyst (three in our series).

Very rarely it occurs as the only hepatic lesion, without portal fibrosis. Some authors believe that the term Caroli's disease should be restricted to these rare cases. None has been seen by us.

Intrahepatic Biliary Hypoplasia

This is characterised by absence or reduction in the number of bile ductules seen in the portal tracts. Two forms have been described: isolated or with associated abnormalies. This is the so-called Alagille's syndrome or syndromic biliary hypoplasia. Alagille's syndrome includes a peculiar facies, peripheral pulmonary artery stenosis, embryotoxon and "butterfly vertebrae".

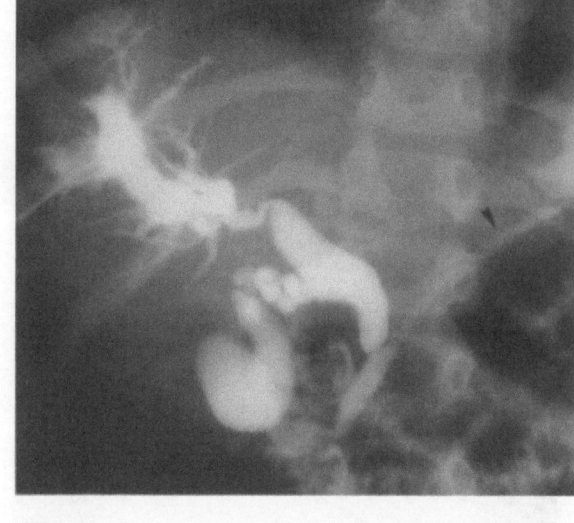

Fig. 5.34. 2 years of age. Choledochal cyst; Percutaneous transhepatic cholangiogram. Moderate dilatation of the CBD. Stenosis at the junction of the common bile duct and the common channel. The common channel is very long and dilated. Wirsung's duct is opacified, slightly dilated (*arrowhead*).

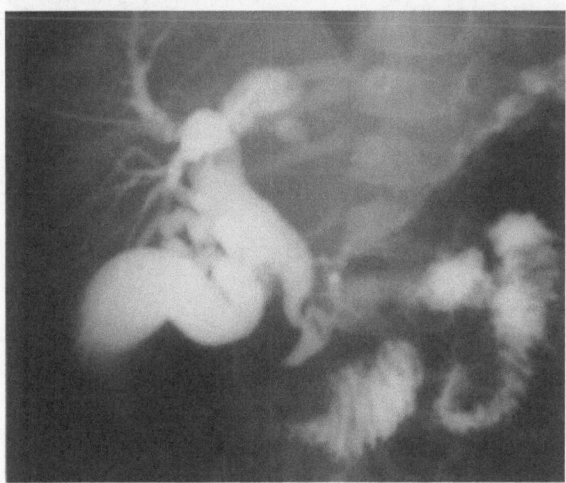

Fig. 5.33. Choledochal cyst; 14 months of age. Percutaneous transhepatic cholangiogram. The common bile duct is dilated. A small filling defect is seen in the common channel (lithiasis). The Wirsung duct is moderately dilated. The left bile ducts are more dilated than the right.

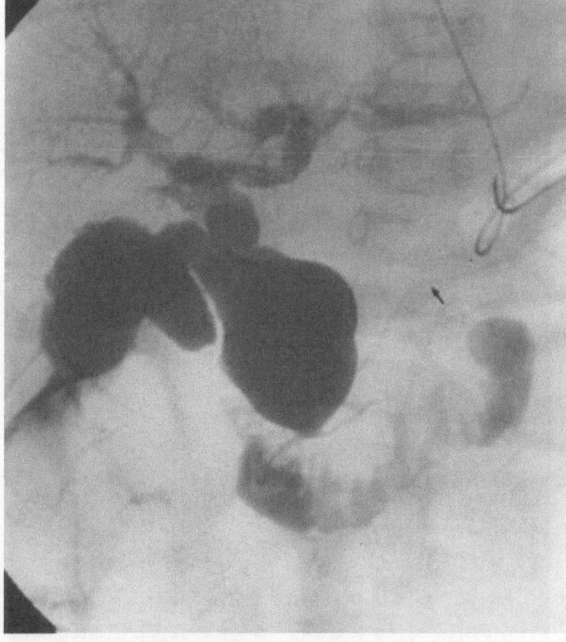

Fig. 5.35. Choledochal cyst diagnosed antenatally; 2 months of age. Percutaneous cholecystography. The common bile duct is cystic. The common channel and the Wirsung duct (*arrow*) are not dilated.

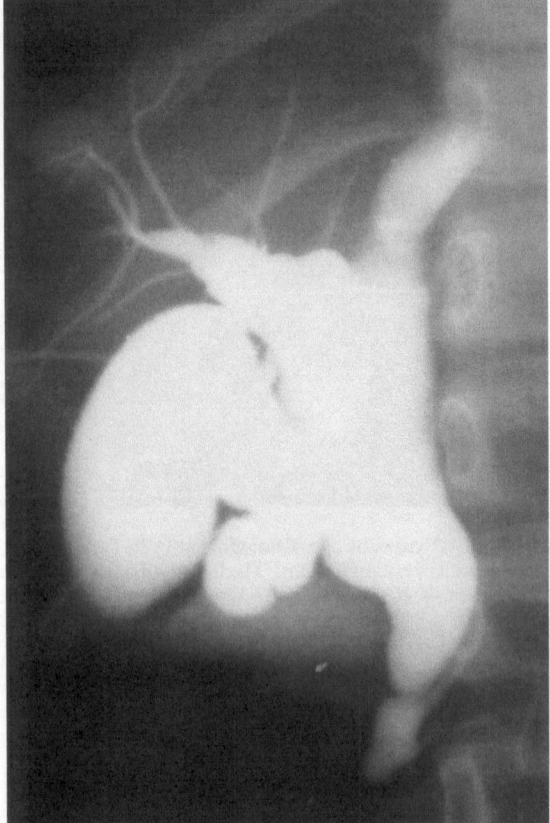

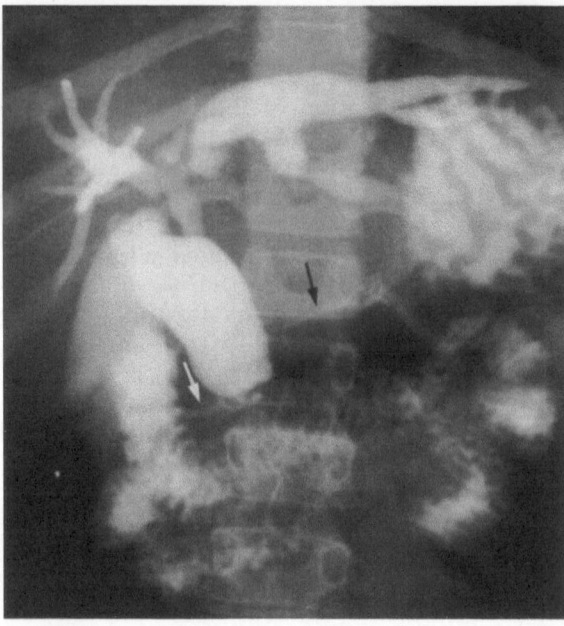

Fig. 5.37. Choledochal cyst; 14 years of age. Percutaneous transhepatic cholangiogram. The intrahepatic bile ducts are large and dilatation is more pronounced on the left. The common bile duct is dilated above a normal diameter common channel (*white arrow*). Wirsung's duct (*black arrow*).

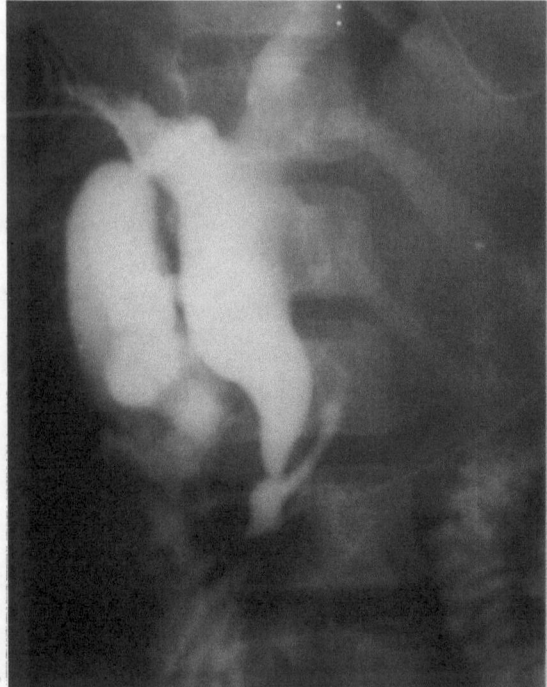

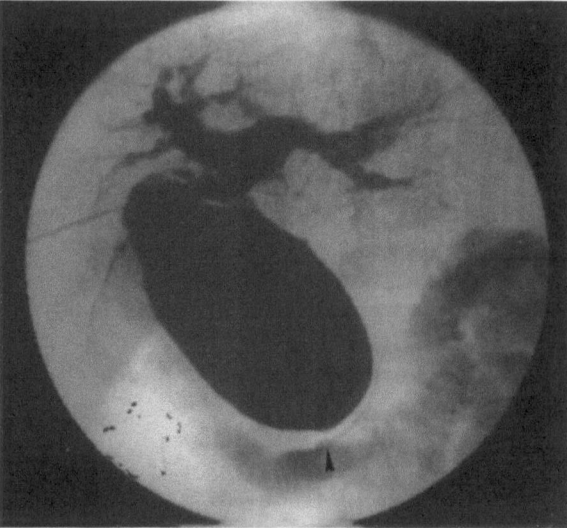

Fig. 5.36. 8 years of age. **a** the common bile duct is dilated, the common channel is large. **b** slightly oblique view: reflux in Wirsung's duct and in an inferior accessory pancreatic duct.

Fig. 5.38. Choledochal cyst; 17 months of age. Transhepatic cholecystography. The common bile duct is large and dilated as well as the intrahepatic bile ducts. The common channel is thin and opens in the third portion of the duodenum (*arrowhead*).

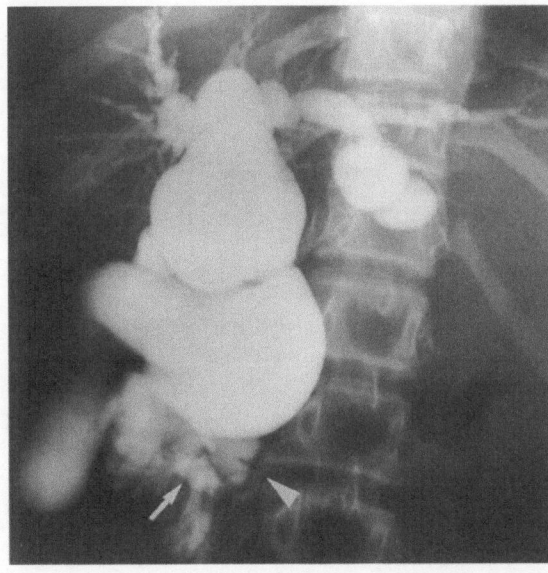

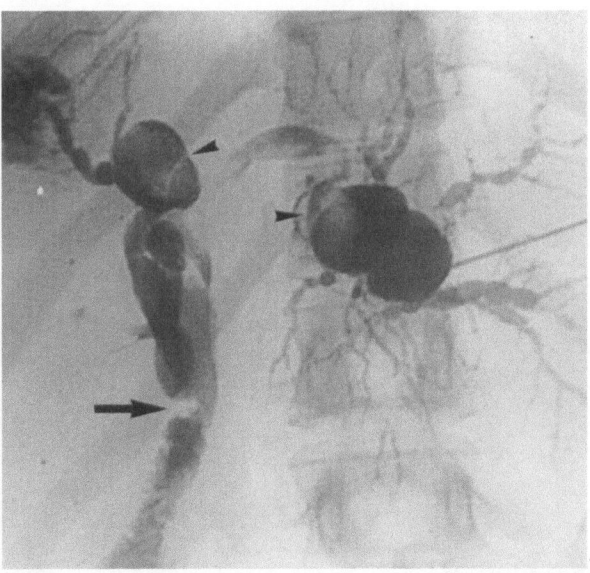

a

b

Fig. 5.39. Choledochal cyst and Caroli's disease; 13 years of age. **a** Percutaneous transhepatic cholangiography. The common bile duct is large and dilated. There are two communicating cysts in the left lobe of the liver. The common channel is dilated. (*arrow*) Minimal reflux in the pancreatic duct (*arrowhead*). **b** After surgery and Roux-en-Y anastomosis, repeated cholangitis. Percutaneous opacification of the left lobe shows persistence of the dilatation of the two communicating cysts. There is a lithiasis obstructing the left lobe bile duct. The bilio-digestive anastomosis is opacified via a right lobe approach. There is also a lithiasis in the ending of the right bile duct. The anastomosis is patent (*arrow*).

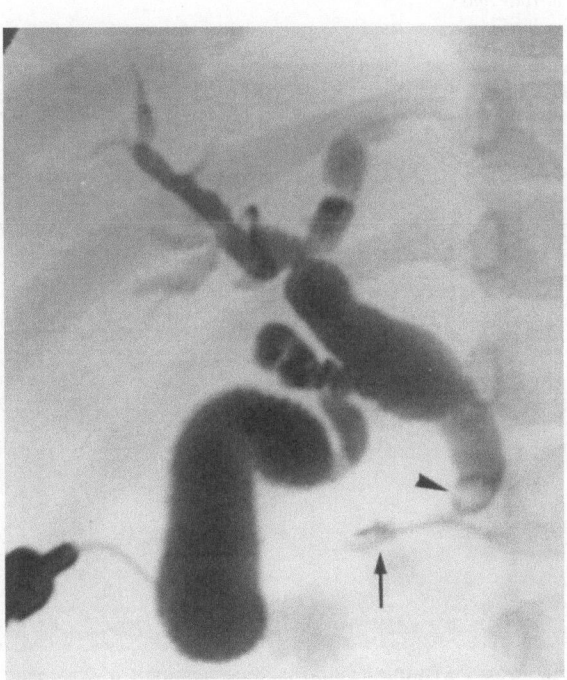

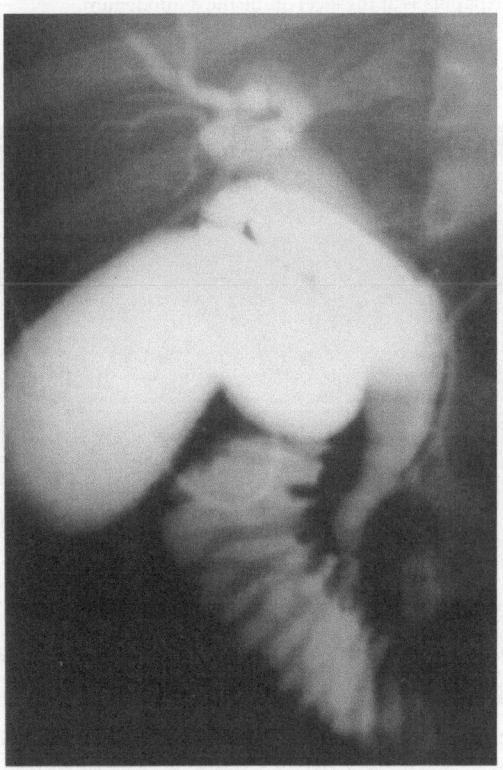

Fig. 5.40. Choledochal cyst; 2 years of age. Percutaneous transhepatic cholecystography. The intrahepatic and extra-hepatic bile ducts are moderately dilated. There is a lithiasis in the terminal portion of the common bile duct (*arrowhead*). The common channel is long but not dilated. Papilla (*arrow*).

Fig. 5.41. Choledochal cyst; 7 years of age. The CBD is moderately dilated. There is an abnormal high junction between the CBD and pancreatic duct. No stenosis is seen on the common bile duct.

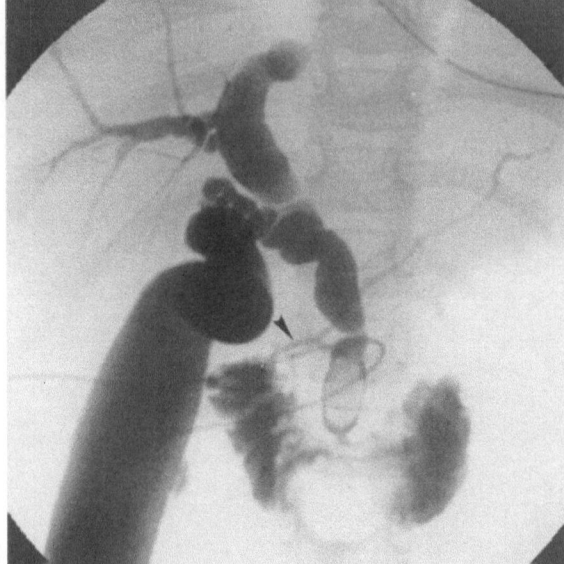

Fig. 5.42. Abdominal pain and fever without jaundice; Pancreatitis; 4 years of age. Percutaneous transhepatic cholecystography. The intrahepatic and extrahepatic bile ducts are moderately dilated. There is a complex malformation with a high junction between the common bile duct and the pancreatic duct. The Santorini duct is patent (*arrowhead*). There is a lithiasis in the terminal portion of the common channel. The papilla is at the level of the third duodenum.

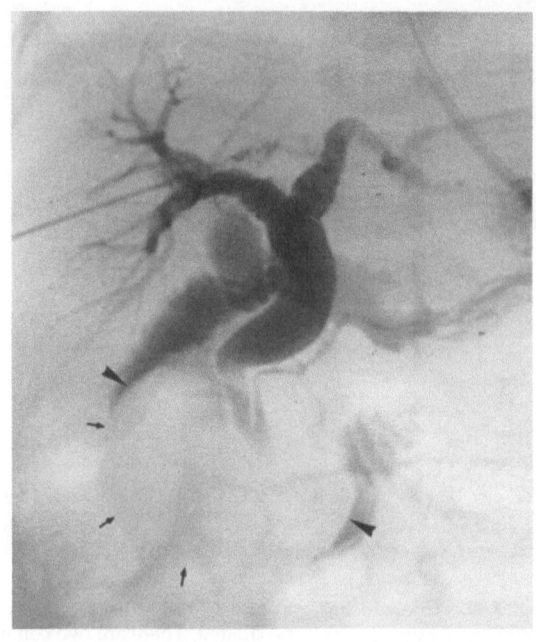

Fig. 5.44. Duodenal duplication; 2-week-old girl with cholestasis and vomiting. On ultrasound there is a bile duct dilatation above a cystic lesion which does not seem to be in continuity with the choledochus. Percutaneous cholangiography shows the extrinsic compression of the distal choledochus by a duodenal duplication cyst (*arrows*) outlined by the passage of contrast medium into the duodenum (*arrowheads*).

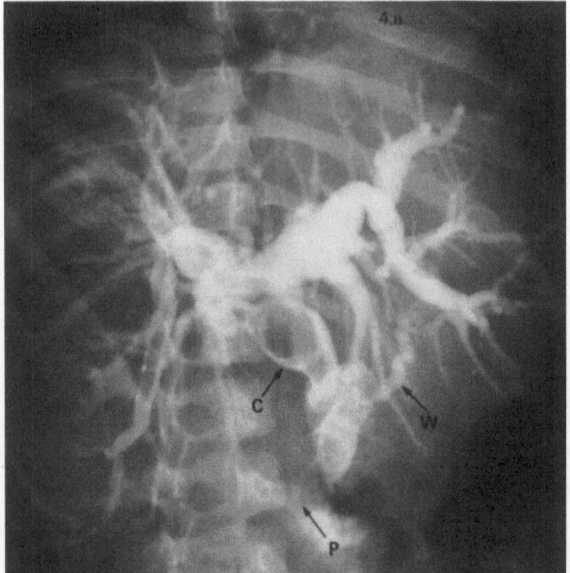

Fig. 5.43. Transhepatic cholangiogram. The intrahepatic bile ducts and the common bile duct are dilated. There is a high junction of Wirsung's duct (W) and the common bile duct (C). The papilla (P) is seen at the level of the second duodenum with a lithiasis at this level. The filling defect in the common bile duct corresponds to thick bile.

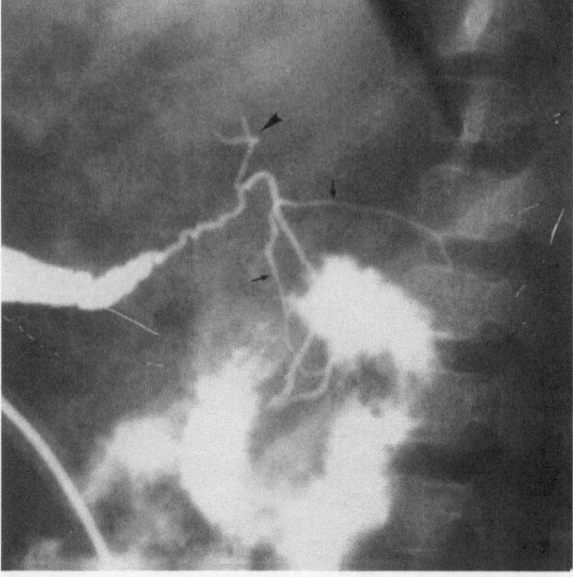

Fig. 5.45. Alagille's syndrome; 10 months of age. The biliary ducts are opacified through the gallbladder, oblique view. The gallbladder is small. There is a patent common bile duct. There is a reflux in Wirsung's duct (*arrow*). The convergence of intrahepatic bile ducts is seen (*arrowhead*), but there is no distal opacification.

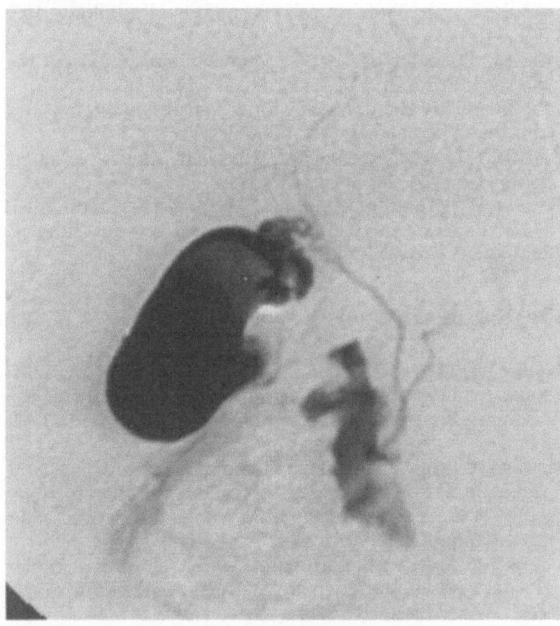

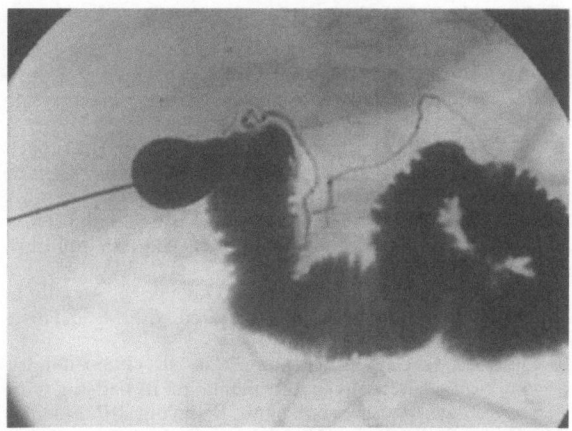

Fig. 5.48. Alagille's syndrome; 5 months of age. Percutaneous cholecystography. There is hypoplasia of the intrahepatic bile ducts. The common bile duct and Wirsung's duct are normal.

Fig. 5.46. A 1-month-old boy with cholestasis. Intrahepatic bile duct hypoplasia; α_1-antitrypsin deficiency. Percutaneous cholecystography. The common bile duct is normal. There is opacification of the convergence of bile ducts, but no opacification of the intrahepatic distal ducts.

Cholangiography (nine cases) (Figs. 5.45–5.48)

Percutaneous cholecystography can be performed when the diagnosis of biliary hypoplasia is uncertain. It demonstrates rarity and tenuity of intrahepatic bile ducts, without irregularities of calibre.

Bibliography

Biliary atresia

Abramson SJ, Treves S, Teele RS (1982) The infant with possible biliary atresia: evaluation by ultrasound and nuclear medecine. Pediatr Radiol 12: 1–5

Brun P, Gauthier F, Boucher D, Brunelle F (1985) Ultrasound findings in biliary atresia in children. Ann Radiol 28: 259–263

Carty H, Pilling DW, Majury C (1986) 123 I BSP scanning in neonatal jaundice. Ann Radiol 29: 647–650

Chaumont P, Martin N, Riou JY, Brunelle F (1982) Percutaneous transhepatic cholangiography in extrahepatic biliary duct atresia in children. Ann Radiol 25: 94–100

Ishïi K, Matsuo S, Hirayama Y et al. (1989) Intrahepatic biliary cysts after hepatic portoenterostomy in four children with biliary atresia. Pediatr Radiol 19: 471–473

Kasaï M, Kimura S, Asakura Y (1968) Surgical treatment of biliary atresia. J Pediatr Surg 3: 665–675

Laurent J, Gauthier F, Bernard O et al. (1990) Long-term outcome after surgery for biliary atresia. Gastroenterology 99: 1793–1797

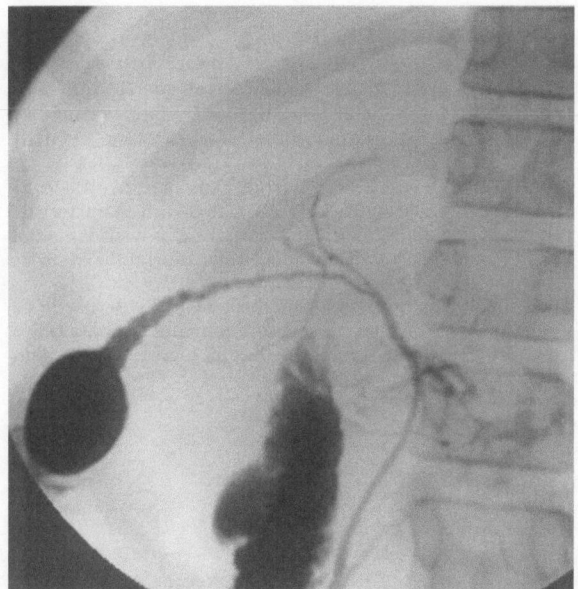

Fig. 5.47. Alagille's syndrome; 14 years of age. Percutaneous cholecystography. The gallbladder is very small. The common bile duct is narrow. There is a typical appearance of hypoplasia of the intrahepatic bile ducts.

Sclerosing Cholangitis

Amédée-Manesme O, Bernard O, Brunelle F et al. (1987) Sclerosing cholangitis with neonatal onset. J Pediatr 111: 225–229

Craig DA, MacCarty RL, Wiesner RH et al. (1991) Primary sclerosing cholangitis: value of cholangiography in determining the prognosis. AJR 157: 959-964

Garel L, Brunelle F, Fischer A, Sirinelli D, Sauvegrain J (1985) Bile duct dilatation and immunodeficiency in children. Ann Radiol 28: 249-225

Leblanc A, Hadchouel M, Jehan P, Odièvre M, Alagille D (1981) Obstructive jaundice in children with histiocytosis X. Gastroenterology 80: 134–139

Letourneau J, Day D, Hunter D et al. (1988) Biliary complications after liver transplantation in patients with preexisting sclerosing cholangitis. Radiology 167: 349–351

MacCarty R, La Russo N, Wiesner R, Ludwig J (1983) Primary sclerosing cholangitis: findings on cholangiography and pancreatography. Radiology 149: 39–44

Pariente D, Bacadi D, Schmit P (1986) Biliary tract involvement in children with histiocytosis X. Ann Radiol 29: 641–645

Sisto A, Feldman P, Garel L et al. (1987) Primary sclerosing cholangitis in children: study of five cases and review of the literature. Pediatrics 80: 918–923

Werlin S, Glicklich M, Jona J, Starshak RJ (1980) Sclerosing cholangitis in childhood. J Pediatr 96: 433–435

Choledocholithiasis

Avni EF, Matos C, Van Gansbeke D, Muller F (1986) Atypical gallbladder content in neonates: ultrasonic demonstration. Ann Radiol 29: 267–273

Bernstein J, Braylen R, Brough J (1969) Bile plug syndrome: a correctable cause of obstructive jaundice in infants. Pediatrics 43: 273–276

Brunelle F (1987) Cholelithiasis in children. Semin Ultrasound, CT, MR 8: 118–125

Brunelle F, Descos B, Bernard O, Valayer J, Chaumont P (1983) Common bile duct calculi in infants. Ann Radiol 26: 147–153

Descos B, Bernard O, Brunelle F et al. (1984) Pigment Gallstones of the common bile duct in infancy. Hepatology 4: 678–683

Haller JO, Condon VR, Berdon WE et al. (1989) Spontaneous perforation of the common bile duct in children. Radiology 172: 621–624

Holgersen LO, Stolar C, Berdon WE, Hilfer C, Levy JS (1990) Therapeutic and diagnostic implications of aquired choledochal obstruction in infancy: spontaneous resolution in three infants. J Pediatr Surg 25: 1027–1029

Keller MS, Markle BM, Laffey PA et al.(1985) Spontaneous resolution in cholelithiasis in infants. Radiology 157: 345–348

Lang EV, Pinckney LE (1991) Spontaneous resolution of the bile-plug syndrome. AJR 156: 1225–1226

Lilly JR (1980) Common bile duct calculi in infants and children. J Pediatr Surg 15: 577–580

Man DWK, Spitz L (1985) Cholelithiasis in infancy. J Pediatr Surg 20: 65–68

Pariente D, Bernard O, Gauthier F, Brunelle F, Chaumont P (1989) Radiological treatment of common bile duct lithiasis in infancy. Pediatr Radiol 19: 104–107

Choledochal Cyst

Babbitt DD (1969) Congenital Choledochal cyst. New etiological concept based on anomalous relationships of the common bile duct and pancreatic duct. Ann Radiol 12: 231–240

Bass EM, Cremin BJ (1976) Choledochal cysts: a clinical and radiological evaluation of 21 cases. Pediatr Radiol 5: 81–85

Caroli J (1973) Disease of the intrahepatic biliary tree. Clin Gastroenterol 2: 147–161

Jequier S, Capusten B, Guttman F (1984) Childhood choledochal cyst with intrahepatic enlarged cyst-like bile ducts. J Can Assoc Radiol 35: 73–76

Reddy KR, Gordon SC, Jeffers LJ (1985) Choledochocele: its clinical spectrum. Gastroenterology 88: 1093–1098

Savader SJ, Benenati JF, Venbrux AC et al.(1991) Choledochal cysts: classification and cholangiographic appearance. AJR 156: 327–331

Schroeder D, Smith L, Crichton Pain H (1989) Antenatal diagnosis of choledochal cyst at 15 weeks' gestation: etiologic implications and management. J Pediatr Surg 24: 936–938

Suarez F, Bernard O, Gauthier F, Valayer J, Brunelle F (1987) Biliopancreatic common channel in childhood. Pediatr Radiol 17: 206–211

Ductular Hypoplasia

Alagille D, Estrada A, Hadchouel M et al. (1987) Syndromic paucity of interlobular bile ducts (Alagille syndrome or arteriohepatic dysplasia): a review of 80 cases. J Pediatr 110: 195–200

Alagille D, Odièvre M, Gautier M, Dommergues JP (1975) Hepatic ductular hypoplasia associated with characteristic facies, vertebral malformations, retarded physical, mental and sexual developmental and cardiac murmur. Pediatrics 86: 63–71

Brunelle F, Estrada A, Dommergues JP, Bernard O, Chaumont P (1986) Skeletal anomalies in Alagille's syndrome. Radiographic study in eighty cases. Ann Radiol 29: 687–690

6 Pancreas

Pancreatic Arteriovenous Malformations (Fig. 6.1)

Arteriovenous malformations were seen in five cases: two involved the region of the pancreas and three the liver as well.

Clinical symptoms include cardiac failure in newborns, Kasabach–Merritt syndrome and portal hypertension. Portal hypertension may be extreme and reversed portal flow may be observed as a result of arterioportal shunting.

Embolisation may be useful to treating the cardiac failure and Kasabach–Merritt syndrome. Intrahepatic arteriovenous malformations are difficult to treat. Surgical hepatectomy cured the condition in one case: two cases had associated trisomy 21.

Pancreatic Tumours

Malignant tumours are rare in children (two cases; one with intrahepatic metastases).

Pancreatic Venous Sampling

Introduction

Pancreatic venous sampling in children is used to differentiate diffuse from local hypersecretion of insulin in hyperinsulinism. When focal secretion is demonstrated preoperative localisation allows selective partial resection. Adenomas and focal hyperplasias are found in these cases. In diffuse forms the entire pancreas exhibit signs of hypersecretion on pathology.

Technique

Anaesthesia

All drugs given to the patient must be stopped before the examination. Parenteral glucose should be given to maintain a normal glucose level 24 h before the anaesthesia. Anaesthesia usually leads to a variable increase of blood glucose level. The examination and samplings should be done during controlled hypoglycaemia. This point is of paramount importance for a correct interpretation of sampling results.

Technique

The portal vein is entered by mid-axillary puncture. Ultrasound can facilitate the right portal vein entry in small babies. Specially designed catheters are used.

Two different shapes of catheters are used to catheterise the pancreatic veins of the head and tail of the pancreas.

Anatomy (Fig. 6.2)

1. Superior pancreaticoduodenal vein: this connects to the right border of the portal

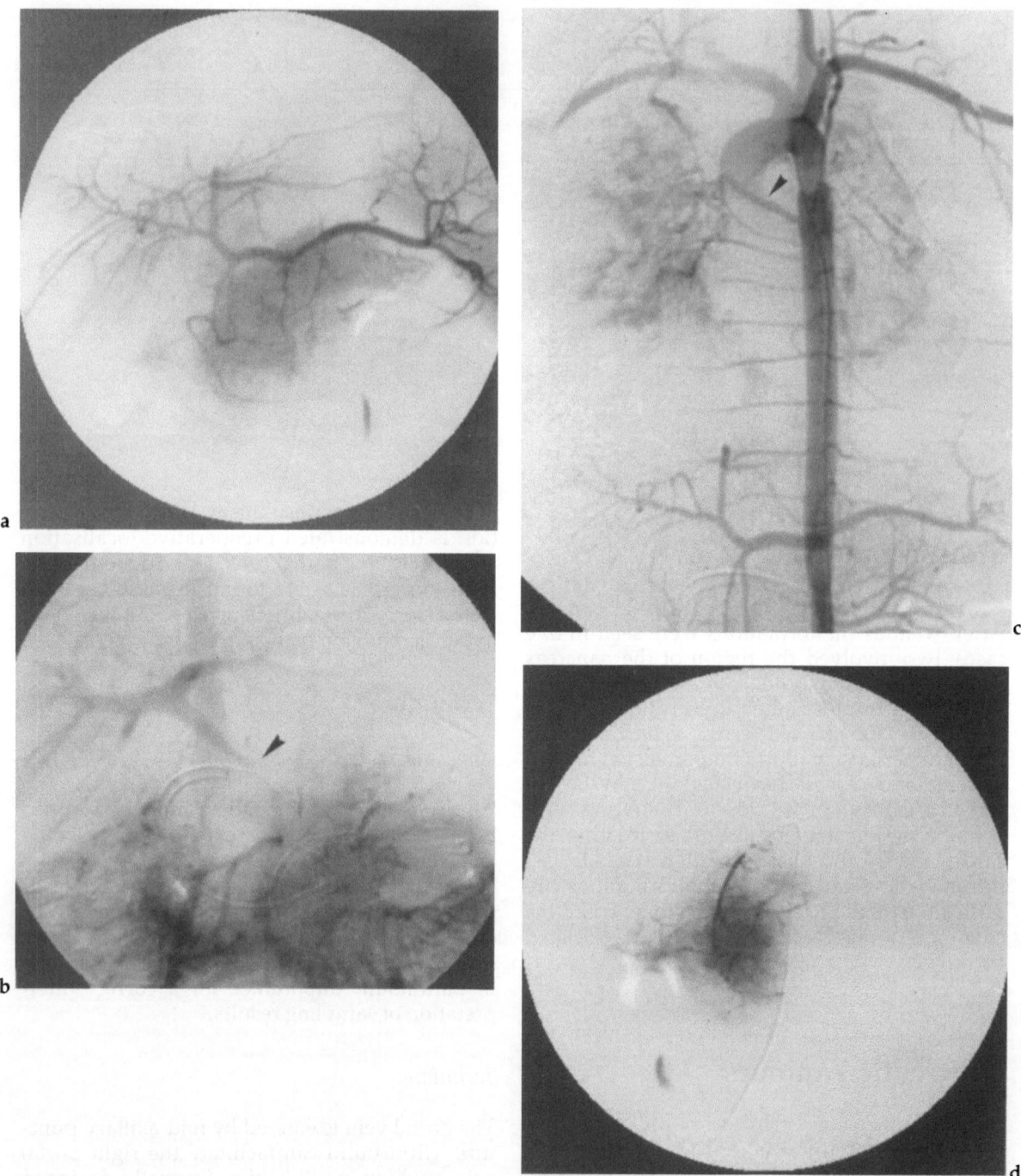

Fig. 6.1. A 1-month-old boy presenting with vomiting, epigastric mass and thrombopenia. The diagnosis of immature angioma is made on surgical biopsy. **a** Coeliac trunk opacification shows an abnormally dense capillary blush of the pancreas. There is no dilated artery and no arteriovenous fistula. **b** The venous phase of the superior mesenteric artery shows a severe narrowing of the portal vein (*arrowhead*) corresponding to the compression by the mass. **c** Thoracic aortogram discloses multiple areas of capillary blushes, mainly supplied by a large right broncho-intercostal trunk (*arrowhead*). **d** Because of increasing signs of compression (cholestasis, vomiting) and of non-response to the medical treatment (corticotherapy and interferon), embolisation was attempted. Selective catheterisation of a branch of the pancreatic dorsal artery, vascularising the head of the pancreas, was performed with Ivalon fragments (50–150 μm). *Continued opposite.*

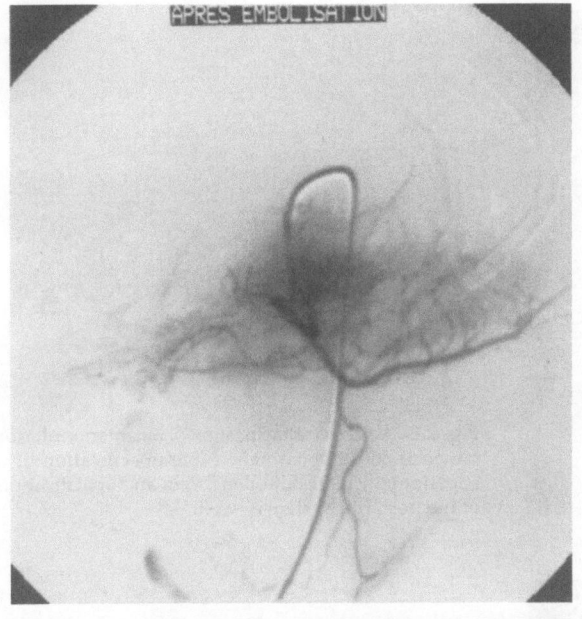

e

Fig. 6.1. A 1-month-old boy presenting with vomiting, epigastric mass and thrombopenia. The diagnosis of immature angioma is made on surgical biopsy. *(continued)* **e** The control after embolisation shows respect of the gastric and duodenal arteries. The enlarged broncho-intercostal artery was also embolised. The evolution was good with rapid increase of platelets and disappearance of the mass.

vein just above or at the level of the first duodenum.

2. Antero-inferior pancreaticoduodenal veins (Fig. 6.3): these connect to the right border of the portal vein above the third duodenum.

3. Postero-inferior pancreaticoduodenal veins: these connect to the left border of the mesenteric veins at the level of the fourth duodenum.

All these veins are linked together by intra-pancreatic collaterals.

4. Isthmic veins. Veins draining the pancreatic isthmus can be opacified. They drain into the splenic vein at the junction with the superior mesenteric vein and anastomose with the transverse pancreatic vein.

5. Transverse pancreatic vein (Fig. 6.4): this drains most of the body of the pancreas and connects to the inferior mesenteric vein or into the splenic vein directly.

6. Dorsal pancreatic veins (Fig. 6.5 and 6.6): although numerous these cannot always be entered.

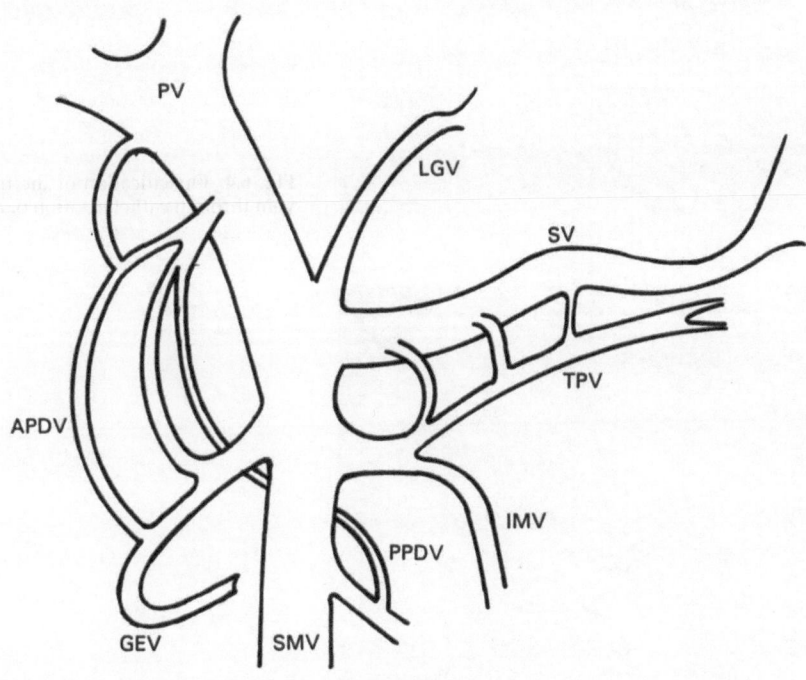

Fig. 6.2. Normal anatomy of the pancreatic veins. PV, portal vein; APDV, anterior pancreaticoduodenal vein; GEV, gastro-epiploic vein; SMV, superior mesenteric vein; PPDV, posterior pancreaticoduodenal vein; IMV, inferior mesenteric vein; TPV, transverse pancreatic vein; SV, splenic vein; LGV, left gastric vein.

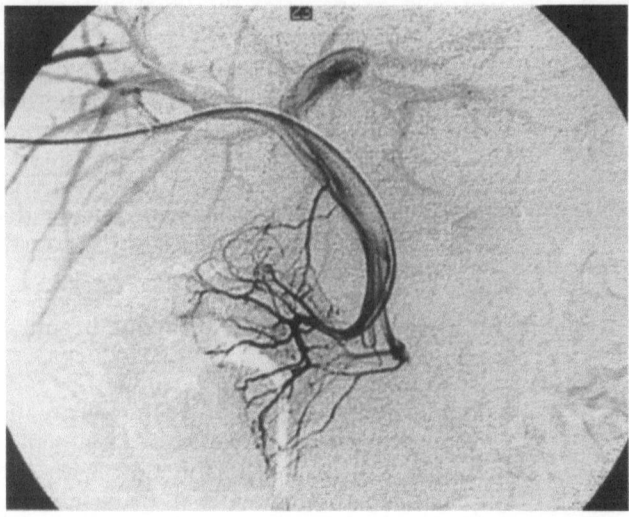

Fig. 6.3. Selective opacification of an anterio-inferior pancreaticoduodenal vein. Note opacification of a superior pancreaticoduodenal vein and opacification of the posterior system as well.

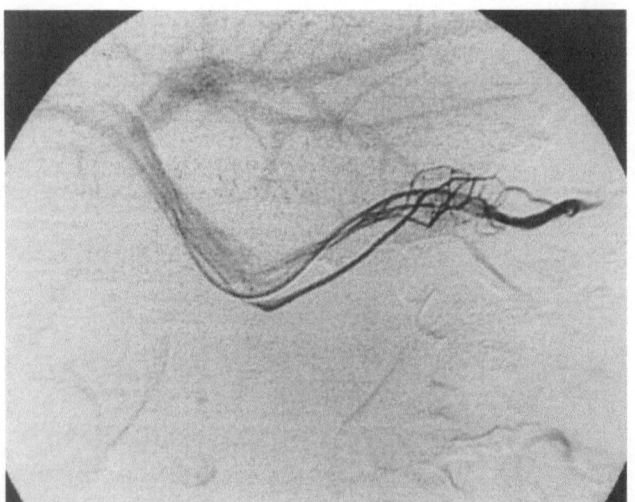

Fig. 6.4. Opacification of the transverse pancreatic vein through catheterisation of a dorsal vein.

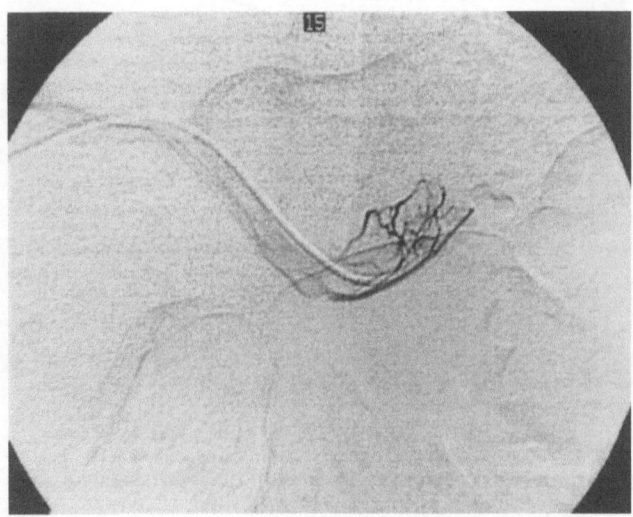

Fig. 6.5. Opacification of a dorsal pancreatic vein. Note opacification of the transverse vein as well.

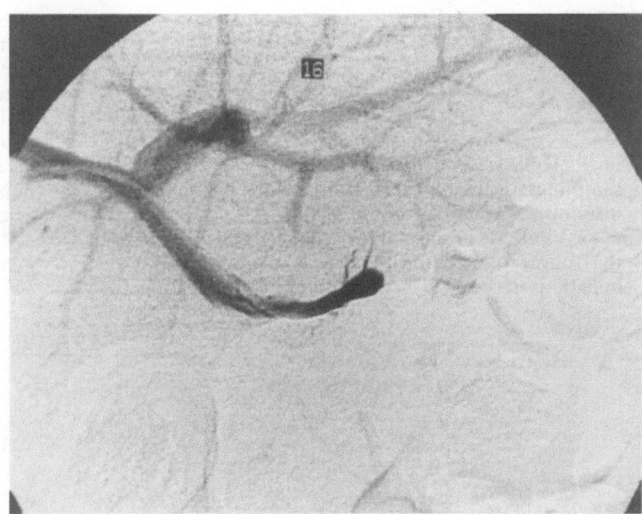

Fig. 6.6. Splenic vein opacification. Two dorsal veins are seen.

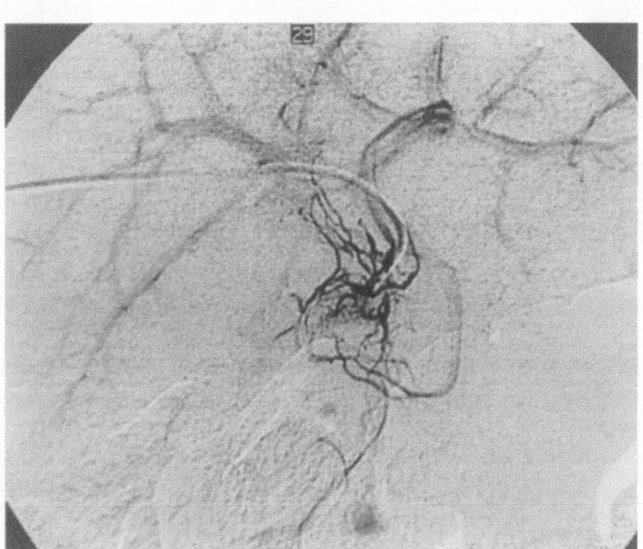

Fig. 6.7. Opacification of a posterio-superior pancreaticoduodenal vein. Note opacification of the peribiliary plexus parallel to the portal vein

Anastomoses

These pancreatic veins anastomose with the left gastric vein, pyloric vein and colic veins. These veins should also be catheterised and sampled (Fig. 6.7).

As the veins are not opacified prior to their entry experience is useful in this type of examination. When a vein is entered opacification should be performed to localise the vein and identify its draining area.

Other collaterals can be seen and then, progressively, all veins can be catheterised and sampled. Films should be taken to compare the anatomy with the level of insulin concentration. High levels of insulin indicate focal secretion.

Bibliography

General

Brunelle F, Negre V, Barth O et al. (1989) Pancreatic venous samplings in infants and children with primary hyperinsulinism. Pediatr Radiol 19: 100–103

Cho KJ, Vinik AI, Thompson NW et al. (1982) Localisation of the source of hyperinsulinism by percutaneous transhepatic portal and pancreatic vein catheterization with hormonal assay. AJR 139: 237–241

Friedman AC, Edmonds PR (1989) Rare pancreatic malignancies Radiol Clin North Am 27: 177–190

Grosfeld JL, Clatworthy HW, Hamoudi AB (1970) Pancreatic malignancy in children. Arch Surg 101: 370–375

Pochard J, Brunelle F, Didier F, Hubert C (1989) Syndrome de Kasabach–Mewitt à localisation pancréatique chez un nouveau-né. Arch Fr Pediatr 46: 443–446

Roche A, Raisonnier A, Gillon Savouret MC (1983) Pancreatic venous sampling and arteriography in localizing insulinomas: procedure and results in 55 cases. Radiology 145: 621–627

7 Liver Transplantation

Introduction

Over the past few years the remarkable results of liver transplantation have changed the management and prognosis of children with liver diseases.

The main indications included biliary atresia, Byler's disease, α_1-antitrypsin deficiency, chronic hepatitis, fulminant hepatitis, tyrosinaemia, glycogen storage disease type 1 and other metabolic disorders.

Over a period of six years, 260 cases of liver transplantation in children have been examined in our department. The rate of survival is approximately 80% with a better prognosis when transplant is carried out electively than on emergency.

Liver transplantation requires extensive use of various imaging techniques especially pulsed Doppler ultrasonography, angiography and cholangiography.

The surgical procedure includes successively five anastomoses: to the suprahepatic vena cava, portal vein, hepatic artery, infrahepatic vena cava and, finally biliary anastomosis (a choledocho-choledochostomy or a choledocho-jejunostomy). Because of the shortage of child donors, adult reduced-sized grafts may be used. The anatomy of these partial livers may complicate the radiological investigation and analysis of the findings.

Preoperative Angiographic Work-up

Preoperative work-up includes evaluation of cardiac and pulmonary status with chest film, echocardiography, scintigraphy and, in some cases, angiocardiography. Increased cardiac output, hypoxia due to pulmonary shunts and pulmonary arterial hypertension are well-known but unexplained complications of cirrhosis and portal hypertension. Their presence may hasten the need for transplantation or even preclude it. Finally, it is essential to evaluate the patency of the inferior vena cava and the diameter of the portal vein, as they represent critical anatomical information for surgical planning. We obtained adequate information in three-quarters of our patients.

Angiography is indicated in four circumstances:

1. When the portal vein is not identified or its diameter less than 4 mm. A decrease in the size of the portal vein is a frequent event in end-stage liver disease, as opposed to dilatation of the hepatic artery. Reverse portal flow can be demonstrated on the late phase of hepatic arteriography or by fine-needle transhepatic portography. Portal vein thrombosis is rare (only one case among about 300 pretransplant work-up), and it no longer pre-

cludes liver transplantation as surgeons are nowadays performing venous anastomoses with venous allografts placed on the superior mesenteric vein or the splenic vein.

2. Angiography is also performed in cases of biliary atresia with the so-called "non-cardiac polysplenia syndrome", as vascular anatomy may be very complex (cf. Chapter 3).

3. Cavography should be performed when the inferior vena cava is not identified or thrombosed (one case). This does not preclude transplantation but the superior caval anastomosis of the graft will be achieved on the inferior part of the right atrium.

4. In cases of previous surgical portosystemic shunt, the size of the portal vein will have decreased and the transplantation will be more complicated.

Postoperative Work-up

After liver transplantation, US with pulsed or colour Doppler is the method of choice for screening for the main complications. However, angiography or cholangiography remains mandatory to confirm and to plan the treatment.

Vascular Complications (Figs. 7.1–7.6)

Hepatic Artery Thrombosis (26 cases)

Clinical Presentation. It is a frequent complication of liver transplantation in children, reported in about 10% of cases and mainly occurs with infant donors or recipients. The greatest risk is during the first 2 weeks, but late occurrence is possible (5 months). It is usually a devastating condition, but its clinical presentation is highly variable and includes fulminant necrosis and septicaemia or delayed biliary complications due to ischaemia of the biliary tract or relapsing fever and bacteraemia.

Angiographic Findings. In the acute phase an aortogram shows the absence of arterial vascularisation of the graft and the occlusion of the hepatic artery which is usually located at the site of anastomosis.

After 2 to 3 weeks there is evidence of an arterial collateral circulation arising from the superior mesenteric artery or parietal arteries. However, this collateral circulation does not seem to prevent delayed biliary complication

and it carries a risk of massive haemorrhage during surgical procedures.

Treatment. In cases of fulminant necrosis retransplantation must be performed on an emergency basis. Biliary complications may be temporarily treated with transhepatic drainage, dilatation or surgical refection of biliary anastomosis but in most cases retransplantation will be necessary.

In all our cases of hepatic artery thrombosis, except one, severe complications have occurred. The best chance to save the graft is probably to remove the obstruction surgically as soon as possible. In this way complications have been avoided in six of 11 cases.

The attemps at *radiological* transluminal thrombectomy have been unsuccessful with recurrent thrombosis, probably because of persistent arterial wall lesions.

Hepatic Artery Stenosis (four cases)

It may be asymptomatic or complicated by biliary problems (biliary fistula or stenosis). Transluminal angioplasty has been successfully performed in two of our cases.

Portal Vein Thrombosis (12 cases)

This is a rarer complication than hepatic artery thrombosis. In 10 cases the portal vein was preduodenal or small before transplantation. In most cases the thrombosis occurred in the first 10 days and was suspected on the pulsed Doppler image.

Angiography was performed in seven cases. The obstruction was at the site of anastomosis in all cases. In four cases the patency of the intrahepatic portal branches was demonstrated with inversion of flow on the late phase of hepatic arteriogram. In three cases a hepatopetal venous cavernoma was evident.

Six children died. Prompt surgical thrombectomy may be undertaken as it was in two of our cases.

Portal Vein Stenosis (one case)

Despite frequently ill-matched anastomosis, symptomatic portal vein stenosis is rare. One child presented with reappearance of the clinical and radiological signs of portal hypertension 9 months after liver transplantation and had to be reoperated on.

Inferior Vena Cava Thrombosis and Stenosis

Inferior vena cava thrombosis in its retrohepatic portion may be encountered (two cases), especially with an adult reduced-sized graft and an ill-matched large inferior vena cava. In most cases, hepatic vein drainage is preserved and no complication occurs.

We have not seen secondary Budd–Chiari syndrome but two cases have been reported in the literature. These were successfully treated by transluminal angioplasty.

Arterial Aneurysm (three cases)

Arterial aneurysm is a very serious complication as it carries a risk of dissection with intractable haemorrhage (one case). It may be secondary to infection ("mycotic aneurysms") or due to severe rejection (one case). It is difficult to depict with ultrasonography or computed tomography and angiography is required. In one case spontaneous disappearance of a mesenteric artery aneurysm was documented 1 year later.

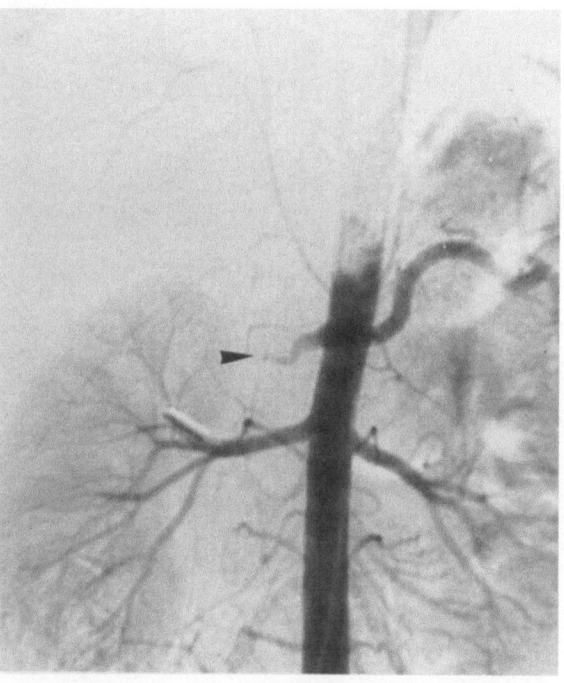

Fig 7.1. Hepatic artery thrombosis: 10 year-old boy with fulminant presentation of Wilson's disease. Transplantation in emergency. No arterial signal is recorded by pulsed-Doppler sonography 35 days after transplantation. Global aortogram shows complete obstruction of the hepatic artery at the anastomotic site (*arrowhead*).

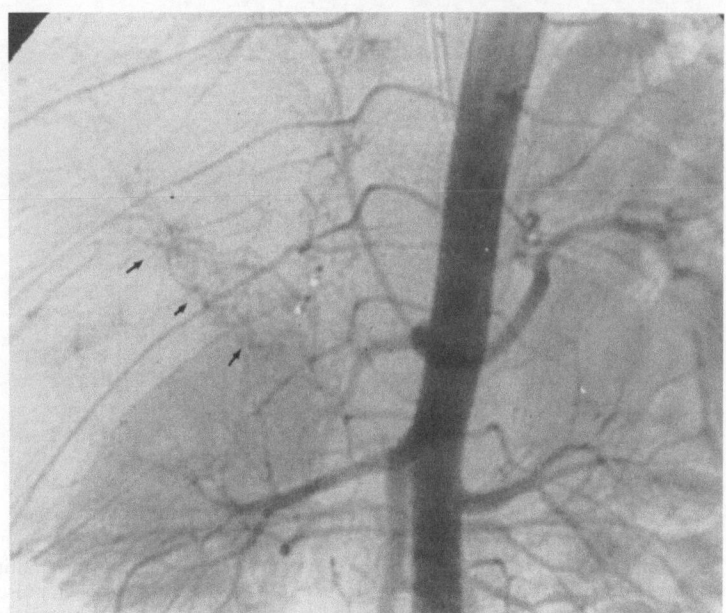

Fig. 7.2. Hepatic artery thrombosis: 9-year-old boy transplanted in emergency for fulminant toxic hepatitis. Cardiac arrest during surgery. The hepatic artery signal is not found on post-operative Doppler sonography. Aortogram performed 2 months later before reoperation for biliary reconstruction: there is a network of arterial collaterals arising from the superior mesenteric artery and the parietal arteries (*arrows*). The biliary reconstruction was so haemorrhagic because of this collateral circulation that the child had to be retransplanted in emergency and finally died shortly after.

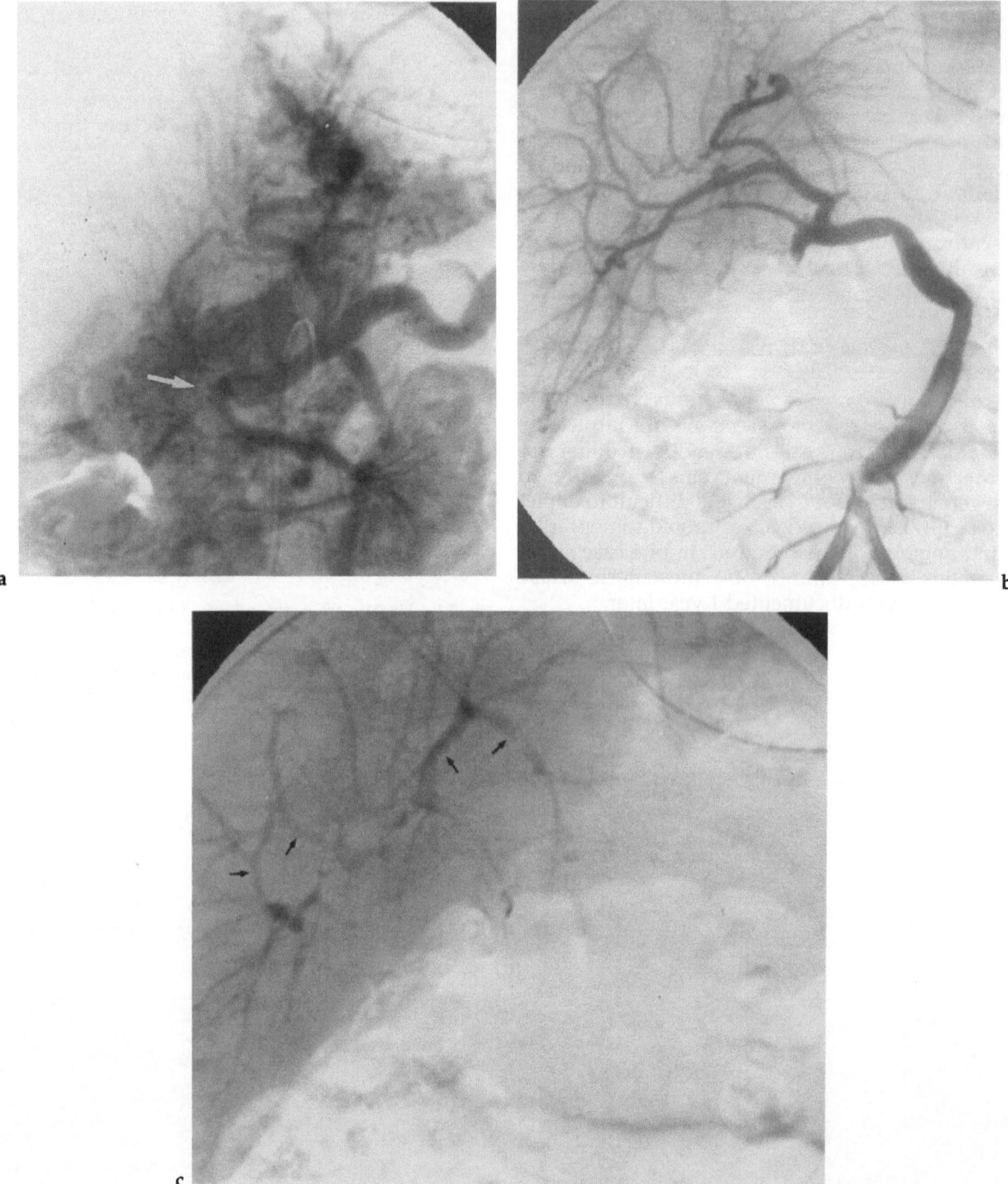

Fig. 7.3. Portal vein thrombosis: 1-year-old boy with cirrhosis secondary to biliary atresia. Incomplete malformative complex including azygous continuation of the inferior vena cava, preduodenal portal vein and multiple hepatic arteries, but no polysplenia. One week after transplantation there was suspicion of portal vein thrombosis on pulsed-Doppler ultrasound. **a** The venous phase of superior mesenteric arteriogram shows absence of opacification of the portal vein with obstruction at the spleno-mesenteric confluence (*white arrow*). **b** Opacification of the hepatic artery: the arterial anastomosis is made with a graft directly placed on the aorta above the iliac arteries. **c** On the late phase of the hepatic arteriogram there is opacification of the intrahepatic portal branches by inversion of portal flow (*arrows*). At surgery the preduodenal portal vein was stretched and flat. The portal anastomosis was reconstructed.

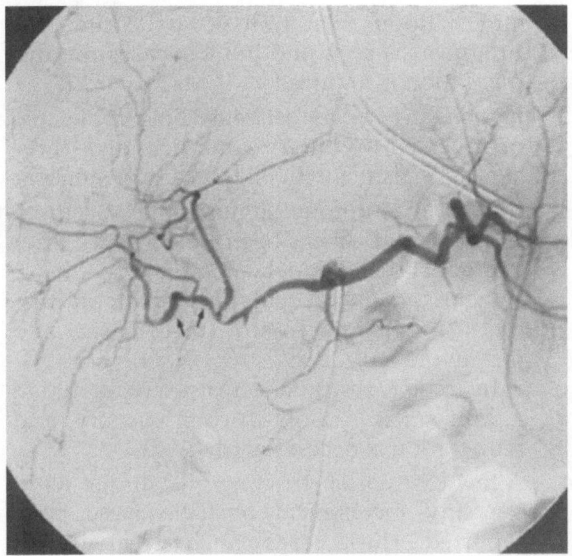

Fig. 7.4. Hepatic artery aneurysms: 3-year-old boy transplanted for biliary atresia. Irreversible rejection (vanishing bile duct syndrome). Hepatic arteriogram shows multiple aneurysmal dilatations of the hepatic artery branches (*arrows*).

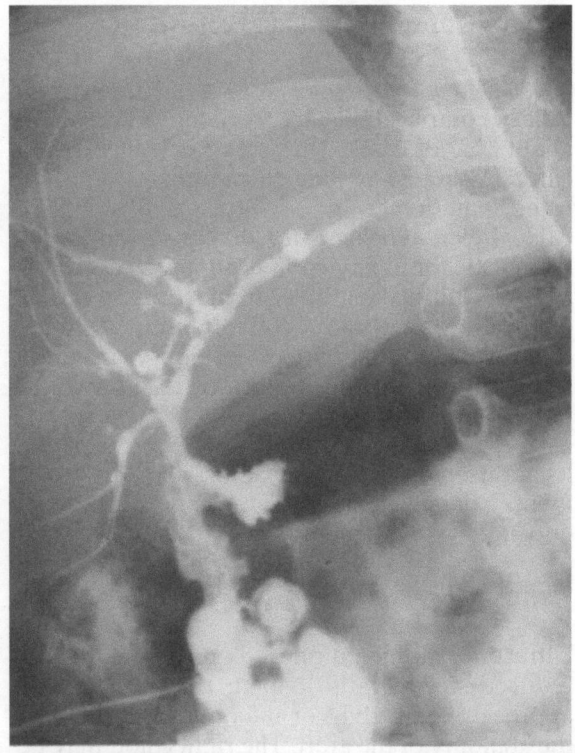

a

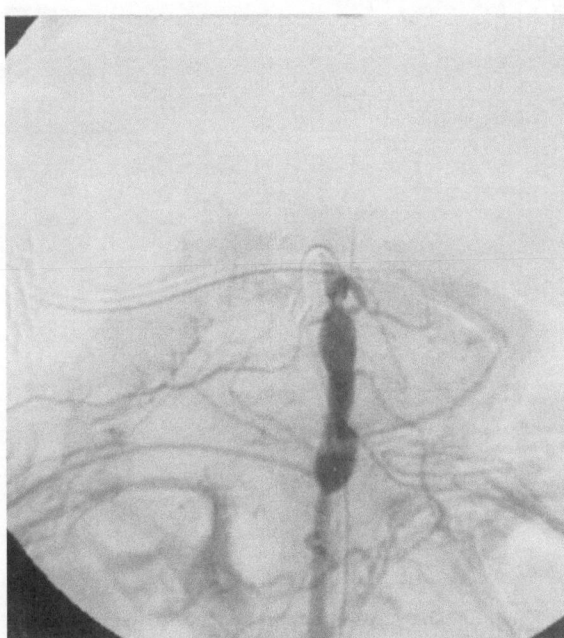

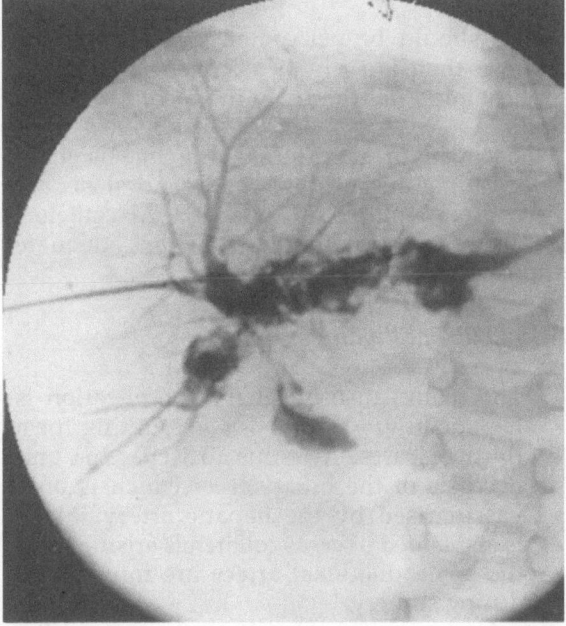

b

Fig. 7.5. "Mycotic" aneurysm of the superior mesenteric artery: 3-year-old girl transplanted for biliary atresia. Complicated postoperative course with multiple episodes of septicaemia. Superior mesenteric arteriogram disclosed an aneurysmal dilatation of the proximal part of the superior mesenteric artery involving the origin of several digestive arteries. No treatment. Spontaneous regression of the lesion 1 year later.

Fig. 7.6. Biliary complication of hepatic artery thrombosis: 2-year-old boy transplanted for biliary atresia. Hepatic artery thombosis on day 5. Surgical de-obstruction attempted. **a** Cholangiography performed 1 month later by the indwelling surgical catheter. There are multiple irregularities of calibre of the intrahepatic bile ducts. **b** Transhepatic cholangiography 1 month later: bile ducts are dilated, with shaggy borders and intraluminal filling defects. This appearance is characteristic of epithelial necrosis. After 3 months of external percutaneous drainage the child was retransplanted.

Biliary Complications (43 cases)
(Figs. 7.7–7.9)

Biliary complications are frequent, occurring in about 15% of cases. These may be encountered early (1–2days) or late (6 months) after liver transplantation.

However, biochemistry of the serum is not diagnostic for biliary complications. Diagnosis is made by ultrasonography in most cases. It may fail in a few cases because of intraluminal sludge or early examination. Liver biopsy in these selected cases may be performed to show intrahepatic cholestasis.

PTC is mandatory to define the cause and location of the lesion and then plan the treatment. The severity of biliary complications is dependent on the aetiology.

Technique

Ultrasonographic guidance is recommended in reduced-sized grafts to plan the transhepatic approach – left, right or inferior – according of the anatomy of the graft. The right colon may be interposed between the lateral abdominal wall and the liver.

PTC should be performed under antibiotic cover, as there is a serious risk of cholangitis and septicaemia in these immunocompromised children.

Placement of an external drainage is mandatory if significant obstruction and stasis are discovered. Multiple side holes 4 or 5 F catheters are usually sufficient to obtain an adequate drainage.

Aetiology and Findings

1. The main cause of biliary complication is hepatic artery thrombosis accounting for a third of cases. It is due to ischaemia and necrosis of the biliary tract which is only vascularised by the hepatic artery in the transplanted liver, as collaterals arising from the gastroduodenal artery are interrupted during surgery.

    Necrosis may occur at any portion of the biliary tract leading to bile leakage, stenosis and dilatation.

    Dilated bile ducts show shaggy borders and large intraluminal defects, very suggestive of epithelial necrosis. Despite multiple surgical procedures, percutaneous drainages

and balloon dilatations (four cases), the prognosis is poor and in most cases retransplantation is required.

2. Hepatic artery stenosis may be complicated or revealed by biliary complications (three cases), i.e. fistula with bile leakage or stenosis.

3. Biliary anastomotic stenosis may occur in isolation. It has been observed after choledocho-choledochostomy or choledochojejunostomy. Percutaneous balloon dilatation may be successful (three cases) and may avoid surgery.

    In some cases this stenosis may be due to a kink or plication during surgery and reoperation is necessary (three cases).

4. A few cases of obstructing bile sludge without any mechanical obstacle have been reported. These cases can be treated with PTC and lavage (three cases). In one case the cause of obstruction was haemobilia secondary to liver biopsy.

5. Formation of a mucocele of the cystic duct remnant is an uncommon event (three cases): it may compress the common bile duct. The treatment is surgical.

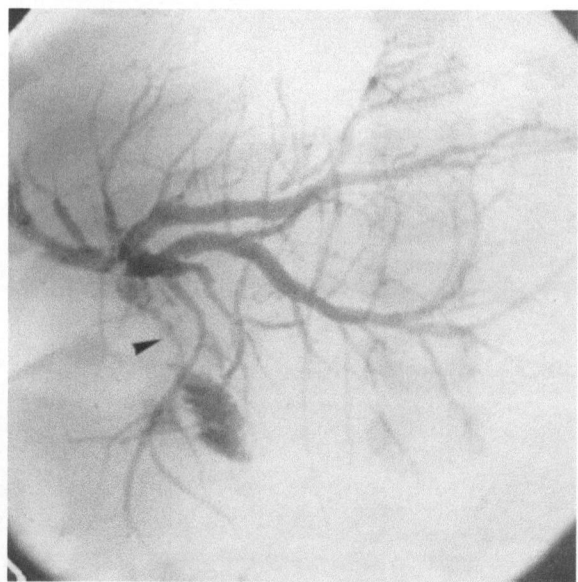

Fig. 7.7. Biliodigestive anastomosis stenosis: 4-year-old boy transplanted in emergency for fulminant virus A hepatitis, with an adult reduced-size graft. Transhepatic cholangiography performed 4 months later, via an epigastric approach under ultrasonic guidance. There is stenosis (*arrowhead*) of the biliodigestive anastomosis and intraluminal sludge in the dilated common bile duct. The child had to be reoperated.

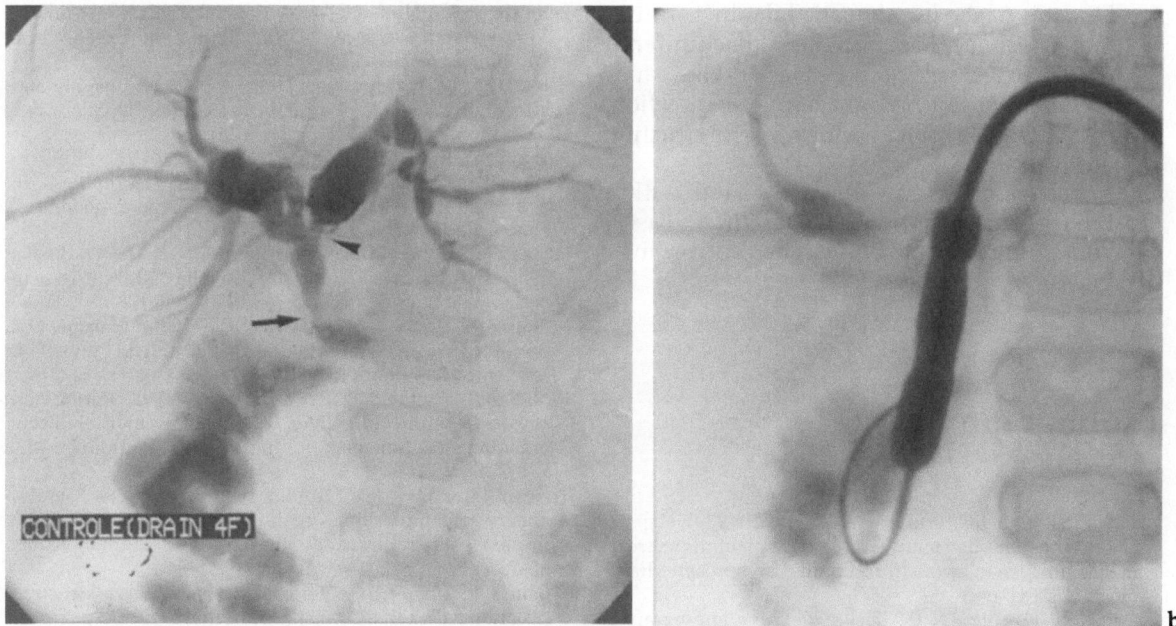

Fig. 7.8. Interventional radiology on biliary anastomosis stenosis: 9-year-old girl transplanted for Byler's disease. **a** Transhepatic cholangiography performed 2 months later shows stenosis of the biliodigestive anastomosis (*arrow*) and of the ending of the left hepatic duct (*arrowhead*). **b** Percutaneous dilatation of both stenoses via a left approach with a 5F balloon catheter. Good result and no recurrence 18 months later.

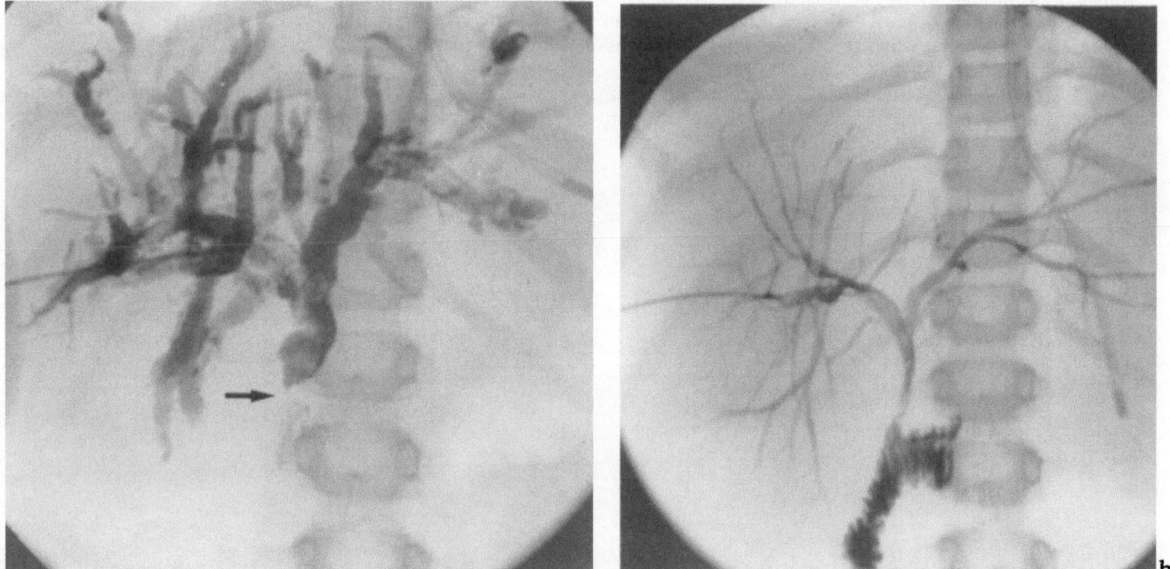

Fig. 7.9. Haemobilia and obstructing sludge: same patient as Fig. 7.1; 2 weeks after second transplantation. Severe bile duct dilatation occurred 2 days after liver biopsy. **a** Transhepatic cholangiography: the bile was dark, probably coloured by haemobilia. There is obstruction of the biliodigestive anastomosis (*arrow*) and intraluminal defects accumulating above. External drainage. **b** After 2 weeks of external drainage the biliary tree and the anastomosis have returned to normal.

6.   Stenosis of the intrahepatic bile ducts of un-
     known cause has also been encountered
     (three cases). Hypotheses as to the cause
     include rejection, cytomegalovirus infection,
     or technical problems during the reduction
     of the graft.
        Rejection may also be associated with a
     biliary anastomotic stenosis (three cases)
     and should always be searched for on liver
     biopsy.

Bibliography

Abad J, Hidalgo EG, Cantarero JM et al. (1989) Hepatic
    artery anastomotic stenosis after transplantation: treat-
    ment with percutaneous transluminal angioplasty. Radi-
    ology 171: 661–662
Cardella JF, Amplatz K (1987) Preoperative angiographic
    evaluation of prospective liver recipients. Radiol Clin
    North Am 25: 299–308
Claus D, Clapuyt Ph (1987) Liver transplantation in children:
    role of the radiologist in the preoperative assessment and
    the postoperative follow-up. Transplant Proc 19:
    3344–3357
Day DL, Letourneau JG, Allan BT, Ascher NL, Hund G
    (1986) MR evaluation of the portal vein in pediatric liver
    transplant candidates. AJR 147: 1027–1030
Flint EW, Sumkin JH, Zajko AB, Bowen AD (1988) Duplex
    sonography of hepatic artery thrombosis after liver trans-
    plantation. AJR 151: 481–483
Hoffer FA, Teele RL, Lillehei CW, Vancanti JP (1988)
    Infected bilomas and hepatic artery thrombosis in infant
    recipients of liver transplants. Radiology 169: 435–438
Letourneau JG, Hunter DW, Ascher Nl et al. (1989) Biliary
    complications after liver transplantation in children.
    Radiology 170: 1095–1099
Letourneau JG, Hunter DW, Payne WD (1990) Imaging and
    intervention for biliary complications after hepatic trans-
    plantation. AJR 154: 729–733
Pariente D, Riou JY, Schmit P et al. (1990) Variability of
    clinical presentation of hepatic artery thrombosis in
    pediatric liver transplantation: role of imaging modalities.
    Pediatr Radiol 20: 253–257
Pariente D, Bihet MH, Tammam S et al. (1991) Biliary
    complications after transplantation in children: role of
    imaging modalities. Pediatr Radiol 21: 175–178
Rollins NK, Andrews WS, Barton RE (1990) Transhepatic
    portal venography in potential pediatric liver transplant
    recipients. Radiology 174: 262–263
Rollins NK, Sheffield EG, Andrews WS (1992) Portal vein
    stenosis complicating liver transplantation in children:
    percutaneous transhepatic angioplasty. Radiology 182:
    731–734
Tobben PJ, Zajko AB, Sumkin JH et al. (1988) Pseudo-
    aneurysm complicating organ transplantation: role of CT,
    duplex sonography and angiography. Radiology 169:
    65–70
Wozney P, Zajko AB, Bron KM (1986) Vascular com-
    plications after liver transplantation: 5 years' experience.
    AJR 147: 657–663
Yandza T, Pariente D, Devictor D et al. (1990) Pediatric
    hepatic artery thrombosis successfully treated by imme-
    diate reoperation associated with selective urokinase in-
    jection. A case report. Clin Transplant 4: 304–306
Zajko AB, Campbell WL, Bron KM et al. (1988) Diagnostic
    and interventional radiology in liver transplantation.
    Gastroenterol Clin North Am 17: 105–143
Zajko AB, Calus D, Calpuyt P et al. (1989) Obstruction to
    hepatic venous drainage after LT: treatment with balloon
    angioplasty. Radiology 170: 763–765
Zajko AB, Bennett MJ, Campbell WL, Koneru B (1990)
    Mucocele of the cystic duct remnant in eight liver trans-
    plant recipients: findings at cholangiography, CT and US.
    Radiology 177: 691–693

8 Miscellaneous

Liver Traumatism

Liver injury is a frequent event in blunt abdominal trauma in children and makes up 25%–30% of visceral injuries.

Diagnosis

Emergency exploratory laparotomy is mandatory in a child with haemodynamic instability unresponsive to aggressive fluid replacement.

In haemodynamically stable children, ultrasonography and/or contrast enhancement CT allow precise identification of the hepatic lesions.

Angiography

Nowadays there is little indication for angiography in liver trauma. Its role is confined to the postoperative patient with continued bleeding and to the occurrence of haemobilia.

Haemobilia (Figs. 8.1 and 8.2) (three cases)

This is a vascular biliary fistula due to an arterial false aneurysm or an arteriovenous fistula. The aetiology is iatrogenic in 50% of cases (percutaneous biopsy or opacification or drainage, or surgery), traumatic in 20%. It is often delayed after the trauma and diagnosis must be suspected when there is adbominal pain, jaundice and gastrointestinal bleeding.

Nowadays, the diagnosis is made with confidence by ultrasonography (pulsed or colour Doppler). We have encountered three cases. Arteriography always showed false arterial aneurysms. In one case there was also arterioportal fistula. All cases were treated by embolisation. A recurrence of haemobilia was observed in one case 6 months later and was treated successfully by embolisation. Embolisation should be the method of choice in the selective treatment of a vascular lesion.

Contusions (eight cases)

Angiography was performed in our early experience before the advent of ultrasonography and computed tomography.

Arterial portal hypoperfusion zones can be seen within the liver. Localised reversal of portal flow may be seen, caused by localised increase in vascular resistance. Hypervascularisation during arterial injection may be seen in the affected territories.

Cholangiography (Fig. 8.3)

Biliary tract lesions are usually associated with highly complex lesions involving the hilum. However, they may be isolated and of delayed identification. They include traumatic rupture of the gallbladder (one case), as well as of the common bile duct at the pancreatic duodenal junction or at the hilum. They may present with acute bile peritonitis or long-delayed biliary obstruction and in this last case cholangiography is indicated.

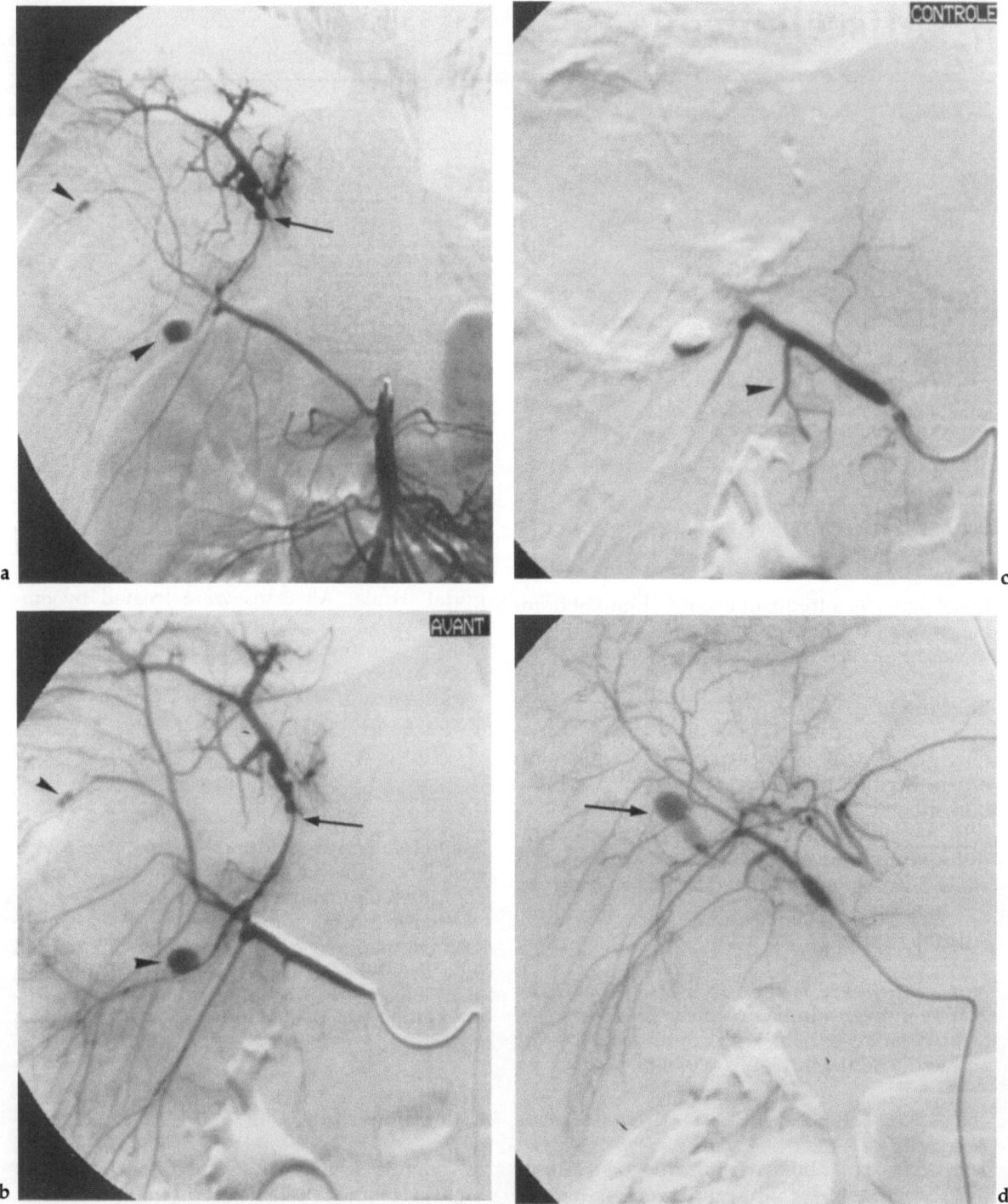

Fig. 8.1. Post-traumatic haemobilia. This 9-year-old boy sustained a severe motor vehicle accident 15 days before. He was treated conservatively. He presented suddenly with abdominal pain, mild jaundice and melaena. Ultrasound disclosed an arterial false aneurysm in the centre of a right lobe contusion. **a** The area of contusion is supplied by a right hepatic artery arising from the superior mesenteric artery. There are three vascular lesions: two arterial false aneurysms (*arrowheads*) and one arterioportal fistula (*arrow*). **b** Selective catheterisation of the right hepatic artery. **c** After embolisation with gelfoam particles, there is no more opacification of the lesions. The cystic artery is still patent (*arrowhead*). **d** 6 months later the child returned with recurrence of haemobilia. Selective catheterisation of the right hepatic artery shows another arterial false aneurysm (*arrow*). Opacification of the hepatic artery arising from the coeliac trunk is now visible, by arterial collaterals in the area of contusion. *Continued opposite.*

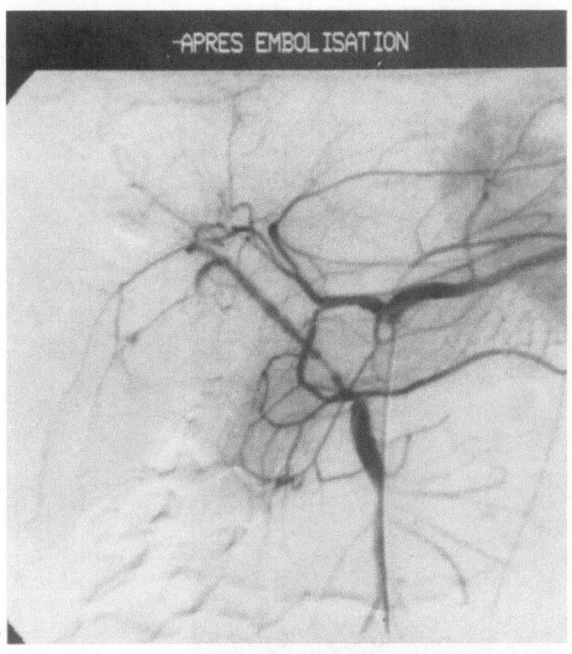

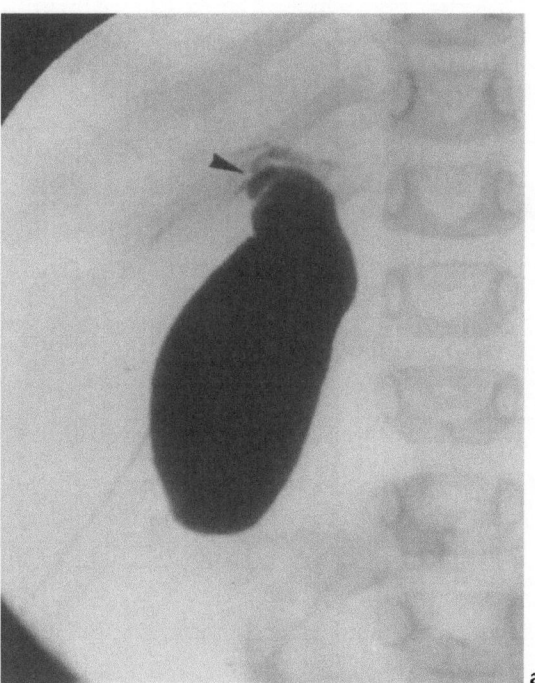

Fig. 8.1. Post-traumatic haemobilia. This 9-year-old boy sustained a severe motor vehicle accident 15 days before. He was treated conservatively. He presented suddenly with abdominal pain, mild jaundice and melaena. Ultrasound disclosed an arterial false aneurysm in the centre of a right lobe contusion. (*continued*) **e** Successful embolisation with a follow-up of 18 months. Control by opacification of the coeliac trunk. Irregularities due to spasm are visible on the right hepatic artery.

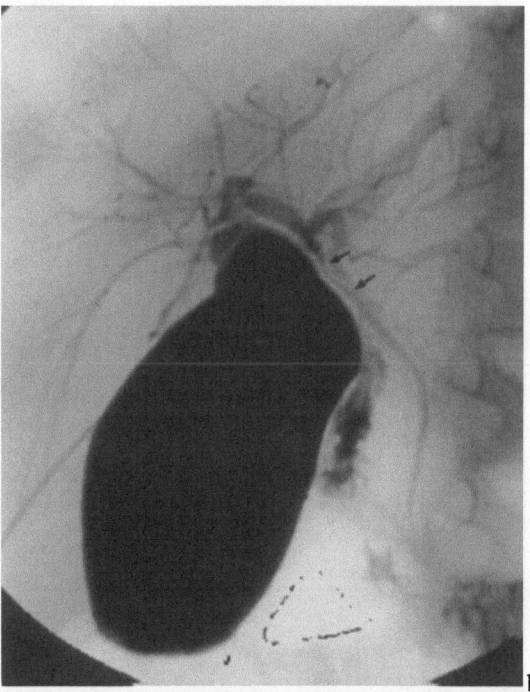

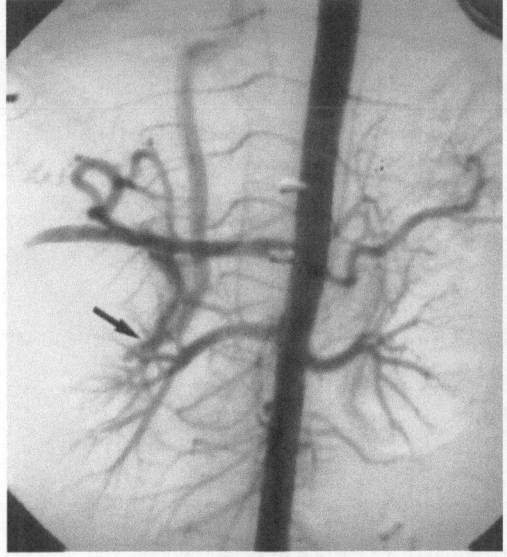

Fig. 8.2. A 10-year-old girl transplanted for fulminant viral hepatitis with a reduced-size adult liver. Global aortogram shows a large arterio-porto-hepatic double fistula (*arrow*) with rapid opacification of the left hepatic vein and of a portal vein branch. This lesion was thought to be secondary to a liver biopsy. It was asymptomatic.

Fig. 8.3. Traumatic rupture of the gallbladder; 4-year-old boy presenting with recurrent episodes of jaundice. An abdominal trauma was noted 2 years before. On ultrasound there was evidence of a hydrocholecyst and mild intrahepatic bile duct dilatation. **a** Percutaneous cholecystography. The gallbladder is markedly enlarged and empties into the right hepatic ducts (*arrowhead*). **b** There is opacification of the left hepatic ducts and of the common bile duct. There is a long segment stenosis of the choledochus (*arrows*). At surgery there was a fibrotic scar involving the choledochus and obstructing the cystic duct.

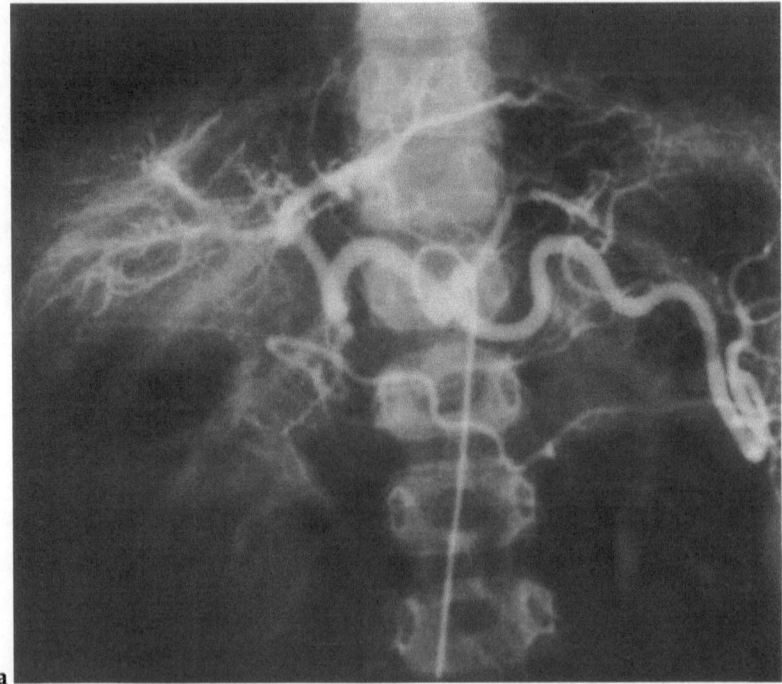

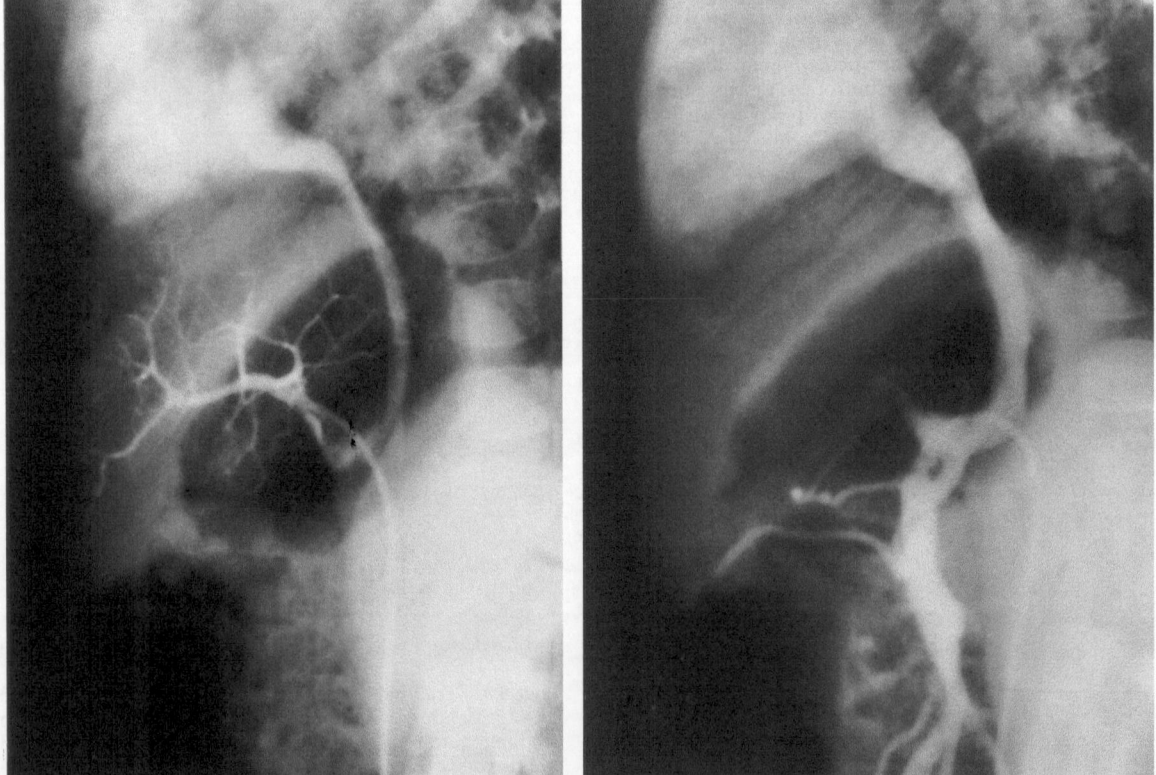

Fig. 8.4. Congenital portocaval anastomosis. Goldenhar's syndrome and splenomegaly. **a** Coeliac artery opacification. The liver is small. The hepatic artery is dilated. **b** Lateral view of a direct catheterisation of the intrahepatic portal system through the portocaval anastomosis. **c** Opacification of the superior mesenteric vein through the portocaval anastomosis. *Continued opposite.*

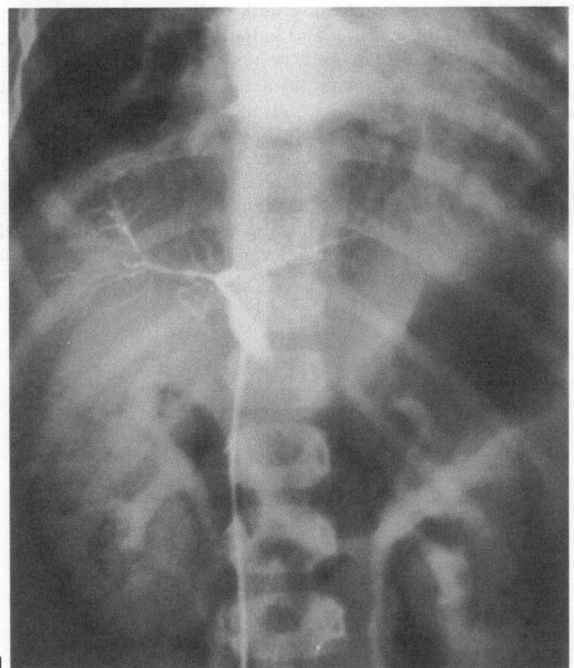

d

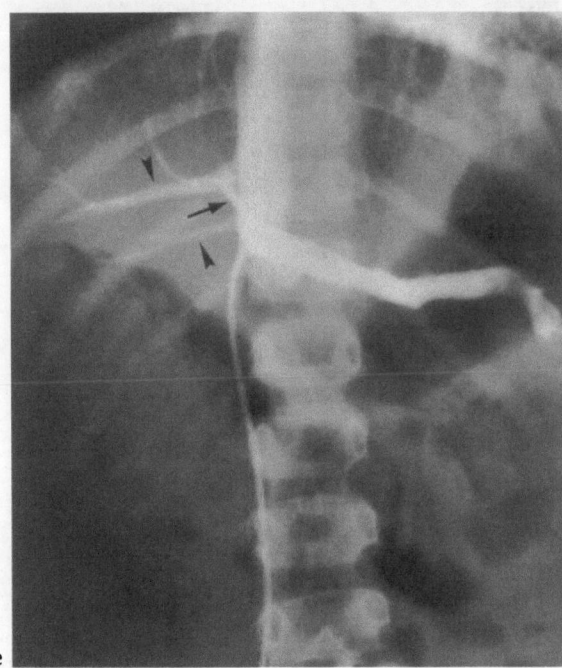

e

Fig. 8.4. Congenital portocaval anastomosis. Goldenhar's syndrome and splenomegaly. (*continued*) **d** Anteroposterior view of the portal opacification. **e** Anteroposterior view of the catheterisation of the splenic vein through the portocaval anastomosis. Reflux opacification of the portal vein (*arrow*) and hepatic veins (*arrowheads*).

Congenital Hepatic Vascular Malformations

These are rare disorders with variable severity and clinical presentation according to the type of abnormal vascular communication. Ultrasonography with Doppler usually accurately demonstrates these malformations.

Spontaneous Portocaval Fistula
(two cases) (Fig. 8.4)

This may be isolated and asymptomatic but can be part of a malformation complex with facial dysmorphism and costal and spinal anomalies. This complex is close to Goldenhar's syndrome which has been reported associated with congenital absence of the portal vein. One of our cases was associated with Budd–Chiari syndrome. On angiography there is a large communication between the portal vein and the inferior vena cava. The intrahepatic portal branches are hypoplastic and the flow in the portal vein is hepatofugal. No treatment is required.

Arterioportal Fistula (two cases) (Fig. 8.5)

This vascular malformation presents with portal hypertension, anaemia and gastrointestinal haemorrhage.

The two cases seen were associated with trisomy 21. There is intrahepatic communication between an enlarged hepatic artery and a dilated portal vein with reversed flow. Treatment may be achieved with embolisation and/or partial hepatectomy.

Localised arterioportal fistula may be seen in malignant tumours, and in angiomas (one case).

Portal Hepatic Venous Malformation
(five cases) (Fig. 8.6)

This has been previously reported in adults: they usually present with encephalopathy and hypoglycaemia.

A few cases have been fortuitously discovered in children by ultrasonography (two cases). No treatment is required. Four of our five cases were associated with hepatic angiomas.

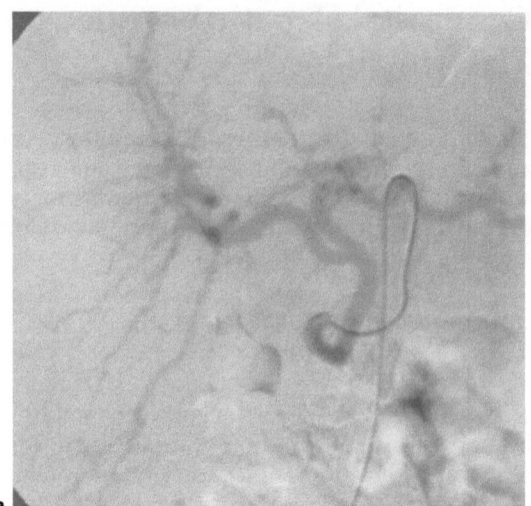

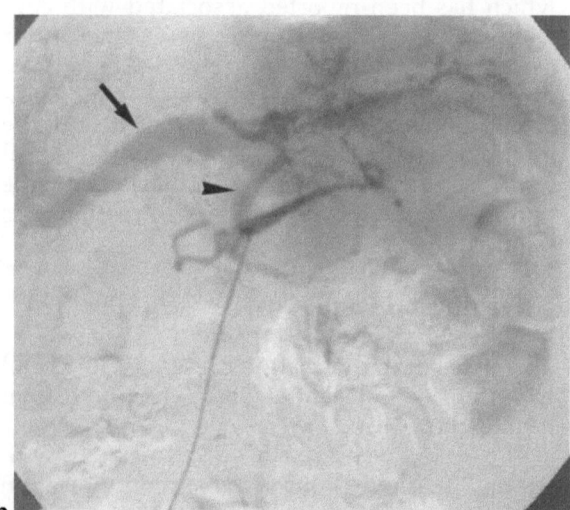

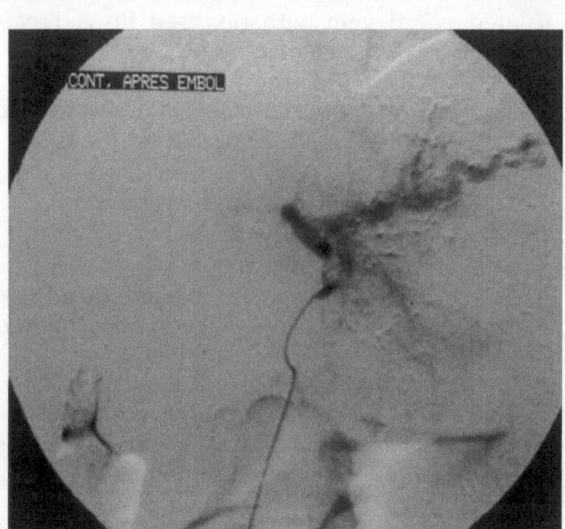

◄ Fig. 8.5. A 5-year-old boy with history of facial angioma treated by embolisation and surgery. Severe thrombopenia. Rectorragies due to juvenile polyposis. Isotopic studies show that the platelets are sequestrated in the liver. **a** Right hepatic artery injection. There is hepatomegaly. The hepatic artery is enlarged and slightly distorted in periphery. **b** The left hepatic artery (*arrowhead*) arising from the left gastric artery, supplies the segment II. There is rapid opacification of the portal vein (*arrow*) due to a peripheral arterioportal fistula. **c** Embolisation of the left hepatic artery was attempted with cyanoacrylate mixed with lipiodol. But the procedure had no effect on the platelet count.

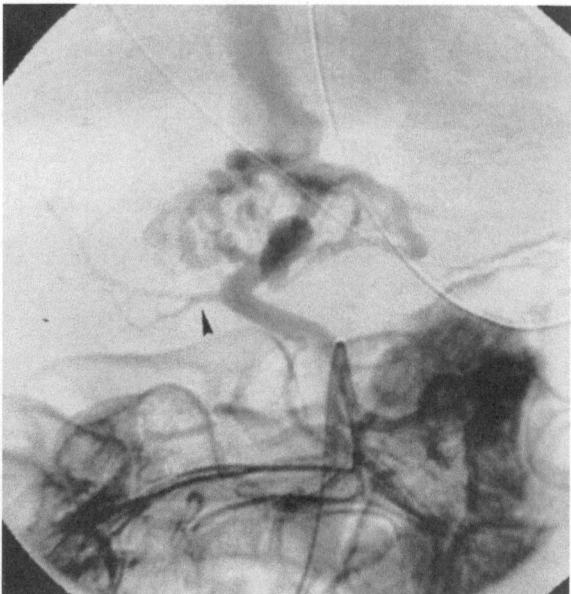

Fig. 8.6. A 2-week-old baby girl presenting with hydrops fetalis, cardiomegaly and hepatomegaly. On ultrasonography the left portal branch and the ductus venous are dilated and multiple tortuous venous structures are visible around them. The venous phase of the superior mesenteric arteriogram shows that there is communication between the left portal branch and the inferior vena cava via a network of tortuous veins. The right portal branch is hypoplastic (*arrowhead*). The baby died a few days later of arterial pulmonary hypertension. This hepatic lesion was not thought to be the cause of the death.

Fig. 8.7. Glycogen storage disease, type I. **a** 5 years of age. Hepatic angiogram. Multiple adenomas slightly (*arrows*) hypervascular are seen in the right lobe of the liver. A large hypovascular mass is seen in the left lobe of the liver (*arrowheads*). **b** 8 years of age. The adenomas in the right lobe of the liver are larger. The mass in the left lobe of the liver is now hypervascular. **c** Note a calcification in the left lobe of the liver on the non subtracted image (*arrowheads*).

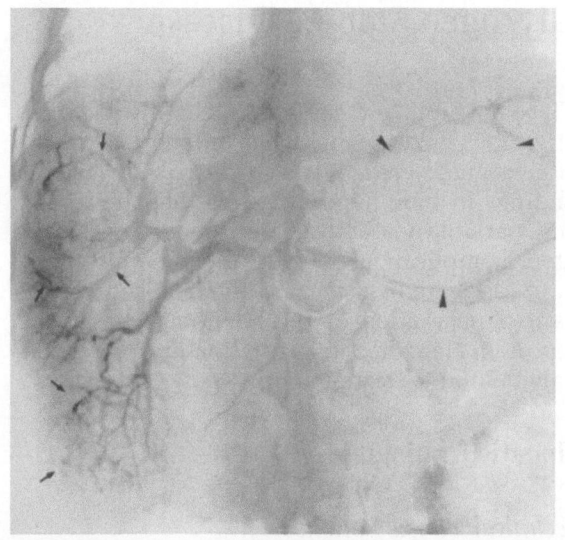

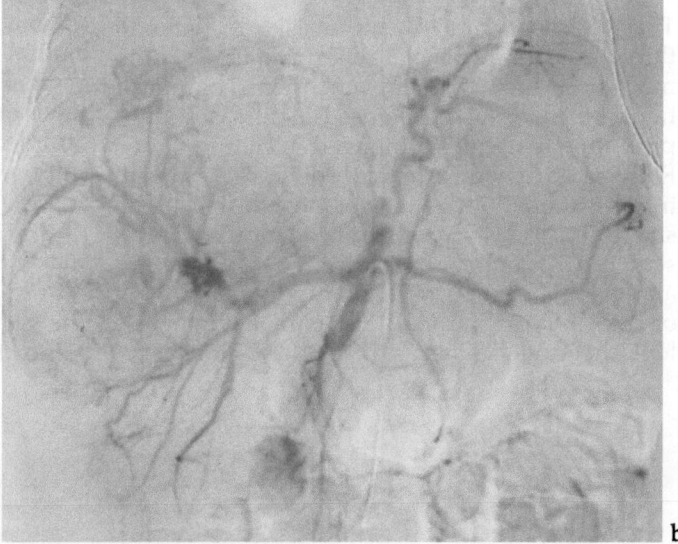

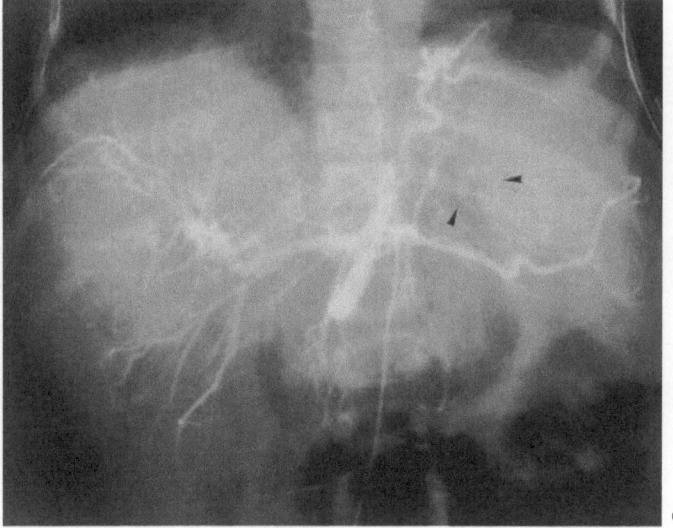

Glycogen Storage Disease

Glycogen storage disease is caused by a deficit of various enzymes involved in the metabolism of glycogen. Several types are described. Clinical findings include hypoglycaemia, hepatomegaly and variable visceromegaly depending of the type. Complications include adenoma in type I. Rare cases are associated with cirrhosis. Malignant degeneration of the adenomas has been reported. Hepatic transplantation represents the only definitive treatment up to now.

Hepatic Angiography

Technical Considerations

These patients are at high risk of femoral thrombosis due to platelet abnormalities. Caution must be exercised to prevent these complications. Heparin should be used in all cases, despite an apparently prolonged bleeding time. Retrograde femoral arterial thrombosis occurred in one patient. Intrahepatic branches are usually small, unless a hypervascular adenoma is present. An uncommonly high number of anomalous right hepatic arteries were seen by us (30% of cases). Opacification of the parenchyma may look heterogeneous, as in Budd–Chiari syndrome, probably because of glycogen infiltration in the liver (Figs. 8.7–8.9).

Portocaval Anastomosis (Fig. 8.10)

Portocaval anastomosis was performed for metabolic reasons in a few cases. In most of them, the portocaval anastomosis was patent. In three cases, hepatopetal collaterals were seen as in portal vein thrombosis, because of a relative stenosis of the portocaval anastomosis.

After portocaval anastomosis, reverse flow occurred in two cases.

Adenomas (seven cases)

Adenomas are usually seen in type I glycogen storage disease. They were hypervascular in four cases and hypovascular in three. One was calcified but probably secondary to a surgical biopsy. They were always multiple. They are angiographically indistinguistable from hepatocarcinomas. α-Fetoprotein levels are routinely sampled for follow-up. No malignant degeneration occurred in any of our cases.

Renovascular Hypertension

One case, presented with renovascular hypertension due to renal artery compression of the kidney by one adenoma.

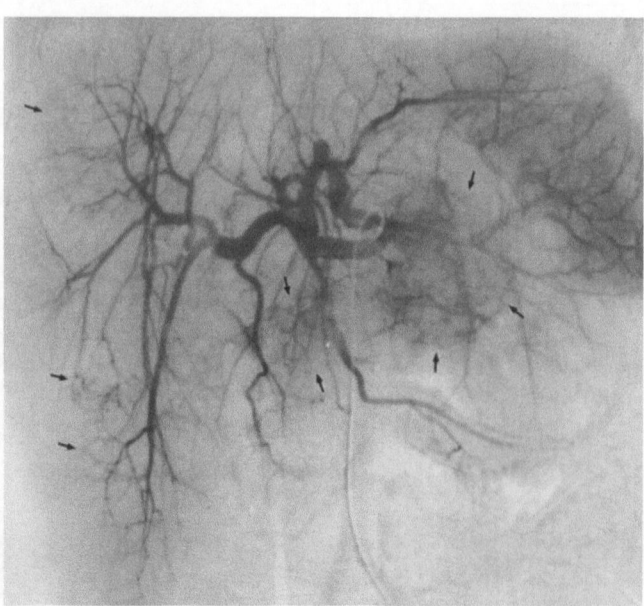

Fig. 8.8. Glycogen storage disease, type I; 10 years of age. Multiple hypervascular masses mainly in the left lobe of the liver (*arrows*). Diagnosis of adenomas.

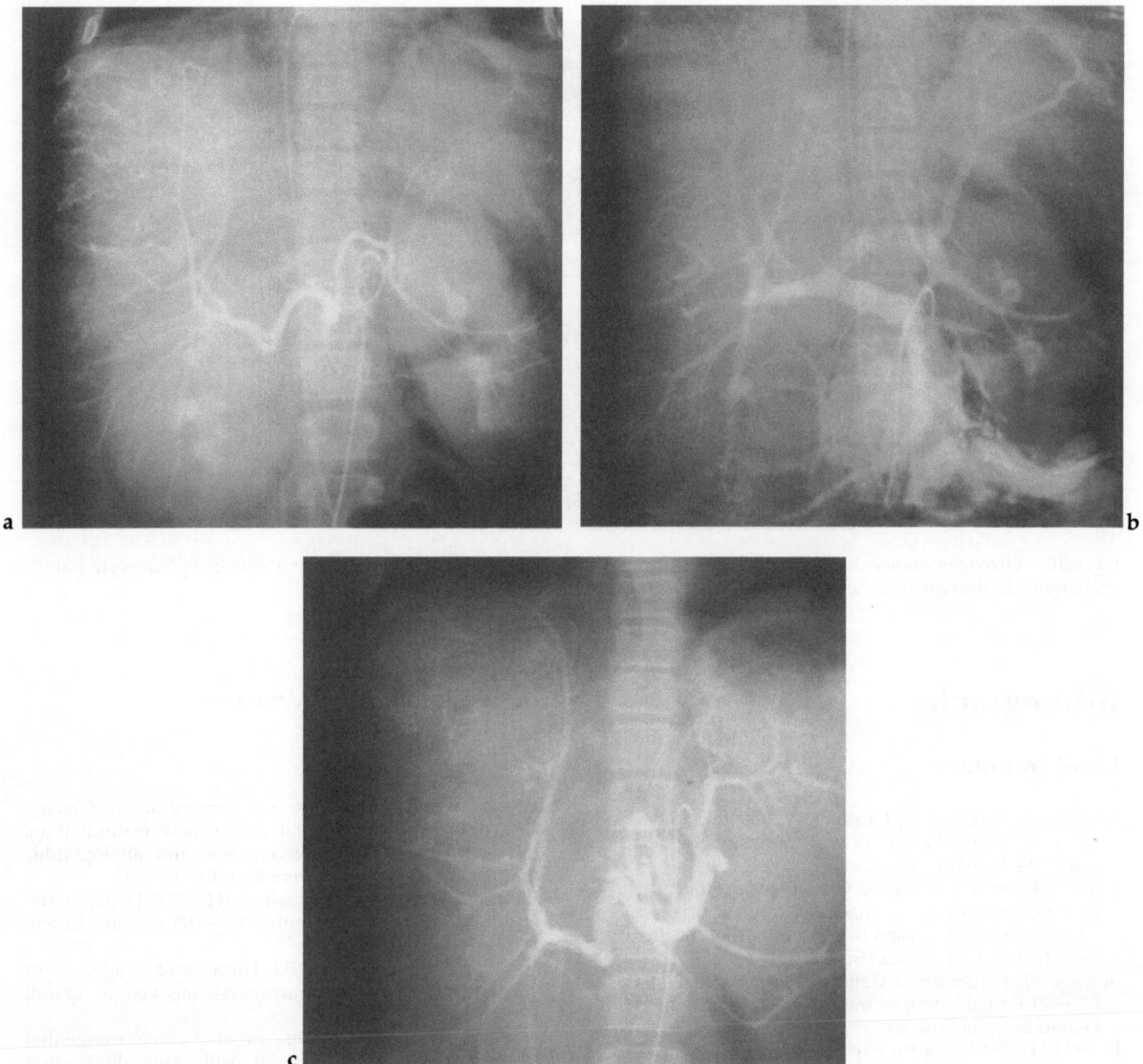

Fig. 8.9. Glycogen storage disease, type I; 15 years of age. **a** Hepatic angiogram shows multiple hypervascular masses in the right lobe of the liver and one large mass in the left lobe of the liver. **b** The venous return of the superior mesenteric artery injection shows distortion of the intrahepatic portal branches without amputation. **c** Same patient, 18 years of age, after portocaval anastomosis, the adenomas are larger as seen on the hepatic artery angiogram. The patient has been transplanted and is well.

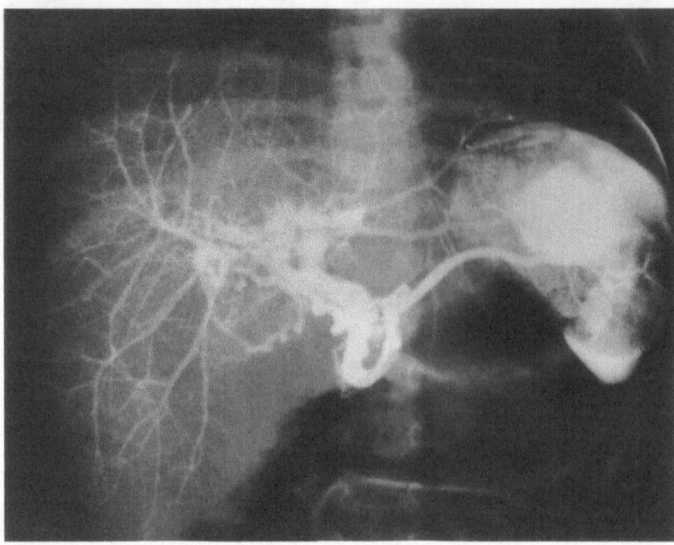

Fig. 8.10.   Glycogen storage disease, type I, after portocaval anastomosis. Thrombosis of the portal vein. Splenoportogram: a cavernoma, in the region of the portal trunk reperfuses the entire liver.

Bibliography

Liver trauma

Brunelle F, Maurage C, Lacombe A, Chaumont P (1985) Emergency embolization in post-tramatic hemobilia in a child. J Pediatr Surg 20: 172–174

Curet P, Baumer R, Roche A, Grellet J, Mercadier M (1984) Hepatic hemobilia of traumatic or iatrogenic origin: recent advances in diagnosis and therapy, review of the literature from 1976 to 1981. World J Surg 8: 2–8

de Lagausie P, Pariente D, Gauthier F, de Dreuzy O, Valayer J (1992) Embolization of traumatic hemobilia in a child. Pediatr Surg Int 7: 61–63.

Evans JP (1976) Traumatic rupture of the gallbladder in a 3-year-old boy. J Pediatr Surg 11: 1033–1034

Kaufman RA, Babcock DS (1984) An approach to imaging the upper abdomen in the injured child. Semin Roentgenol 19: 308–320

Kendall RS, Chapoy PR, Busutil RW, Koladny M, Ament ME (1980) Acquired bile duct stricture in childhood related to blunt trauma. Am J Dis Child 134: 851–854

Sandblom P, Saegesser F, Mirkovitch V (1984) Hepatic hemobilia: hemorrhage from the intrahepatic biliary tract. World J Surg 8: 41–50

Veyrac C, Couture A, Baud C (1987) Les traumatismes des organes intrapéritonéaux. In: Le traumatisme chez l'enfant. Cliniques de pédiatrie, Vigot (ed). Paris, p 138

Congenital Hepatic Vascular Malformations

Charnsangavej C, Chin-Shiung Soo, Bernardino ME, Chuang VP, Wallace S (1983) Portal hepatic venous malformation: ultrasound, computed tomographic and angiographic findings. Cardiovasc Intervent Radiol 6: 109–111

Helikson MA, Shapiro DL, Seashore JH (1977) Hepatoportal arteriovenous fistula and portal hypertension in a infant. Pediatrics 60: 921–924

Jabra AA, Taylor GA (1991) Ultrasound diagnosis of congenital intrahepatic porto systemic venous shunt. Pediatr Radiol 21: 529–530

Morse SS, Taylor KJW, Strauss EB et al (1986) Congenital absence of the portal vein in oculo auriculovertebral dysplasia (Goldenhar syndrome). Pediatr Radiol 16: 437–439

Park JH, Cha SH, Han JK, Han MC (1990) Intrahepatic porto-systemic venous shunt. AJR 155: 527–528

Glycogen Storage Disease

Brunelle F, Chaumont P (1984) Hepatic tumors in children: ultrasonic differentiation of malignant from benign lesions. Radiology 150: 695–699

9   Complications

Eighteen complications were encountered on about 1500 studies (1.2%).

Complications of Arteriography

Femoral Artery Thrombosis (three cases)

Seen early in our experience, femoral artery thrombosis is now exceptional, due to the use of heparin and small catheters.

It has to be emphasised that two of the cases had glycogen storage disease. The hypercoagulability state of these patients may be a predisposing factor. The risk of femoral artery thrombosis is greater when the femoral artery diameter is small, especially in infants with hypervascular tumours. The use of digital subtraction angiography has greatly improved the situation. In our experience the occurrence of femoral artery spasm and thrombosis is not related to the duration of the examination.

Complication of General Anaesthesia
(one case)

One death occurred during induction of general anaesthesia in a child with Budd–Chiari syndrome. It was probably secondary to severe compression of the inferior vena cava. Since then no patient with Budd–Chiari is ever examined under general anaesthesia.

Complications of Embolisation

Hepatic Abscesses (two cases)

Two cases occurred after focal nodular hyperplasia embolisation. It can be prevented by antibiotic therapy. It can be related to the fact that this benign tumour is supplied by the hepatic artery.

Incidental Splenic Embolisation (one case)

This occurred during embolisation of the hepatic artery in a patient with hepatic angioma and was associated with pain and fever. The patient made a full recovery.

Gallbladder Necrosis (one case)

This followed a hepatic artery embolisation with absolute alcohol. The gallbladder was resected and found to be atrophic.

Complications of Splenoportography

Death

One death occurred in the 1970s 8 hours after a splenoportography in a child presenting with ascites and cirrhosis. Ascites and disorders of the coagulation must be considered as contra-indications. However, there is one exception, namely isolated thrombopenia due to hyper-splenism.

Splenic Subcapsular Haematoma (two cases)

Contrast medium was seen around the spleen in two cases. Recovery was uneventful. In one case an intraperitoneal contrast leak was seen during splenoportography but this had no after-effects.

Complications of Percutaneous Cholangiography

In patients with liver disease general anaesthesia is used not only for radiological investigations but also for liver biopsy and endoscopy. It is the rule to perform abdominal ultrasound subsequently to detect any complications.

Intraperitoneal Contrast or Bile Leak

Minimal leak of contrast medium can be seen without further consequence after percutaneous transhepatic cholangio- and cholecystography.

Intrahepatic Haematoma (two cases)

This occurred in two cases after percutaneous cholangiography, and was diagnosed by ultra-

sonography and had no clinical significance.

Haemobilia (two cases)

This was observed in two cases of liver transplantation, with a low platelet count. One child had to be operated a few hours after the examination.

Infectious Shock (three cases)

This occurred in three cases of liver transplantation, secondary to fulminant cholangitis. Antibiotic cover of the PTC and external drainage are mandatory especially in immunocompromised children.

Further Reading

Alagille D, Odièvre M (1978) Maladies du foie et des voies biliaires chez l'enfant. Flammarion Médicine, Sciences Paris

Doyon D, Roche A, Chaumont P (1978) L'angiographie digestive chez l'adulte et l'enfant. Masson, Paris

Mowat AP (1987) Liver disorders in childhood 2nd edn Butherworths, London

Saadoon K (1991) Atlas of normal and variant angiographic anatomy, WB Saunders, Philadelphia

Silverman A, Roy CC (1983) Pediatric clinical gastroenterology, 3rd edn, CV Mosby, St Louis

Stanley P (1982) Pediatric angiography. Williams and Wilkins, Baltimore

Stringer DA (1989) Pediatric gastrointestinal imaging. BC Decker, Toronto, Philadephia

Index